ROUTLEDGE LIBRARY EDITIONS:
HEALTH, DISEASE & SOCIETY

Volume 13

THE EXPERIENCE OF
ILLNESS

THE EXPERIENCE OF ILLNESS

RAY FITZPATRICK, JOHN HINTON,
STANTON NEWMAN,
GRAHAM SCAMBLER and
JAMES THOMPSON

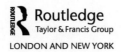

Routledge
Taylor & Francis Group

LONDON AND NEW YORK

First published in 1984 by Tavistock Publications

This edition first published in 2022
by Routledge
4 Park Square, Milton Park, Abingdon, Oxon OX14 4RN

and by Routledge
605 Third Avenue, New York, NY 10158

Routledge is an imprint of the Taylor & Francis Group, an informa business

British Library Cataloguing in Publication Data
A catalogue record for this book is available from the British Library

ISBN: 978-0-367-52469-2 (Set)
ISBN: 978-1-032-25562-0 (Volume 13) (hbk)
ISBN: 978-1-032-25565-1 (Volume 13) (pbk)
ISBN: 978-1-003-28396-6 (Volume 13) (ebk)

DOI: 10.4324/9781003283966

Publisher's Note
The publisher has gone to great lengths to ensure the quality of this reprint but points out that some imperfections in the original copies may be apparent.

Disclaimer
The publisher has made every effort to trace copyright holders and would welcome correspondence from those they have been unable to trace.

Ray Fitzpatrick · John Hinton
Stanton Newman · Graham Scambler
James Thompson

The Experience of Illness

Tavistock Publications · London & New York

First published in 1984 by
Tavistock Publications Ltd
11 New Fetter Lane, London EC4P 4EE

Published in the USA by
Tavistock Publications
in association with Methuen, Inc.
733 Third Avenue, New York, NY 10017

Typeset by Nene Phototypesetters Ltd
and printed in Great Britain by Richard Clay
(the Chaucer Press) Ltd, Bungay, Suffolk

British Library Cataloguing in Publication
Data

The Experience of illness. – (Social science
  paperbacks; 272)
  1. Medicine and psychology
  2. Medicine Psychosomatic
  I. Fitzpatrick, Ray   II. Series
  616'.001'9   R726.5
  ISBN 0–422–78530–X

Library of Congress Cataloging in
Publication Data

Main entry under title:
The Experience of illness.
  Bibliography: p.
  Includes indexes.
  1. Medicine and psychology.   2. Sick –
Psychology.   3. Social medicine.
I. Fitzpatrick, Ray.
R726.5.E96   1984   616'.001'9   84–14909
ISBN 0–422–78530–X (pbk.)

Contents

Acknowledgements

The other authors would like to acknowledge the support and encouragement of Professor John Hinton who, as head of the Academic Department of Psychiatry, was responsible for fostering the collaboration between the authors out of which this book emerged.

The following are thanked for providing helpful comments on particular sections of the book: David Armstrong, Margaret Ballard, Mary Boulton, Mike Bury, Susan Lonsdale, and Anthony Williams.

The authors of Chapter 4 would like to thank the King Edward's Hospital Fund for London for providing financial assistance in the collection of materials for the chapter, although the King's Fund is not responsible for the authors' conclusions.

The help of Pat Hinton, Sine McDougal, and Amanda Owen in typing and general assistance was invaluable and very much appreciated.

1   Introduction

In the twentieth century health care in the developed world has changed dramatically. Rapidly growing basic medical sciences have provided an ever more complex understanding of the body in health and illness. At the same time increasingly sophisticated diagnostic and therapeutic facilities have become available. Knowledge and technique have combined to transform medicine from the status of a craft to that of a technological science. Recently the growth has also occurred of ways of approaching health care which complement the dominant idiom of technology. The focus of this approach is upon psychosocial aspects of illness and treatment.

Two kinds of change within health care have made the development of a psychosocial perspective an urgent imperative. On the one hand it has become increasingly apparent that the traditional 'craft' skills of health care may be jeopardized if the training of health workers concentrates exclusively on the technological and biomedical dimensions of health care. On the other hand changes in the kinds of goals which are set for medicine require new forms of health care practice in which a psychosocial perspective is of particular importance. Both changes require elaboration.

2 The Experience of Illness

The traditional skills of health care

It is understandable how, in a society dominated by technological values, the occupations of health care, especially medicine, might be entranced by the technical forms of diagnosis and therapy which have come to the fore in the recent history of medicine. This process could involve diminishing importance being attached to such social skills as listening, eliciting, recognizing, and explaining. The contribution of the behavioural sciences is partly to demonstrate that an appreciation of the interpersonal components of health care may be acquired in the same way as the health professional learns a framework of biological knowledge relevant to the provision of health care. This view can best be discussed in terms of specific examples. One obvious primary task of the clinician is the identification of the patient's problem. There is evidence from such diverse settings as paediatric clinics (Korsch, Gozzi, and Francis 1968), neurological clinics (Fitzpatrick and Hopkins 1981b), general medical wards (Maguire *et al.* 1974) and general practice (Marks, Goldberg, and Hillier 1979) that a large proportion of the concerns and problems experienced by patients are not recognized by their clinician. The role of the behavioural sciences in response to such evidence is threefold:

1 First and foremost to provide a framework of concepts and evidence to enable more attention to be given to the complexities of patients' presentations. Only by elaborating a language and network of ideas from evidence about patients' experiences can the psychosocial factors in illness be made as 'visible' as the physical factors emphasized in the rest of training.
2 It behoves the behavioural sciences to show that the ability to recognize psychosocial aspects of health problems can develop from training and sensitizing. Evidence that this is so is now beginning to appear (Goldberg *et al.* 1980).
3 There is evidence, such as the study of paediatric clinics cited above (Korsch, Gozzi, and Francis 1968), that the recognition by health workers of patients' broader concerns with regard to the problems that they present is associated with substantial benefits to the patient. Research needs to build on such evidence, further discussed in Chapter 2, to explore the ways in which the health worker's support, personal interest and sensitivity to patients' concerns may directly influence the outcomes of health care.

Another central task of health care is providing reassurance and comfort to those who are in distress with illness. The behavioural sciences have begun to provide a framework for coping with patients' concerns regarding illness (Chapter 2) and the anxieties surrounding the experience of surgery (Chapter 7). The dynamics of reassurance in such circumstances are not commonsensical (Kessel 1979). In more serious, particularly terminal, illness there is a limit to the comfort or reassurance that is possible and, as is suggested in Chapter 11, there are good reasons for scepticism about the appropriateness of rigid nostrums and policies in the care of the dying. Nevertheless careful research can make clearer to those responsible for the care of the dying some of the common trajectories that patients will experience (Kübler-Ross 1970), or the patterns of communication within families of the dying (Chapter 11).

A third task of health care has always been to provide an explanation for illness and instructions to the patient as to how to deal with it. At the extreme, illness may be so devastating and unexpected that it is very difficult for the doctor to provide any really satisfactory explanation. However, for many health problems, information can be given regarding the likely causes, course, prognosis, and therapy of the illness. Giving such information may be the most crucial task performed by the doctor for many problems presented to him. Yet as indicated in Chapters 5 and 8 it is the area of health care which causes most dissatisfaction amongst patients. The evidence also shows that giving appropriate health information is a social skill which can be improved.

Thus these core tasks of health care offer their own intellectual challenges and require a framework through which skills may be acquired and some of the dilemmas and limitations of health care recognized.

New challenges in health care

A range of new problems confront medicine. They arise partly out of the increasing demands upon the patient resulting from the more complex medical treatments now available and partly because of changing patterns of ill health and changing priorities in health care.

Many modern medical treatments, if they are to be at all successful, require of the patient a very long-term commitment to often arduous regimes. The careful control of diet by the diabetic clearly illustrates a form of treatment which makes arduous, long-term demands of the patient. Drug control of hypertension is now a potentially very effective form of therapy. The patient's adherence to the regime is crucial. Appreciation of the patient's perspective and of the problems of adherence has been shown to be an important influence upon the doctor's ability to help such hypertensive patients adhere to their medication (Inui, Yourtee and Williamson 1976).

As disease prevalence and health priorities change, infectious diseases have given way to chronic and degenerative problems. With such chronic mental illnesses as schizophrenia or physical disorders such as severe arthritis, health care has come to focus on quite modest and more realistic goals such as achieving for the patient a level of satisfactory functioning within the constraints set by the disorder. Such targets necessitate greater attention to the economic, social, and psychological circumstances of a patient. The health worker must make decisions that go beyond the primary physical disorder of the patient and beyond the immediate crisis period of medical intervention. The behavioural sciences have contributed towards making such decisions more soundly based. Thus Vaughn and Leff (1976) have shown that very specific aspects of emotions in the family are associated with a poor prognosis for schizophrenic patients after discharge from hospital and that careful consideration by the clinician of such factors can considerably reduce the chances of relapse back into hospital. The long-term consequences of stroke and head injury, reviewed in Chapter 9, require a broader attention to a range of physical, psychological, and social problems.

An equally important challenge stems from the growing recognition that much illness is preventable, even if the extent of practical prevention is still a subject of debate (Doll 1983). One needs to recognize that prevention may concern either avoiding the onset of disease or avoiding the re-occurrence or deterioration of a health problem. A large part of avoidable disease suffered in modern societies may be traced to aspects of behaviour. Two familiar and commonly cited examples are smoking and overeating. Increasingly it is argued that the health worker is, or should be, at the centre of influencing behaviour (Tudor Hart 1981). Whilst health workers such as general practitioners accept this role of health educator in principle, they may in practice feel uncomfortable and uncertain and avoid intervening in this way in consultations (Boulton and Williams 1983). These difficulties may partly account for the modest, although crucial, effects general practitioners have in altering patients' smoking habits (Russell *et al.* 1979). Nevertheless, according to bodies such as the Royal College of General Practitioners (1981) this constitutes a most vital role for primary care and evidence regarding the constraints and opportunities of communication (Chapters 5 and 6) will be of increasing importance.

Focus of the book

The purpose of this book is to outline the contributions of the behavioural sciences to the understanding of experience of illness and treatment. The focus throughout the chapters is upon social and psychological processes that shape the experience of illness presented to health care and the responses of patients to treatment for their problems. We have limited our attention to problems taken to health care. In writing this book, we are primarily directing ourselves therefore, to the health professionals concerned with the care of patients, together with those social scientists who are involved in research and teaching in the health field. With this set of concerns in mind the contributions are organized into three sections. In the first section – 'Illness and Help Seeking' – the emphasis is upon the social and psychological factors that influence the presentation of health problems. The process of defining illness and seeking help is clearly one which is considerably influenced by a range of cultural, social and economic factors.

The second section of the book concentrates on 'The Experience of Treatment'. Here the focus is upon patients' responses to treatment, whether in terms of the anxieties provoked by illness and treatment or in terms of patients' evaluations of the quality of their treatment and of the appropriateness of the health worker's actions. The influence of the health worker is a central issue of the section.

In the last section – 'Chronic and Terminal Illness' – the more devastating and demanding effects of long-term and terminal illness are discussed. It is apparent that, in the range of health problems discussed in this section, the intimate connections of biological, psychological, and social factors are of particular importance. The distress of illness involves not only the patient but his or her family and social network.

The book is intended therefore as a contribution toward the kind of psychosocial perspective upon illness which must increasingly become a core part of the thinking of the health worker. Others before us have advocated such an integration. Engel (1977) has clearly argued that the 'biomedical model' of disease must be radically supplemented to become a 'biopsychosocial model' to incorporate social, psychological, and behavioural dimensions of illness. He proposes that medicine should adopt a systems approach in which it is recognized that disease can be understood by means of several hierarchically organized levels or sub-systems from the cell through levels such as the person, the family, and ultimately society. Others (Katon and Kleinman 1981) have attempted to develop his ambitious 'biopsychosocial' perspective by means of illustrative clinical case material. Katon and Kleinman, for example, discuss a patient with duodenal ulcer. They explore the different levels of explanation of the problem from the biological through to the social, showing the variety of treatment options from drug therapy, through dietary advice and family therapy to intervention at the level of social stressors. Kleinman, Eisenberg, and Good (1978) have advocated what they call a clinical social science. They argue that an integrated bio-psychosocial perspective needs to be fostered by institutional arrangements such as having social scientists and health workers sharing elements of training, working closely together within a department of clinical social science, and carrying out teaching and research from immediate clinical experience.

Whether progress is envisaged in terms of the theoretical integration of disciplines by means of systems theory, or in terms of the institutional integration of social scientists and clinicians in particular academic or health care settings, writers such as Kleinman acknowledge the difficulties of bringing a psychosocial perspective to bear in health care. There are prior problems which have perhaps received less attention. The social science to which reference is made is in reality not one unitary discipline but composed of many sometimes conflicting approaches.

A psychosocial perspective would presently reveal a diversity of methods, acceptable forms of evidence, differing problems, and practical interests. This heterogeneity is explained by the diversity of academic disciplines which contribute to the perspective. One major contributor is psychology which in turn is diverse in focus and interests. It has developed a variety of concepts relevant to the experience of illness, from personality and other forms of individual variation through models of coping and decision-making and more social-psychological analyses of exchanges in health care. It has also traced many intimate connections between the cognitive and the emotional aspects of the experience of illness. Sociology has particularly examined notions such as power, conflict, and divergence of interests in examining relations in health care. Social administration and social medicine have been concerned with issues such as the use of health services by different social groups. Social anthropology has increasingly focused on health care as a cultural belief system. Medical specialties such as psychiatry and general practice have, in the work of authors such as Eisenberg (1977) in America and Balint (1957) in Great Britain, contributed new conceptual frameworks for clinical use in identifying and responding to patients' problems and motivations.

Inevitably the variety of concerns – from identifying problems in the use of health services through to providing models of clinical relevance to the doctor – have led to a diversity in fundamental assumptions that have sometimes reduced the frequency of exchanges across the disciplines that constitute a psychosocial approach.

In addition, institutional pressures within academic settings reinforce disciplinary boundaries between branches of the social and behavioural sciences. The ways in which health professionals are introduced to the subjects strengthen tendencies for disciplines to be perceived as separate. The wide scope of material presented in introductions to medical sociology (from 'the health care services' to 'social causes of illness') or to medical psychology (from 'human development' through to 'perception' and 'memory') require an emphasis on the disciplinary distinctiveness of each subject, to present a coherent perspective to students in a short space of time. Indeed some respect for a discipline's distinctive origins is important. Yet for health care practitioners and those involved in health care research the intellectual challenges reside in the directions set by Engel's programme for a 'biopsychosocial model', a prior step towards which must be the quest for links and relations between the different social sciences.

This is a productive and demanding approach. Where human actions are concerned, a number of different levels of explanation are involved which, if they are to be treated systematically, require a variety of forms and sources of evidence. To take one kind of behaviour – compliance with medical regimes – one would at least imagine the measurement of the problem itself to be uncomplicated. Even if patients' accounts of their drug consumption are deemed unreliable, one could resort to measurement of drug levels in the blood or urine. However, even the latter are not simply and reliably associated with drug ingestion. Moreover the prior and more important problems for the behavioural sciences are the reasons for and causes of patients not complying with medical regimes. Attempts to explain any particular human action such as drug consumption can in principle involve an ever-widening network of factors, from stable properties of the individual's personality, coping style or attitudes, through transient aspects of perception, motives, beliefs, emotions, or relations with health care, to more structural factors such as cultural background or economic circumstances. It is not possible to say in advance which level is adequate for the investigation of any particular problem. The forms of evidence are correspondingly varied in the behavioural sciences, from experiment through questionnaire and interview to observation. No single lines of evidence can be sufficient for the diversity of problems to be addressed.

Thus, in urging that the health worker should take account of a wider range of factors regarding illness, one is also maintaining that he or she accept the rich diversity of sources of evidence that constitute the social sciences. Part of our aim in writing this book has been to gather together some of this evidence, so that it should not simply fall to individual health professionals to do the task on their own.

Part 1
Illness and help seeking

2 *Lay concepts of illness*

Ray Fitzpatrick

The elementary but important principle of this chapter is that human illness occurs, of necessity, within a particular culture that fundamentally shapes and influences the way the illness is experienced. This chapter examines the concepts and beliefs about illness that form one important part of such cultural influences. Illness beliefs shape the responses to symptoms by the sufferer and his or her social network. If health care is sought, the definitions that the lay person brings to bear on his or her illness constrain the kinds of help sought and the perceptions of benefits gained from treatment. This chapter explores the evidence that has recently accumulated about lay concepts of illness and then discusses their significance for providers of health care.

The anthropological investigation of beliefs

Anthropologists in particular have drawn attention to the ways in which cultural beliefs profoundly influence experience and behaviour. They have documented enormous differences in culture from one society to another and, by analysing beliefs that seem very strange and exotic to modern western readers, they make possible a more critical awareness of one's own more familiar and taken for granted beliefs. Illness is one realm of life in which anthropology has vividly demonstrated cultural variation between societies, often documenting beliefs that appear on the surface to be most bizarre and irrational. One of the best-known examples of strange beliefs held in relation to illness is the widespread explanation of illness in terms of witchcraft.

Evans-Pritchard (1937) examined the beliefs of a simple agricultural society in the Sudan – the Azande – amongst whom beliefs about witchcraft were prevalent. For a wide variety of misfortunes, from crop failures to personal accidents and illnesses, the Azande would some-times seek a more basic reason for their occurrence, in addition to more immediate causes such as a pest or a physical hazard. On these occasions a Zande might suspect the possibility that a neighbour had acted as a witch and brought the pest or hazard by despatching the soul or spirit of his witchcraft. To test the hypothesis a number of different kinds of oracle were available which, if consulted by means of appropriate rituals, were believed capable of identifying the source of the witchcraft. If the oracle confirmed that someone had acted as a witch by causing an illness, that individual could be confronted with the charge and requested to withdraw their influence. If necessary, vengeance could be obtained from the guilty party by practising magic in retaliation.

Lest these ideas seem too remote and exotic to be of any relevance to understanding more western communities, Snow (1974) describes simi-lar beliefs amongst working-class blacks who have grown up in the rural southern regions of the United States. He argues that their explanations of illness fall into three general categories: natural and environmental hazards, punishments from God, and spirits and witchcraft. Similar ideas have been described (Fabrega 1974) in Latin American peasant communities who may explain illnesses as due to the 'evil eye' (*mal ojo*) of an enemy.

For present purposes several important lessons emerge from anthro-pological investigations of such exotic belief systems. Clearly they demonstrate the survival of forms of explanation of illness that differ completely from interpretations found in western science. More impor-tantly such beliefs can be seen to form a coherent pattern of ideas in terms of which illness is explained. Ideas, which on the surface seem bizarre, can be seen to make sense when considered more carefully. Evans-Pritchard showed that Azande beliefs about witchcraft and oracles formed a closed, coherent set of ideas that made good sense of reality. Thus if a particular consultation with an oracle produced contradictory or unconvincing results, the individual was not led to question the entire system of beliefs. Instead the particular poison or ritual procedures employed were thought to be at fault. Hypotheses of witchcraft put to the oracles tended to be confined to immediate social networks, amongst whose members enmities and rivalries were more likely to exist, which would confirm the sense of the oracle's decision.

More generally the system of beliefs provided a coherent philosophy of misfortune. The immediate cause of a serious accident would be interpreted in the same way by a Zande and western observer – a branch falling from a tree. However the more fundamental explanation of why the event occurred at a particular moment and to a particular man standing beneath the tree would be found in terms of quite different underlying processes at work in the two observers.

Zande beliefs form a coherent mode of making sense of misfortunes such as illness. Of course in western societies the dominant mode of explanation of illness is quite different and in its most organized form – the science of medicine – is based upon a highly complex and integrated set of concepts of disease aetiology and organic mechanisms in the functioning of the body. Nevertheless there is substantial evidence that this mode of interpreting illness is not uniformly shared by members of western societies and takes different forms in different social groups. The task of this chapter is to review the form and content of lay concepts in western communities, and to examine the extent to which there are substantial differences in lay compared with medical professional concepts and the significance for health care of such differences.

The cultural shaping of illness

First of all it needs to be appreciated that culture, understood here as a connected pattern of language and beliefs, enters into the very nature of illness. An important conceptual distinction is frequently made in this context between disease and illness. Eisenberg discusses the distinction thus: 'patients suffer "illnesses"; physicians diagnose and treat "disease" . . . illnesses are experiences of disvalued changes in states of being and in social function: diseases are abnormalities in the structure and function of body organs and systems' (Eisenberg 1977: 11). Illness therefore here refers to all the *experiential* aspects of bodily disorder which are 'shaped by cultural factors governing perception, labelling, explanation of the discomforting experience' (Kleinman, Eisenberg, and Good 1978: 252).

A useful paradigm for thinking about the influence of cultural and social context upon bodily experience is provided in experiments by the social psychologist Schacter (1975). Subjects were injected with epinephrine which stimulated the sympathetic nervous system, resulting in symptoms such as increased perspiration. Some were then informed of the likely effects of the procedure; others were misinformed or given no information. Subjects were then left in a room with another individual, who, unknown to the subjects, was acting as an assistant to the experiment. These assistants were instructed to act in a variety of moods such as with anger or humorously. Schacter then investigated the subjects' definitions of their own feelings. He found that those who had not been appropriately informed of the physiological implications of their injection were considerably influenced by the mood or example to which they had been exposed; interpreting for example their arousal as anger more often if they had previously been in the company of the assistant instructed to display anger. A control group injected with saline which did not generally stimulate physiological arousal were less influenced by their social context. Schacter developed a theory in which the nature and quality of emotions is determined in an interaction between physical state and cognitive perceptions which are in turn influenced by social context. His demonstration also offers a model for thinking about disease and illness: the cognitive meaning assigned to abnormal bodily states is socially and culturally shaped and in turn constitutes the experience for the sufferer.

The example of depressive disorders can be used to develop the point. In many non-western cultures, for example in China and the Middle East (Fitzpatrick 1983; Katon, Kleinman, and Rosen 1982) depression and other neurotic disorders are presented with a greater concentration of physical symptoms than are found in western psychiatric clinics. Often patients from such societies, although displaying depressed affect, may report few symptoms relating to internal mood states, concentrating rather on various physical symptoms. Kleinman (1980) found in his clinics for Chinese psychiatric patients in Taiwan that the majority that he diagnosed as suffering from depression presented physical symptoms as their main complaint. He points out that the languages of Taiwan are rich in terminology relating to the body but have few terms corresponding to the wide variety of western internal psychological states.

White (1982) examined the notion of cultural differences in concepts of illness by means of a sample of students in Hawaii, half of whom were Hong Kong Chinese, the other half Caucasian American. The students were given a list of psychosocial problems such as 'difficulty sleeping', 'feeling anxious and tense', 'headaches' and 'feeling lonely'. They were asked to give in as much detail as possible the likely causes of each problem. Coders classified the students' explanations. For both somatic problems such as 'headache' and psychosomatic problems such as 'appetite loss' the American students were more likely to give explanations in terms of internal emotional states. For psychological problems such as 'sadness' and for somatic problems, the Chinese students were more likely to cite external pressures such as the family or the demands of academic studies. Thus the two cultures offered different conceptual emphases in the causes of problems: American culture focusing upon internal feeling states, Chinese culture emphasizing external situational causation.

The content of western lay beliefs

In recent years investigators have begun to consider the form and content of beliefs about illness of modern western communities. The most striking result of such studies is the variety and importance of ideas about the causes of illness. Blaxter (1983a) interviewed a sample of working-class, middle-aged women in Scotland about their ideas of health and illness. The women were free to discuss whichever disorders they wished in unstructured interviews focused upon the health of their families. The sample discussed 587 examples of episodes of disease and the issue of cause was mentioned in 74 per cent of examples. Blaxter then classified the causes cited by the women. Infection was by far the most common category of cause invoked. Next most frequent was heredity, followed by environmental hazards, secondary effects of other diseases, stress, childbearing and the menopause, and trauma and surgery. Less common as a category of cause was the notion of a self-inflicted disorder through neglect or behavioural choices. Blaxter observes that the search for causal patterns in their health histories was extremely important to the women and she refers to a 'positive strain towards accounting for their present bodily state . . . by connecting together the relevant health events' (Blaxter 1983a: 67).

A similarly designed study by Pill and Stott (1982) allows some comparison with another region of Great Britain – South Wales. The authors report interviews conducted with women aged 30–35 years who were selected from a social background of skilled manual workers. In these interviews infection or germs were again the most commonly cited cause of illness, after which, in decreasing order of frequency, were cited life-style, heredity, and stress. Approximately half the women in this sample employed concepts of cause that involved behavioural choice and some degree of individual responsibility for illness. These women were more likely to be home owners and to have had more education, and their feeling of control in their lives may account for the greater sense of responsibility compared with Blaxter's respondents.

Although the methods of investigation in the two studies were not identical, some common themes emerged which can be put into a comparative perspective. Chrisman (1977) provides a framework from a review of cross-cultural evidence of folk ideas about illness in which he identifies different modes of thought about the causes of illness. He calls such modes of thought 'logics' and identifies four basic kinds:

1   A logic of degeneration in which illness follows the running down of the body.
2   A mechanical logic in which illness is the outcome of blockages or damage to bodily structures.
3   A logic of balance in which illness follows from disruption of

harmony between parts or between the individual and the environment.

4   A logic of invasion which includes germ theory and other material intrusions responsible for illness.

These logics may be viewed as dominant themes or metaphors which permeate beliefs about illness and vary in importance from one culture to another. Thus the logic of balance is fundamental to traditional Latin American beliefs about the implication of 'hot' and 'cold' factors in illness and is also important in classical Indian ideas of the balance between 'humours' determining health. As shall be seen in the work of Herzlich (1973) such thinking may also be involved in western folk beliefs in illness as an outcome of relations between man and an 'unnatural' environment.

Ideas of degeneration were not frequently cited in the studies by Blaxter or Pill and Stott as causes of specific diseases, although disorders such as rheumatism were sometimes seen as a natural part of ageing. Clearly in modern Britain the logic of invasion is an important mode of thinking about illness and must partly be seen as the cultural result of the impact of microbiological developments in western science in the last part of the nineteenth century. The theme of heredity, frequently expressed in both Blaxter's and Pill and Stott's samples, is less easily traced back to earlier modes of medical thought and, as Blaxter observes (1983a: 63), there appears to be a greater readiness to invoke genetic causation in lay culture than in medical science. Patterns of shared illness in families offer a powerful source of ideas of inheritance. However it is unclear how universal such interpretations are. A review (Janzen and Prins 1981) of traditional African systems of explaining illness makes little mention of heredity as a form of cause.

Probably one of the most characteristically western modes of interpreting illness can be found in the variety of related concepts such as 'stress', 'worry', and 'tension'. Yet it has often been argued (Eisenberg 1977; Engel 1977) that the dominant approach to health and illness in modern western society is one which seeks the explanation of disease in reductionist physical principles and operates with a mind–body dualism, that is a perspective in which the two realms are distinct and separate. Engel terms this approach the 'biomedical model':

'The dominant model of disease today is biomedical, with molecular biology its basic scientific discipline. It assumes disease to be fully accounted for by deviations from the norm of measurable (somatic) variables. It leaves no room within its framework for the social, psychological and behavioural dimensions of illness.'

(Engel 1977: 196)

It is therefore at this point that there may exist some of the sharpest differences between popular, lay ideas and those enshrined in the culture of medical science.

The structure of lay beliefs

One of the most striking qualities of lay concepts of illness is their very complexity. Both Blaxter and Pill and Stott were impressed by the complex, multifactorial approach that their respondents frequently employed in explaining illness. This quality becomes most apparent when some systematic effort is invested in obtaining a number of respondents' ideas about one particular disease. Blumhagen (1980), as an example of such research, investigated the views about their disorder of 103 patients attending a clinic for hypertension in the United States. The members of the sample cited an average of thirteen separate items each in their view of what constituted the causes, pathophysiology and prognosis of hypertension. Blumhagen lists ten different kinds of causal factors that were commonly cited, ranging from chronic external stress to heredity, salt, water, and food generally. Thus Blumhagen argues that the folk concept of hypertension is complex, involving a large number of elements and numerous connections between elements. It is interesting that in this study too stress plays a major part in beliefs about causation. Half the sample cited chronic external stress as implicated in hypertension, either in terms of 'the build up of normal stresses of life' or 'job stresses' in particular. Specific acute stresses were also seen by more than half the sample as involved in hypertension. In fact psychosocial factors were so central to the patients' understanding of the disorder that Blumhagen sees 'Hyper-Tension' in the sense of 'excessive tenseness' as being the essence of the idea of the disorder for many patients by contrast with the professional medical model of hypertension as a systemic circulatory problem.

Although such research suggests a good deal of complexity in the patterns of ideas about illness reported by lay individuals, it may be misleading to talk of such ideas, as some writers have (for example Pill and Stott 1982: 45) as lay *theories*. The term 'theory' implies a high degree of consistency, order, stability, and rationality, properties that may not be essential to lay concepts. Blumhagen, for example, reports that some respondents gave unrelated, parallel models of hypertension at different stages in their interview. When confronted with the differences, the patients did not feel that the inconsistencies between different parts of their explanations were problematic. In relation to the illogicalities and inconsistencies that are a part of lay belief systems in every culture, Kleinman points out that 'laymen are not concerned with their theoretical rigor so much as the treatment options they give rise to' (Kleinman

1980: 93). In other words lay concepts are pragmatic, and are rarely publicly produced for critical scrutiny.

For the same reason, in so far as lay ideas are seldom formalized and normally only emerge as an element of decision-making about actual illness episodes, they are expressed extremely tentatively. Thus Pill and Stott describe their respondents as 'unsure of themselves and less articulate when discussing aetiological topics' (Pill and Stott 1982: 46). The tone of interviews became more hesitant and statements were more often qualified by such phrases as 'I suppose'. People may be quite uncomfortable about expressing and organizing ideas which normally remain tacit background resources to be drawn upon when coping with their own or other peoples' illnesses. Stoeckle and Barsky argue for the importance to doctors of eliciting patients' concepts in their consultations but acknowledge that 'On initial contact patients may be reluctant to divulge their ideas for fear these will be regarded as unsophisticated, foolish or so irrational that they themselves will be met with amusement, disrespect or even reproach' (Stoeckle and Barsky 1981: 225).

Another way in which such ideas differ from theoretical knowledge is that they are *syncretic* in origin, that is, deriving from a variety of originally disparate and distinct sources. Ideas are selectively drawn upon from a variety of different traditions and adjusted according to the current concerns of the individual. This is most easily shown in the interpretations people make of illness in a society such as Sri Lanka in which a number of separate medical systems survive with quite independent traditions such as Ayurvedic practice, western scientific medicine, and folk, spiritist healing. Amara Singham (1980) describes a family in Sri Lanka attempting to make sense of the onset of mental illness in their daughter and to obtain practical help. They turn from one kind of healer to another and although they are offered explanations and treatments that are theoretically incompatible with each other, they nevertheless selectively retrieve elements from each that help to make sense of the alarming experience. The study shows how active, constructive, and selective is the process of making sense of illness, in which ideas from a variety of sources are drawn upon and reworked. It is the syncretic nature of lay ideas about illness which explains why it is frequently observed (e.g. Blaxter 1983a: 67) how difficult it is to disentangle the sources (whether the media, social networks, or doctors) that people draw upon in their ideas.

One particular way in which lay ideas differ from formal forms of thought is the flexible manner in which ideas respond to experience. Anthropologists and other social scientists normally portray the culture of a society, of which beliefs are an element, as a stable and relatively enduring means by which the society copes with its environment. In terms of general, fundamental themes, cultural beliefs about illness are quite stable. Nevertheless there is a danger of what might be termed *reifying* lay explanations of illness and viewing them as fixed frameworks in terms of which health and illness are experienced. This is the risk attached to any approach to explaining human action which focuses on beliefs and ideas: the very investigation of the beliefs may make them appear more solid and inflexible than in reality they are. One way in which this point can be illustrated is by looking at the impact that incurring an illness may have on beliefs about the nature of the particular disorder. Linn, Linn, and Stein (1982) asked two groups of patients in an American hospital about their beliefs about the causes of cancer. One group were end-stage cancer patients; the other patients suffered from other chronic diseases such as diabetes. Although both groups cited smoking and work as causes of cancer, the cancer sufferers were much more likely to cite what the researchers term 'God's will' or inheritance compared to the other patients who attributed more importance to other environmental factors such as diet. More importantly, the cancer patients were less firm in their convictions about causes than the other group. The authors suggest that the non-cancer sufferers may respond in terms of stereotypes of risk factors to which the media have drawn attention. For persons afflicted with a life threatening disease, the need to make sense of personal misfortune is immense. Publicly available ideas about causes provide only partial sense of why the individual and not others also at risk have been afflicted. Cultural beliefs about causes may therefore be a less salient part of the experience and more transcendental explanations come to the fore.

Beliefs as a 'system'

Some anthropologists take seriously the term 'system' when they talk of a community's belief system with regard to health and illness. Essentially they argue that the beliefs about illness identified in a community should be analyzed in terms of a system in the sense that beliefs are held to be interconnected and structured elements of a whole, rather than a random set of items that a group of people happen to believe in common. An example of the application of this approach to the experience of illness is the work of Helman (1978) who as a general practitioner and anthropologist has examined patterns of ideas about infectious illness in a north London community. Helman argues that a folk classificatory system, with origins quite distinct from medical science, can be detected behind a variety of ideas about illnesses which are commonly viewed as departures from normal body temperature. Patients distinguish the subjectively hot illnesses which are fevers from the cold illnesses which are classified as chills or colds. From a knowledge of which category a set of symptoms indicate, it is possible to read off a set of causes, typical kinds of course, appropriate treatment and also the degree of individual blame attached to the sufferer in contracting the illness. Colds and chills are viewed as the product of the individual's relations with the natural environment and lower temperatures in the environment can, through dampness, cold winds and draughts, penetrate particularly vulnerable surfaces of the body such as the head and the feet. Transitions from hot to cold such as 'going into a cold room after a hot bath' can leave an individual particularly vulnerable. Treatment involves restoring temperature equilibrium by hot drinks or a warm bed. The individual may often be to blame for incurring the illness by irresponsible actions such as going out with wet hair. Fevers are due to invisible entities – 'germs' or 'bugs' – transmitted from individual to individual. One important treatment is fluid which 'flushes out' germs. The individual is less personally responsible for fevers as they are unavoidably transmitted through social relationships. Helman points out that germs are spoken of in similar ways, and have a similarly hypothetical nature to the spirits thought responsible for illness in many simple agricultural societies.

Helman suggests that this system of beliefs is, at present, unstable: in particular, younger patients tend to view both colds and fevers as due to germs and viruses and less as a result of their own responsible actions. These changes in beliefs are partly due to changes in medicine, especially the growth in availability of antibiotics.

The derivation of such a *system* of beliefs by anthropological techniques involved interpretive methods of detecting patterns and themes behind a number of respondents' expressed views. It may well be that no individual could explicate all of the distinctions and principles that the observer would claim to exist in a community's beliefs. This is an important point because in clinical practice, or where a researcher discusses the views of a single respondent, it may be difficult to identify patterns of the kind that Helman has examined. The elements of an individual's views about illness may be more limited, tentative, inconsistent and less elaborately worked out. Young (1981) warns of the dangers of a 'Rational Man' assumption in this field if one too enthusiastically looks for cognitive patterns behind statements. Results may be the peculiar product of the exchange between researcher and respondent rather than reflecting ideas that are important to the respondent in actual episodes of illness.

Images and associations in concepts of illness

So far lay concepts of illness have been discussed as if they paralleled scientific medicine in concentrating upon the symptoms, causes, and therapies of illness entities. Certainly studies such as those of Blaxter, Blumhagen, and Helman suggest that such focuses are important.

However a different approach suggests that illness concepts, in addition to naming an alternative set of entities and causes to those of medicine, also operate as condensed symbols that refer to a wider variety of experiences contained in a culture. Lay concepts of illness do not merely name entities in the body but are powerful images associated with other realms of life. Good (1977) offers an analysis in these terms of a commonly reported complaint in traditional Iranian communities that he translates as 'heart distress'. It is particularly common in working-class women and frequently presented to the doctor. It is viewed as a disturbance in the heart caused by emotional distress. Traditional Iranians believe the heart to be the source of heat and vitality and the driving force of the body in contrast to western emphasis on its role in the circulation of blood. At the same time the heart is used linguistically to express emotions. Thus physical sensations of the heart and emotional feelings are intimately connected in traditional thinking. The complaint of 'heart distress' conveys a wider series of associations in Iranian society. Firstly the contraceptive pill is thought by many Iranian women to cause 'heart distress' and is also associated with ageing and infertility. Other associations link the contraceptive pill with menstrual flow and ritual pollution. Good argues that 'heart distress' is therefore a powerful idiom to express many female concerns with sexuality and fertility. Another set of associations link heart distress with on the one hand grief and melancholy from the loss of relatives and on the other hand with the anxiety of interpersonal problems and poverty of working-class life. One respondent explained to Good: 'We are poor, we don't have any money, we all have heart problems' (Good 1977: 47).

Thus Good argues that 'heart distress' in Iranian culture is not a neatly defined category referring to a specific disorder and may convey any of a variety of symptoms, illnesses, or problems. 'Heart distress is an image which draws together a network of symbols, situations, motives, feelings and stresses which are rooted in the structural setting in which the people of Maragheh live' (Good 1977: 48). Western-trained doctors are likely to misunderstand patients presenting with heart distress, examining the heart and offering reassurance that there is nothing wrong.

The importance of research by anthropologists such as Good is that we are reminded that lay concepts of illness may have powerful symbolic significance which cannot conveniently be expressed in so many words by the patient or informant but which form an essential element of the meaning of illness experience. They also suggest that we too narrowly limit the search for meaning if we only look for references to bodily symptoms or causes in lay ideas of illness.

Herzlich argued that there was a need for 'a modern anthropology of the facts of health and illness' (Herzlich 1973: 6) that would identify the images and symbols that are the counterparts in modern society to those investigated by anthropologists such as Good. She interviewed a sample of professional and middle-class French subjects about their ideas of health and illness. One of the dominant themes that emerged was the influence of 'the way of life' upon illness. Mainly respondents connected urban life-styles and illness. To some extent individual differences in reserves of health were thought to influence resistance to the impact of one's way of life, but the latter was paramount. City life was associated with a variety of other concepts: 'unhealthy', 'constraining', 'abnormal', 'chemical', 'unnatural', and 'hurried pace of life'. The toxic influences of city life were linked to an intermediate state between health and illness – a feeling of physical and mental fatigue – which rendered the individual vulnerable to illness. The unnatural and unhealthy features of urban life contrasted with the natural, the rural and past ways of life in which man was more in harmony with his environment. Herzlich's respondents viewed the unnatural as the product of modern, technological society.

The contrasts drawn between, for example, the natural and the unnatural were seldom given precise meaning and, as Good also argues, gain sense from condensing powerful associations within the culture of the respondent. Herzlich points out (1973: 26) that they are images daily reproduced by the media and require little effort or original thought when applied by individuals to their own lives. Nevertheless they provide an important vocabulary in terms of which illness is explained and one which has only superficially been replaced by the language of physiology or bodily processes. Herzlich's respondents do present particular health problems in terms of localized symptoms involving particular organs, especially when presenting to doctors, but they look for patterns and interpretations in terms of a wider set of themes.

Patients' ideas of particular illnesses can be considered in the same way to uncover their multiple associations. For example nervous tension is a frequent theme in Herzlich's study. 'Nerves' have played an important role in pre-modern medical theories of disease long before the development of neurological models of the structure and function of nervous tissues. Thus the nerves played a central explanatory role in the theories of disease of the influential Edinburgh medical school in the eighteenth century (Lawrence 1979). Since then the meaning of the concept has undergone many transformations from the development of psychoanalytic theory as well as from changes in physiological science. Thus lay ideas might be expected to reflect many of these developments. 'Nerves' are one of the categories of illness reported by Blaxter's sample of women. It is a common form of illness presentation in British general practice (Stimson and Webb 1975: 62), and one of the most common ways in which patients currently taking psychotropic drugs define their problem (Helman 1981: 524). Descriptions of nerves suggest combinations of emotional states such as agitation with such physical symptoms as a 'tight stomach'. Nerves may also cause other health problems. One-third of a sample of sufferers of rheumatoid arthritis explained their disorder in these terms (Markson 1971: 164). This damaging property of nerves clearly parallels eighteenth-century medical ideas as well as contemporary psychosomatic research. On the other hand nerves especially as a diagnosis from a doctor may be interpreted as a dismissive term, especially where it is diagnosed from only superficial acquaintance with the patient (Blaxter 1983a: 64). Here the term has associations with failure to cope with normal demands in life, resulting in trivial symptoms. The images and associations of lay concepts are not easily delineated and the context of their use is most likely to give greater specificity to the intended meaning. It is quite clear that they are above all flexible and capable of a range of referents.

The 'gulf' between lay and medical concepts

Underlying the chapter has been a question as to how different are the concepts of patients and of medicine with regard to illness. In order to draw attention to and make sense of problems of communication between health professionals and the public, social scientists have sometimes portrayed in quite dramatic forms the distance between the two modes of thought. The view of Freidson for example is that 'the separate worlds of experience and reference of the layman and the professional worker are always in potential conflict with one another' (Freidson 1974: 286). This clash of perspectives is most evident when one considers the beliefs of ethnic minority groups in modern western societies who have remained least integrated into the majority culture. There are many instances in the United States. The beliefs in spiritual causation of illness of some black rural communities have already been cited. Harwood (1971) describes the 'hot'–'cold' concepts of Puerto Ricans, by which illnesses are classified as 'hot' or 'cold' and are treated by medications that are classified as their opposite. Such examples suggest possibilities of profound problems in communication between western medicine and those folk belief systems with different cultural origins.

However the analysis of writers such as Freidson is often used to portray a profound gulf between scientific medicine and the majority of lay persons, especially because of the reliance by medicine upon scientific technology to the neglect of those social and psychological aspects of disorders which concern patients. Clearly this view finds support in the work of Engel (1977) and others who would wish to modify the biomedical model in medicine.

Yet there is a risk that the notion of a cultural gulf between lay and professional modes of thought be exaggerated or misunderstood. In the first place those who have sharply contrasted the medical model with lay perspectives may have failed to recognize the major differences that exist between medicine enshrined in textbooks and clinical practice. Lock (1982) examined the approaches of medicine to the menopause. The subject as treated in textbooks is formal, complex, and replete with unresolved technical controversies. When Lock interviewed practising gynaecologists, their views about menopause were simpler, based on fewer scientific principles, and selective. Also there was a wide variety from very biomedical to very psychosocial approaches amongst clinicians. Lock argues that the doctors' views were best understood as folk models to contrast them with formal textual models. Medical folk models have to be simpler to deal with the practical exigencies of clinical work. There is evidence (Gaines 1979) that doctors retain many lay assumptions and ideas about illness acquired before training and that these assumptions play an important role in clinical practice alongside formal scientific principles.

General practice may be more directly influenced by lay or folk concepts and may be thought of as a system of thought midway between hospital medicine and lay ideas. Helman (1978) argues that general practice depends to a large extent on the doctor moving some distance towards the categories that are important to his patients. This is clear, he argues, in the case of the fevers and colds presented to the general practitioner. Cough mixtures are frequently prescribed even where scientific evidence suggests that they are of negligible pharmacological benefit. Yet they do make sense in terms of a folk model that sees cough mixtures as washing out the germs of fevers. Similarly antibiotics are given inappropriately for viral conditions because the doctor is responding to the patient's presentation of 'germs' which are not differentiated in the folk model. He concludes:

> 'Biomedical concepts are tailored to fit in more closely with the patient's model in the consultation; partly to avoid "cognitive dissonance" in the interpretation of the illness; partly because most conditions in the Fevers/Colds/Chills model are self limiting – so that treating them symptomatically the GPs are less concerned to be biomedically "scientific" than they would be in more dangerous conditions.'
>
> (Helman 1978: 132–3)

Thus for various reasons an uncritical assertion of 'two worlds of experience' may be misleading. Gulfs of a different kind used to be implied in many early studies of communication between doctors and patients which identified the causes for failures of communication in patients' ignorance of medical terms and in the gaps in knowledge between the two parties. Although much depends on how knowledge is measured, the simple stereotype of the ignorant patient has had to be modified in the light of research. Segall and Roberts (1980) examined the levels of understanding of twelve medical terms in a sample of patients attending clinics in a Canadian hospital. The proportion of respondents giving what the researchers accepted as correct interpretations varied from 95 per cent for 'cerebral' and only 28 per cent for 'tendon'. The average level of correct understanding was 76 per cent. The items used were the same as a study reported in 1961 and a comparison showed higher levels of correct answers in the more recent sample.

Segall and Roberts also asked the doctors concerned to estimate the proportion of their patients who would correctly understand each item. For some items the doctors seriously underestimated their patients: for example 83 per cent of doctors underestimated patients' abilities to understand 'cerebral'. Overall 47 per cent of doctors were accurate, 12 per cent overestimated and 41 per cent underestimated patients' comprehension. It is possible that the stereotype of the patient with little or no ability to comprehend medical language is self-perpetuating; in other words that doctors, assuming a poorly informed patient, avoid extended discussion in consultations as a result of which their stereotypes are perpetuated (McKinlay 1975). The point argued here is that the idea of unbridgeable gulfs, whether in terms of knowledge versus ignorance or a more cultural theory of separate worlds of experience, may be misleading or damaging. Indeed the major weakness of such views is that they are unable to do justice to the complex processes at work in communication.

Active 'sense-making'

The most important feature of communication between lay and professional models of illness in western societies such as Great Britain and the United States is that, on the majority of occasions, there is *some* common ground of language and meanings. The work of Segall and Roberts and other studies (Plaja, Cohen, and Samora 1968) show this. But this shared ground may be misleading to both parties as well as to the observer.

It is becoming increasingly apparent that communication of any kind is an active and constructive process in that the parties to communication have to make up and fill out the sense behind the information they receive. This constructive 'sense-making' is achieved by means of the actor's own assumptions, beliefs, and ideas. Perhaps the most dramatic, if bizarre demonstration of the active work involved in making sense of information is reported by Garfinkel (1967). Students were informed that as a way of improving a student psychotherapy counselling service, a pilot project was being tried in which students in the consulting room were to express their queries and problems in a form that allowed an answering service to reply either 'yes' or 'no': no other response would be available. Unknown to the volunteers in the experimental form of counselling, the service was constructed to produce randomized answers which would bear no relation to the questions posed by those consulting. Students interviewed after their sessions with this strange service showed remarkable abilities to make sense of the series of replies they received to their questions and inferred patterns of meaning behind the random yesses and noes that they had heard. This ability to see patterns and sense in other people's expressions is an essential element of human communication. When the terminology is the same, it is all too easy to imagine that the meaning intended by both parties overlap completely. Blumhagen graphically summarizes the problem for medicine from his own research: 'Plain folk say "Hyper-Tension"; the experts say, hypertension and each thinks the other is talking about the same thing' (Blumhagen 1980: 224). Instead his research shows significant differences in meaning that doctors and patients bring to bear. In the following quotation, a general practitioner draws out, from the doctor's point of view, the problems that are hidden by the apparent familiarity of patients' complaints such as 'biliousness', 'indigestion', 'eye strain', and 'fibrositis'.

> 'The familiarity of such ideas blinds many physicians to the fact that they are rooted in a system of folk medical concepts and are alien to the cosmopolitan medical system. It is so easy to translate from a patient's description of himself as "bilious" into the attendant symptoms of nausea, anorexia, abdominal discomfort and maybe eructation . . . into a diagnostic category of cosmopolitan medicine, that most physicians perform the translation unconsciously.
>
> '. . . it must not be assumed that identical terms have identical referents in the two systems . . . when a patient speaks of "rheumatism" he is not usually referring to one of the rheumatic diseases recognized by doctors.'
>
> (Stevenson 1980: 1)

All of the same cautions about being misled by familiar terms might just as easily be given to patients! The ease of translation, so essential to communication, is also the problem for both parties in medical consultations. Thus Kleinman (1980), Good (1977), and others argue that it is a constant and essential task of health care professionals to clarify the meaning behind presented problems and to monitor the ways in which patients interpret and assimilate important information which they have been given.

It is now essential to address directly the view that patients' ideas may be relevant to the practice of health care, and to review evidence of the therapeutic benefits of a concern for patients' concepts of their health problems.

The therapeutic significance of lay concepts of illness

IDENTIFYING THE PROBLEM

Patients present problems rather than diseases. There is a considerable amount of selection by patients of how problems are to be presented to the doctor (Stimson and Webb 1975: 22–36). 'In perceiving his symptoms, the patient attempts to interpret them and in explaining these symptoms both to himself and to the doctor, he is defining, categorizing and causally linking them to other factors which he feels may be related' (Stimson and Webb 1975: 40). Stimson and Webb suggest there is almost a ritual order governing the form in which problems are actually presented in the consulting room, for example with priority being given to physical symptoms, leaving fears about serious disease unexpressed until the end of a consultation. The clinician's task is not only to arrive at a diagnosis of the diseases in terms of abnormal physical or mental functioning (and in many instances no diseases can be found) but also to identify the illness – the concerns and perceptions that organize and motivate the patient's consultation. The evidence is familiar and convincing that consultations are less successful from the patient's point of view where the illness as well as the disease is not dealt with by the doctor (Balint 1957; Zola 1973). A constant concern with the ideas behind presented problems is one way of paying attention to illness as well as disease.

MONITORING THE IMPACT OF DIAGNOSTIC INFORMATION

One of the most important functions of the doctor is to provide a name for problems and an explanation of the name. It is rare that this information is the sole source for patients who are discovering the meaning of their health problems. It is important to be aware of the meanings that patients come to assign to the diagnoses that they receive. Haynes and colleagues (1978) showed that one of the unforeseen consequences of a programme for identifying and treating patients with high blood pressure was that a number of men, previously unaware of any health problem, subsequently defined themselves as ill and absented themselves from work. The degree of handicap that they associated with their condition may well have been unnecessary and could have been redressed by the doctor. Bloom and Monterossa (1981) identified a group of individuals who had been in a screening survey of blood pressure in a low-income community in California. They had been told in the survey by a physician that they were hypertensive but were later judged on the basis of three more measures to be normal. They were found to have more depressive symptoms and to report a lower state of general health than a comparison group, which could only be attributed to the impact upon them of being labelled as hypertensive. Both studies suggest a different set of interpretations of the medical label from those of either medicine or Blumhagen's Hyper-Tension. There is every reason to think that addressing the meanings assigned to such labels could be beneficial in reducing such secondary handicaps.

REASSURANCE IN RELATION TO 'NON-DISEASE'

A high proportion of the work of medicine involves reassuring patients who have become concerned about symptoms which prove to have no basis in disease. Mayou (1976) observes that, although estimates of the frequency of such worries amongst patients are very high, little is known of their prognosis after medical treatment. The firm 'don't worry, it's quite normal' from the doctor does not necessarily produce reassurance and indeed may well be counterproductive in its insensitivity. Reassurance is clearly more complex. In a study (Fitzpatrick and Hopkins 1981a) of patients presenting at out-patient clinics with headaches, none of which were found, on investigation, to be due to serious structural lesions, 60 per cent of patients were assessed prior to their clinic consultations as having worries about serious diseases such as, for example, brain tumour. Of the patients with such worries, 40 per cent continued to express such concerns when interviewed three weeks afterwards.

There would appear to be at least two essential elements to successful reassurance which this study illustrates. Firstly patients who were dissatisfied with communication at the clinics were less likely to be reassured. As Kessel observes, 'An important requisite of reassurance is information. A patient needs to know what his condition is and that knowledge should allow him to appreciate what his symptoms signify' (Kessel 1979: 1130). Before that, however, it is important, following the terms of a discussion of reassurance by Sapira (1972) to elicit the 'affective meaning of symptoms'. From the patient's point of view reassurance is more convincing if the doctor has understood his or her perspective as an individual. Kessel summarizes this essential element:

> 'The doctor may wish to consider the patient's condition within medical terms of reference – that is pathological process. The patient's terms of reference embody what he is actually going through and he will not be reassured unless he believes that the doctor is sensitive to and understands that.'
>
> (Kessel 1979: 1131)

Frequently doctors infer the feelings and ideas patients have about their symptoms from indirect cues such as tone of voice. This may not always be the most successful strategy. In the study of patients with headache, 39 per cent of those worried about their illness were not recognized as such by the specialist. Sapira and Kessel both recommend simple strategies directly to elicit patients' thoughts, such as: 'Tell me more about the way this symptom worries you.' In any case eliciting the patients' ideas gives the doctor a clearer view of the worries that he needs to address and is likely to give the patient the sense that subsequent steps to reassure are personally appropriate.

OBTAINING CO-OPERATION WITH LONG-TERM TREATMENT

Chronic illnesses are now the biggest form of health problem confronting medicine. Longer periods of time in which the sufferer lives with his or her illness also mean more time in which to reinterpret the significance of symptoms and their treatment. The doctor has therefore a greater task in maintaining the co-operation of treatments especially where, as in long-term drug therapy, the patient administers the treatment. A study by Inui, Yourtree, and Williamson (1976), again in relation to hypertension, suggests the importance of bringing to the fore patients' own concepts of illness in fostering co-operation with treatment. They report the results of giving a group of doctors a single training session about the nature and importance of patients' health beliefs. These doctors were encouraged to elicit patients' beliefs and, where necessary, to modify them to be more appropriate to co-operation with long-term drug therapy. The single session had the desired effect in that study doctors allocated more time to discussing patients' ideas. Subsequently their patients were found to be more compliant with drug regimes and to have better control of their blood pressure than patients in a control group.

Mazzuca (1982), reviewing a large number of such studies evaluating the benefits of health education upon chronic illness, concludes that a standard presentation of medical information (on such matters as health risks) is less effective than interventions designed to address the variety of individuals' particular problems of coping with long-term treatment. Indeed a more recent investigation (Morisky et al. 1983) of the efficacy of health education in the treatment of hypertension showed impressive results from incorporating the following into the intervention: firstly a brief consultation in which the individual's own concerns in relation to therapy were discussed in a short consultation; secondly a session involving discussions with a key family member regarding perceptions and problems with the treatment of the hypertensive and thirdly a group discussion of hypertensive patients on problems of treatment. In their five-year follow-up hypertension related mortality was 53 per cent less than a normally managed control group. The open discussion of patients' concerns and ideas is therefore an essential first step to offering personally appropriate health information.

The value of an awareness of lay concepts of illness is suggested in a different way in the study by Harwood (1971), cited earlier. The metaphorical classification of illnesses and treatment into 'hot' and 'cold' amongst New York Puerto Ricans presents a particular problem in the case of pregnant women who may avoid iron or vitamin supplements which are classified as 'hot' and thought to cause rashes and irritations (both 'hot') in their babies. Fruit juice however is 'cold'. Doctors may therefore suggest that fruit juice be taken with supplements in order for the 'cold' to neutralize the 'hot'.

More generally, sensitivity to patients' concepts of illness may be essential to a continuing awareness of the wide variety of treatments used, especially by the sufferers of chronic illness, which may make good sense from within lay concepts of a disorder and its treatment but may be viewed as problematic by the doctor concerned with possible inter-actions with his own therapy. How common such alternative treatment may be is illustrated in a study of sufferers of rheumatoid and osteo-arthritis which found that no less than 94 per cent had used 'alternative' therapies, with an average of more than three different items each (Kronenfeld and Wasner 1982).

SUPPORTING THE PATIENT

Stoeckle and Barsky (1981) provide an important discussion of the relevance for clinicians of patients' illness 'attributions' which is their term for the concepts that patients have about symptoms. They observe:

'Patients are more likely to feel genuinely supported when they sense that the doctor's behaviour expresses a concern based on a personal understanding of them than when it only shows authoritative medical competence. Because attribution is a sensitive indicator of the patient's perceptions, its recognition is one demonstration of that understanding.'

(Stoeckle and Barsky 1981: 225)

Eliciting patients' views on their illnesses may be an important means of expressing concern and providing support. Some evidence for the direct therapeutic value of this form of support comes from the study of patients presenting at clinics with headaches already cited (Fitzpatrick and Hopkins 1981b; Fitzpatrick, Hopkins, and Harvard-Watts 1983). Those patients who were satisfied that their consultation with the specialist had been appropriate to their personal concerns and problems were found one year later to have significantly less severe symptoms than patients who had found their consultation superficial or inappropriate. These beneficial effects were separate from the influence of reassurance already discussed. The relationship was also quite independent of any specific treatment such as medication which had only modest therapeutic effects. The study illustrates the powerful non-specific therapeutic effects in Stoeckle and Barsky's concept of personal support. Similarly Mumford, Schlesinger and Glass (1982) review thirty-four controlled studies of the effect of psychological intervention in patients recovering from surgery or post heart-attack hospitalization. Giving information to patients clearly enhances the speed of recovery, but it is more effective when matched to the particular concerns and ideas of the individual patient. Again, it is suggested that the eliciting of patients' ideas is an essential requisite of successful support.

Conclusions

The evidence of this chapter suggests that patients' interpretations of their symptoms are governed by concepts and ideas of considerable complexity and variety. More attention still needs to be given to the ways in which such ideas are brought to bear in coping with specific health problems. This new field of study has of necessity presented a somewhat preliminary, global, and static view of the role of concepts in coping with illness, and their dynamic relations in patients suffering illness and seeking treatment needs further investigation. Nevertheless there are firm grounds for arguing that attention to patients' interpretations of their health problems has been shown to be clinically fruitful and can be successfully incorporated into the practice of health care.

3   *The illness iceberg and aspects of consulting behaviour*

Graham Scambler
and Annette Scambler[1]

Introduction

The study of health-related behaviour has mushroomed in the last twenty years and the published literature is now massive, detailed and disparate. Not surprisingly there have been many attempts during the same period to distinguish different categories of such behaviour. One early and useful attempt was that of Kasl and Cobb (1966), who suggested the following three-fold classification. They defined 'health behaviour' as any activity undertaken by individuals who see themselves as healthy for the purpose of preventing disease or detecting it in an asymptomatic stage; 'illness behaviour' as any activity undertaken by individuals who perceive themselves as ill for the purpose of defining their state of health and discovering an appropriate remedy; and 'sick-role behaviour' as any activity undertaken by individuals who consider themselves to be ill for the purpose of getting well. This chapter focuses largely on illness behaviour, thus defined, although some reference is also made to health and sick-role behaviour.

1 Annette Scambler is currently a researcher in the Department of Psychiatry, St George's Hospital Medical School, London.

Another distinction worth making at the outset is one that has become commonplace in the last few years and which is utilized elsewhere in this volume, that between 'disease' and 'illness' (see Chapter 2). Disease refers to a medical conception of pathological abnormality diagnosed by means of signs and symptoms; and illness refers to the subjective interpretation of problems which are perceived as health-related (Kleinman, Eisenberg, and Good call illness 'the human experience of sickness' (1978: 251)). Disease and illness do not stand in a one-to-one relationship. It is quite possible for individuals, on the one hand, to have a disease without defining themselves as ill, and, on the other, to define themselves as ill without having a disease. In as far as what follows has to do with 'illness' behaviour, it essentially concerns *lay* rather than medical concepts and actions.

Kasl and Cobb claim that the fundamental problem of illness behaviour is: in the presence of symptoms, what will individuals do and why? As two pioneers of the systematic investigation of illness behaviour, Mechanic and Volkart, point out: 'Two persons having the same symptoms, clinically considered, may behave quite differently; one may become concerned and immediately seek medical aid, while the other may ignore the symptoms and not consider seeking treatment at all' (1961: 52). The study of why this should be so is important for anyone engaged in health work for at least two reasons: first, effective medical treatment almost always depends upon the initiative of 'patients' in seeking diagnosis and treatment; and second, the medical understanding of many diseases is based on populations of self-referred sick patients, and unknown systematic biases in self-referral can seriously distort comprehension of the disease processes (i.e. treated cases might not be typical of all cases).

In the first part of this chapter the significance of the concept of the 'illness iceberg' is considered; the second introduces different approaches to the study of illness behaviour and gives examples of psychological and sociological 'models'; the third dwells on the role played by lay referral systems and social networks in help-seeking; and in the final part attention is given to the study of illness behaviour in women, special reference being made to perceptions and responses to menstrual symptomatology.

The concept of the 'illness iceberg'

Early studies conducted in the 1940s and 1950s, and many since, have shown that the majority of illness symptoms are either ignored or receive non-medical attention. Last (1963) has used the term 'illness iceberg' to refer to the fact that most symptoms do not lead to a medical consultation. Research using symptom recall techniques suggests that only about a third of those with symptoms refer themselves for medical advice. In one recent prospective study, seventy-nine women aged 16–44 were invited to complete six-week health diaries and were subsequently interviewed (Scambler, Scambler, and Craig 1981). Symptoms were recorded on an average of one day in three. When the same symptom was entered on consecutive days this was defined as one 'symptom episode', the episode ending on the day on which it was last recorded. Occasions when a symptom was entered on one day only were also defined as symptom episodes. Only one diarist, a married woman aged twenty-eight, reported no symptoms. The ten most frequently recorded symptoms are given in *Table 1*, which also shows how many times these precipitated medical consultations and the ratio of medical consultation to symptom episodes. Headache and changes in energy or tiredness accounted for a third of the symptom episodes but precipitated only 6 per cent of the medical consultations. At the other extreme, rashes, itches, and skin problems accounted for only 1 per cent of the symptom episodes but were responsible for a quarter of the medical consultations. Overall, there was one medical consultation for every eighteen symptom episodes. These results were strikingly similar to those obtained by Morrell and Wale (1976) in their comparable study of women aged 20–44.

From the vantage point of the health worker it might reasonably be assumed that most of those symptoms untreated by doctors are mild, unobtrusive and not indicative of conditions or diseases requiring medical intervention. There is some support for this in the work of Ingham and Miller (1979), who made comparisons of symptom severity between attenders and non-attenders who had reported one or more of seven selected symptoms. They found symptom severity to be significantly greater in attenders than in non-attenders. However, other studies have shown that general practitioners are not being consulted about many diseases that would undoubtedly respond to treatment. In one particularly impressive study, the medical officer for the London borough of Southwark, using a mobile health clinic, undertook a survey investigation of the health status of a sample of individuals aged 16–60 living in the borough (Epsom 1969). Social and medical histories were taken from participants in the study; an extensive battery of tests administered – haemoglobin estimation, blood pressure, urine testing, vision, measurement of height and weight, cervical smear for women aged over twenty-five and X-ray of the chest; and a comprehensive general medical examination was given. Many diseases that had been untreated were revealed. Indeed, 57 per cent of the 3,160 seen in the mobile health clinic were referred to their family doctors for further investigation and possible treatment. Among the major diseases detected were seven cases of pre-invasive cervical cancer, one active case of pulmonary tuberculosis and one confirmed case of carcinoma of the breast. A follow-up survey was carried out with a 25 per cent sample of

Table 1 *Symptom episodes and medical consultations recorded in the health diaries*

main types of symptoms recorded	*number of symptom episodes*	*percentage of total number of symptom episodes*	*mean length of symptom episodes (days)*	*number of occasions on which symptom episode precipitated medical consultation*	*ratio of medical consultations to symptom episodes*
headache	180	20.9	1.3	3	1:60
changes in energy, tiredness	109	12.6	1.4	0	—
nerves, depression, or irritability	74	8.6	1.7	1	1:74
aches or pains in joints, muscles, legs or arms	71	8.2	1.6	4	1:18
women's complaints like period pain*	69	8.0	1.7	7	1:10
stomach aches or pains	45	5.2	1.5	4	1:11
backache	38	4.4	1.6	1	1:38
cold, flu, or running nose	37	4.3	4.1	3	1:12
sore throat	36	4.2	2.4	4	1:9
sleeplessness	31	3.6	1.5	1	1:31
others	173	20.0	1.9	21	1:8
totals	863	100.0	1.7	49	1:18

*Stomach aches and pains and backache were classified as period pains if so defined by the women themselves.
Source: Scambler, Scambler, and Craig (1981).

those referred to their general practitioners, and it transpired that 38 per cent of the survey findings had not previously been known to general practitioners, and that 22 per cent of the findings made known to general practitioners for the first time were judged to be sufficiently serious to warrant referral to hospital or specialist services.

Even if resources were made available, simply extending the primary care services in the hope of attracting individuals with untreated but treatable diseases would not solve all the problems. For example, one common complaint by general practitioners concerns the high proportion of 'trivial' consultations. In the 1960s, Cartwright (1967) found that 26 per cent of a national sample of general practitioners felt half or more of their surgery consultations were 'trivial, unnecessary or inappropriate'; when a similar study was done in the 1970s, this proportion was virtually the same at 24 per cent (Cartwright and Anderson 1981). Considered in conjunction with the discussion above, these results suggest marked disjunctions between lay interpretations of illness and medical perspectives on disease.

The study of illness behaviour

APPROACHES

In a recent study of self-referral, Hannay (1980) asked a random sample of patients registered with a Scottish health centre to complete a questionnaire which included a checklist of symptoms; each positive symptom was then graded by the patient for pain, disability and perceived seriousness. He found that 26 per cent of those with symptoms, who either defined the pain or disability associated with one or more of them as severe or considered one or more of them serious, did not refer themselves for professional advice. Conversely, 11 per cent of those with symptoms who had no pain or disability and did not think any symptoms serious referred themselves to their general practitioners. The existence of such 'incongruous' referral behaviour provides further confirmation of the now well-documented view that illness behaviour is rarely explicable in terms of straightforward accounts of patients' perceptions of symptoms (the exceptions, Mechanic (1969) contends, being cases involving such symptoms as temperature of 105 degrees, fractured leg, broken back, severe heart attack and extreme psychosis). In fact, numerous different kinds of factors have been shown to exert an influence on illness behaviour.

In a general review of studies of health care utilization, which is pertinent also to the broader consideration of the literature on illness behaviour, McKinlay (1972) identifies six analytically distinct orientations or approaches:

1 The *economic:* in which attention is concentrated on the impact of financial barriers to help-seeking.
2 The *socio-demographic:* in which the emphasis is on the significance of gross characteristics like gender, age, and education for utilization.
3 The *geographic:* in which the focus of attention is the association between the geographical proximity of health services and utilization.
4 The *social-psychological:* in which the emphasis is on the link between individual motivation, perception and learning, and utilization behaviour.
5 The *socio-cultural:* in which the orientation is towards examining associations between the values, norms, beliefs, and life-styles of different socio-economic groups and utilization.
6 The *organizational or 'delivery system':* in which the focus of attention is on the effects of aspects of health care organization on use of services.

McKinlay stresses that the purpose of these distinctions is heuristic, and adds: 'Seldom do researchers in the area of utilization behaviour adopt only one approach to the exclusion of all others, although one may be given greater emphasis' (1972: 140). Most relevant to this chapter are the 'social-psychological' and 'socio-cultural' orientations. In a selective review of studies of illness behaviour, Bloor (1970) distinguishes in an almost parallel fashion between the 'psychological' and 'sociological' schools of social psychology. His interest is in the contrasting theoretical models of illness behaviour produced by members of these schools (although he is aware that these need not be mutually exclusive and that researchers have tended to be fairly eclectic).

THE HEALTH BELIEF MODEL

Models generated by the psychological school might be termed 'individualistic' (Dingwall 1976). The most obvious example is the still evolving Health Belief Model (HBM), formulated initially in connection with health behaviour but since extended to embrace illness and sick-role behaviour. In early versions there were two main variables: 'readiness' to take a particular action; and 'perceived benefit', the belief that the action would have beneficial consequences. Readiness to act was based upon perceived susceptibility to a health threat and upon the perceived seriousness of that threat. Beliefs about perceived benefit also incorporated perceived barriers to the proposed action. Consideration of these factors allowed an estimate of the likelihood of the action being taken. In addition, it was recognized that 'cues to action' (or 'triggers') were necessary to precipitate the action. These cues could be 'internal' (e.g. pain) or 'external' (e.g. interference with occupational tasks). In recent years a fourth class of factors, usually termed 'modifying factors' and said to influence all the other factors, has been incorporated in the HBM. These include 'demographic' factors like gender, age, and ethnicity; 'social-psychological' factors like social class and personality; and 'structural' factors like knowledge about disease and prior experience of it.

Stone (1979a) has characterized the HBM as follows:

> 'In essence, the theory says that the likelihood of taking a particular action is a function of perceived threat and perceived benefit. Perceived threat is a function of perceived susceptibility, a subjective probability, and of perceived seriousness, a value. Perceived benefit is the probability that threat will be reduced (by some amount) minus the perceived cost of the action, which must itself be reduced to a set of probabilities times values. The theory does not specify what the functions are that relate these variables, nor how the values of the variables arise and change. Therefore, it does not make quantitative predictions but relative predictions, such as: "If perceived threat is increased (or higher for one group than another), likelihood of action will increase (or be higher for the appropriate group)".'
>
> (Stone 1979a: 73)

Many of the criticisms of the HBM stem from its high level of abstraction. Indeed it is perhaps more appropriately described as a conceptual framework for thinking about illness behaviour than as a 'model'. As Stone notes, its advocates have little or nothing to say about the weight to be attached to any of the key variables. Moreover, some of these variables seem extremely elusive. Writing of Rosenstock's (1966) concept of psychological readiness, for example, Dingwall asks: 'How are we to recognize a "state of readiness to act", apart from deducing it *post hoc* from some observed conduct? If we can recognize it only by this *post hoc* linking of consequent and supposed antecedent, how can it have any predictive status?' (1977: 3). Despite these and other limitations, however, the HBM continues to provide a productive focus for social-psychological research and is still subject to scrutiny and amendment (Rosenstock and Kirscht 1979).

FREIDSON AND LAY REFERRAL SYSTEMS

If theoretical models of illness behaviour deriving from the psychological school of social psychology are primarily individualistic, those originating in the sociological school tend to be 'collectively oriented': they emphasize that patterns of behaviour appropriate to specific situations are 'learned' through socialization into particular cultures and subcultures. One example of such a model is Freidson's (1970). This model will be described in some detail as it leads on to a consideration of lay reference groups and lay referral. Freidson argues that an individual's actions are only explicable in terms of the meaning that he or she attributes to them, and that these meanings are culturally transmitted:

'In the process of imputing meaning to his experience, the individual sufferer does not invent the meanings himself but rather uses the meanings and interpretations that his social life has provided him. Thus, one can predict the behaviour of a collection of individuals without reference to their individual characteristics, by referring solely to the context of the social life in which they participate.'

(Freidson 1970: 288–89)

It is lay culture, in Freidson's view, that creates 'illness' as a social meaning (just as the medical profession creates 'disease' as a social meaning). Lay definitions of illness therefore need to be seen as historically and culturally relative: 'what the layman recognizes as a symptom of illness is in part a function of deviation from the culturally and historically variable standard of normality established by everyday experience' (1970: 285). If an individual perceives himself to be ill and in need of medical help, he is likely to find agreement and support within his cultural milieu only if 'he shows evidence of symptoms the others believe to be illness and if he interprets them the way the others find plausible' (1970: 289).

Once the need for health care is acknowledged, help-seeking is 'organized' by what Freidson calls the 'lay referral system'. This consists of two elements: 'lay culture', which may be more or less congruent with that of the medical profession, and a 'network of personal influences' which Freidson terms the 'lay referral structure':

'the structure or organization of the lay community is a factor influencing utilization, in that it organizes the process of becoming ill by pressing the sufferer into or away from the professional consulting room. The organization of lay referrals can enforce a particular orientation toward illness, or it can be so loose as to leave the individual fairly free of others' influence, to make decisions contrary to that of his peers without having to suffer their ridicule or scorn.'

(Freidson 1970: 292)

Thus the lay referral structure not only provides lay consultants to whom the individual can turn for advice, but also influences the extent to which the lay culture determines his actions for him. This analysis leads Freidson to the model presented in *Table 2*.

He points out that in circumstances where the lay referral system inhibits the utilization of health services, the exploration of alternative forms of care – for example, self-care or treatment by 'folk' practitioners – tends to be encouraged. This, Bloor suggests, means Freidson's work can be regarded as offering a comprehensive model of illness behaviour.

Table 2   *Predicted rates of health care utilization by variations in lay referral systems*

lay culture		
lay referral structure	congruent with professional	incongruent with professional
loose, truncated	medium to high utilization	medium to low utilization
cohesive, extended	highest utilization	lowest utilization

Source: Freidson (1970).

Freidson's model, like the HBM, is of course open to criticism. Many commentators have described it as simplistic; Ignu refers to it almost apologetically as 'a very useful general idea' (1979: 446). Bloor notes that although there would seem to be a measure of empirical support for Freidson's model from studies like Suchman's (1964) and McKinlay's (1973), these studies examine social networks in 'stable' cultural milieux, where social and geographical mobility is low. In areas where mobility is relatively high, then people's illness behaviour will presumably need to be explained in terms of the norms of both past and present social networks, and this may lead to significant problems of methodology. Recent ideas and work on lay referral systems and social networks are sufficiently interesting, however, to justify closer consideration.

Lay referral systems and social networks

LAY CONSULTATIONS, REFERRALS, AND INTERVENTIONS

It is helpful to distinguish between lay 'consultations', lay 'referrals', and lay 'interventions'. It is clearly routine for individuals who perceive themselves to be ill to 'consult' other lay persons, to discuss symptoms and to seek advice. Suchman (1964) found that three-quarters of those symptoms referred to a physician had first been discussed with a lay person (usually a relative). Scambler, Scambler, and Craig (1981) report the same finding; and they add that over the period of six weeks that their sample of women kept health diaries, an average of eleven lay consultations were registered for every one medical consultation (a ratio which they have reason to believe understates the frequency of lay consulting). Of the total of 547 lay consultations recorded, 50 per cent were with husbands, 25 per cent with female friends, 10 per cent with mothers, 8 per cent with other female relatives and 7 per cent with various others (e.g. fathers or boyfriends). During the diary period almost all married women consulted their husbands and about half of them consulted female friends; single women and women who were separated or divorced were most likely to consult, first, their mothers, and second, female friends. The nature of the symptoms seemed to have little effect on who was consulted.

Relatives or friends who are consulted about symptoms, or who offer unsolicited opinions about them, may refrain from prescribing a particular course of action or may 'refer' the sufferer either to a doctor or to some other non-medical agency. Zola (1973) found lay referral to be one of the key 'triggers' or precipitants of medical consultations, a phenomenon he called 'sanctioning'. In certain circumstances, of course, lay persons take it upon themselves to 'intervene' to initiate medical consultations. This is most likely to occur when symptoms are perceived to be serious or threatening or when the victim is rendered temporarily incapable of self-help. In his study of epilepsy, Scambler (1983) found that in 79 per cent of cases, first contact with the medical profession was arranged by someone other than the sufferer. In his analytical account of 'acute illness behaviour', based on two studies of acute coronary artery disease, Alonzo (1980) posits a 'lay evaluation phase' commencing when lay others become aware of the emerging crisis and ending with medical involvement. He writes:

> 'It cannot be over emphasized that lay others – family, neighbours, friends, workmates or strangers – play an inordinately significant role in care-seeking during acute life-threatening illnesses. In instances of acute coronary artery disease others frequently represent the only means of summoning assistance if the individual becomes unconscious or otherwise incapacitated.'
>
> (Alonzo 1980: 519)

Alonzo also found, like Salloway and Dillon (1973), that lay others who are not members of the victim's family are less likely than those who are to tolerate delays in help-seeking resulting from the normalization or denial of symptoms. Calnan speculates that this may be because non-kin face 'a dilemma between feeling morally obliged to help the sufferer but not wanting to become too involved as this might disrupt plans and commitments'; the dilemma is resolved by (anonymously) calling for an ambulance (1983; 27). Finlayson and McEwen (1977) have graphically described how the wives of some men tried, and failed, to persuade them to see a doctor in the hours preceding myocardial infarction.

SOCIAL NETWORKS

It is one thing to establish that lay consultations, referrals and interventions commonly occur and constitute an important dimension of illness behaviour, and quite another to generate social scientific theories or models that take account of this. Most of those who have attempted to do so have taken their cue from Freidson and concentrated on properties of people's social networks. Both Liu and Duff (1972) and Granovetter (1973) distinguish between 'strong' and 'weak' network ties. With the former there is either a high degree of interdependence or consultation with a relatively small number of individuals; and with the latter there is either little interdependence or consultation with a wider range of diverse individuals. There is some evidence in the United States and Britain that strong network ties tend to be most common in stable working-class environments; and these have been associated with an extended process of lay referral and delayed help-seeking. Weak network ties have been linked with vague and contradictory lay counsel and with early medical consultation (Reeder, Marcus, and Seeman 1978).

McKinlay (1973) studied the influence of the family and kinship and friendship networks on the use of maternity care services by eighty-seven lower working-class women in Aberdeen. In the course of a recent review of the literature, he summarizes his findings in the following way:

'Differences emerged between the utilizers and underutilizers regarding aspects of the kin and friendship sectors of their social networks, and from questions concerning lay consultation and lay referral for various hypothetical but commonly occurring problem situations. It appeared that *utilizers made greater use of friends and husbands* and less use of mothers or other relatives, and tended to consult a *narrower range* of lay consultants. These findings were consistent with, and perhaps reinforced, observed differences in their network structure. Underutilizers appeared to rely more on a variety of *readily available relatives and friends as lay consultants*. There appeared to be only *one* large *interlocking network* within which the underutilizers obtained the majority of their advice. Utilizers, on the other hand, had separate or *differentiated kin and friendship networks*. There was a lack of reliance on relatives on the part of utilizers, but no evidence in the data that kin lay consultation was replaced to any large extent by friendship lay consultation. Utilizers appeared to be relatively independent of both kin and friends, and frequently took no prior lay advice from the members of their networks, or consulted only their husbands.'

(McKinlay 1981: 88–9, his emphasis)

As mentioned earlier, these findings are compatible with Freidson's model, even if they do not confirm it.

A number of social scientists have developed clear distinctions between kinship and friendship networks in trying to understand illness behaviour. Salloway and Dillon (1973), for example, found that large family networks tend to inhibit medical consultation and large friendship networks to precipitate it. McKinlay (1981) gives his provisional endorsement to the view expressed by several authors that kinship and friendship networks have essentially different functions. He quotes Horwitz's (1978) study of the influence of the family and kinship and friendship networks on psychiatric help-seeking. Horwitz argues that kinship and friendship networks have 'special spheres of competency'.

> 'Kin members tended to provide services such as financial assistance and living quarters which imply long-term commitments, permanent ties and invoke a norm of reciprocity. Friends were better suited to provide knowledge of professionals outside the primary group. The general pattern for kin is to attempt to maintain individuals within the informal network, while the tendency of friends is to connect the individual to a wider outside network of professionals.'
>
> (McKinlay 1981: 90)

Not all research, however, seems consistent with these conclusions. Scambler, Scambler, and Craig (1981) looked at various properties of women's social networks – for example, size, composition, and location – and use of general practitioner services in the previous year. The most convincing links with use involved *active* networks. An active network was defined as comprising everyone aged sixteen or more whom a woman either met or spoke with on the telephone at least once a week. Although there was no association between size of active network and service use, when the active network was divided into active kinship and friendship networks, a rather different picture emerged. Large, active kinship networks were associated with high use, and large, active friendship networks with low use. These results are presented in *Table 3*. The authors hypothesize that discussion of symptoms with kin may be intense and protracted and lead to kin referrals to general practitioners (i.e. Zola's 'sanctioning'). On the other hand, discussion with friends may be more casual and unfocused and result in symptoms being re-defined as unimportant and not in need of medical attention.

Apparently contradictory findings in this area may yet prove theoretically reconcilable. To date, the very different populations, methodologies and foci of published studies make genuine comparisons extremely difficult. McKinlay (1981) wisely calls for further refinement in the explication of characteristics of social networks and in their operationalization. Hammer (1983) argues that it is unimaginative to focus exclusively, as most have done, on people's 'core' networks – consisting only of those with whom they have direct and regular contacts. She suggests that attention should also be paid to their 'extended' networks – consisting possibly of several hundred others with whom there is some direct or indirect association. 'What happens to the core network over time in terms of loss and recruitment of members, and thus in terms of its functional adequacy for the individual, must be strongly affected by the

Table 3   Sizes of active kinship and friendship networks by service use in the year prior to the study

use during the previous year	size of active kinship network*				size of active friendship network**			
	small (0–3)		large (4+)		small (0–2)		large (3+)	
	%	n	%	n	%	n	%	n
low (0–4 consultations)	61	22	37	16	32	8	56	30
high (5+ consultations)	39	14	63	27	68	17	44	24
totals	100	36	100	43	100	25	100	54

*Q = +0.45; x^2 = 4.48; d.f. = 1; p = <0.05.
**Q = −0.45; x^2 = 3.79; d.f. = 1; N.S.
Source: Scambler, Scambler, and Craig (1981).

Table 4   Sex differences in office visits to physicians by reason for visit, United States, 1977–78*

reason for visit	ages 15–24			ages 25–44			ages 45–64		
	females	males	sex difference	females	males	sex difference	females	males	sex difference
all visits	2,787	1,545	1,242	3,442	1,891	1,552	3,729	2,800	930
pregnancy	558	—	558	427	—	427	7	—	7
gynaecological exam, Pap smear, family planning	195	1	194	255	20	235	115	3	113
symptoms and diseases of the genito-urinary system and breast	275	45	230	337	69	268	271	100	171
general examination	79	38	41	129	59	71	177	138	39
weight gain	36	3	34	94	18	75	70	13	58
psychological symptoms such as anxiety, depression, etc., social problem counselling	60	46	14	183	118	64	134	88	46
injury	79	209	−131	84	149	−66	96	118	−22

*Rates of office visits per 1,000 population per year. Sex differences shown are female minus male rates. In some cases there are slight discrepancies between the differences shown and the female v. male rates due to rounding.
Source: Waldron (1983).

characteristics of the larger, extended network in which it is embedded' (Hammer 1983: 411). What does already seem clear, however, is that social networks are highly pertinent to the better understanding not only of illness behaviour, but also of health and sick-role behaviour, and that they might one day be utilized fairly routinely by health workers as therapeutic aides. Indeed, 'clinical network intervention' in the field of mental health is beginning to attract quite a lot of attention, especially in the United States (Greenblatt, Becerra, and Serafetinides 1982).

Women, illness behaviour, and menstruation

In all modern industrialized societies, male mortality rates are higher than the rates for females. Yet in all societies for which data are available, women report more acute illness than men and make more use of health services (Nathanson 1977). Few would contest this general statement, but there is little agreement about how it should be interpreted. Some writers give the impression that *any* attempt at interpretation is premature: 'there is a way in which there can be no adequate, systematic theory-building as of yet because of the conceptual indeterminacy in the definition and problems in the measurement of illness and gender' (Clarke 1983: 77). Waldron (1983) has provided one of the most cautious and well-informed reviews of official statistics and academic studies in this difficult area. Consider, for example, use of health services. One major reason why women show a higher rate of utilization than men, she claims, is the nature of their reproductive systems. In the United States consultation for pregnancy, gynaecological examinations, and symptoms or diseases involving the genito-urinary system and breast accounted in 1977–78 for 79 per cent of the female excess between the ages of fifteen and twenty-four, 60 per cent between the ages of twenty-five and forty-four and 31 per cent between the ages of forty-five and sixty-four (see *Table 4*).

Women also seem to experience higher rates of symptoms than men, which may be another important reason for their higher utilization. As Waldron points out, however, the sex difference in symptoms may reflect sex differences in perceptions as well as sex differences in actual somatic condition (1983: 1115). This explicity raises issues of illness behaviour. Hibbard and Pope (1983) found that women – probably as a result of socialization – have a greater interest and concern with health than men, and claim that this has important implications for both their perceptions of symptoms and their utilization rates. Citing other studies to add weight to their findings, they speculate that 'males and females do not differ in symptom reports for specific diseases where symptoms tend to be powerful and obvious. However, obligations and expectations associated with female gender roles may contribute to the inclination to give attention to and evaluate ambiguous or mild body cues as symptoms of illness' (Hibbard and Pope 1983: 137). They contend that this partially accounts for the greater morbidity reports and higher rates of utilization of health services among women. Several other variables, like the fact that women are less likely than men to be employed and therefore supposedly have more time for medical consultations, have of course also been linked with higher utilization, but Waldron finds the evidence to be generally inconclusive.

EXPERIENCING MENSTRUATION

Clare (1983) notes that the greatest disparity between male and female use of health services occurs during the years when women are actively menstruating, and that this has led some commentators to look at menstrual symptomatology with a view to assessing its contribution to women's higher utilization rate. Fry (1979) has estimated, in fact, that in a practice population of 2,500 persons, sixty-eight women are likely to consult annually for menstrual disorders. In their investigation of the prevalence and severity of menstrual symptoms, Kessel and Coppen (1963) asked 465 respondents aged 18–45 to rate any pain, irritability, depression, anxiety, nervousness or tension, and headaches they experienced on a four-point scale – nil, slight, moderate, and severe. The prevalence of all symptoms was high. Forty-five per cent reported moderate or severe (12 per cent) pain, 32 per cent moderate or severe (11 per cent) irritability, 23 per cent moderate or severe (6 per cent) depression, anxiety, nervousness or tension, and 22 per cent moderate or severe (11 per cent) headaches. In addition, 72 per cent reported some swelling and 16 per cent said their periods were so irregular that they did not know when the next would come.

Recent unpublished work by Scambler and Scambler supports the view that menstrual symptoms are common and often perceived as distressing. As part of their study cited earlier (1981), they invited their sample of seventy-nine women to complete a modified version of the Moos Menstrual Distress Questionnaire (Moos 1977). The original forty-seven symptoms were reduced to thirty-four in accordance with a procedure adopted by Clare (1980). Women were asked to rate each symptom for 'an average period' on a six-point scale – nil, barely noticeable, mild, moderate, strong, and acute. Any symptoms rated as strong or acute were defined as distressing. *Table 5* gives the rank order of the twelve symptoms most frequently defined as distressing during the seven days prior to menstruation, during the menstrual flow, and during either or both of these phases. In all, 82 per cent of the women rated at least one symptom as distressing; 15 per cent suffered distress in the premenstrum only, 9 per cent during the flow only, and 58 per cent during both phases. Despite these figures, only 28 per cent of the total sample had consulted a doctor about menstrual symptoms in the six months before interview. Twenty-six per cent said they had never sought medical advice or help for menstrual symptoms. This reinforces Kessel and Coppen's conclusion that there is a considerable menstrual illness iceberg.

Snow and Johnson (1977) have shown in a small study of forty women attending a public clinic in Michigan that 'folk' beliefs and negative attitudes towards menstruation can affect body image, perception of disease, diet, willingness to take medicine and contraceptive use and failure. They found that over half had no knowledge of menstruation prior to menarche and did not know where menstrual blood comes from or why periods begin and stop when they do. They also discovered a wide range of menstrual folk beliefs: a third thought women should avoid water and cold air during menstruation, nearly a quarter that they should change their diet, and one in eight that menstruating women may be attacked by reptiles. These findings are partly explicable in terms of the fact that the sample was multi-ethnic and the women relatively poorly educated. The study does, however, emphasize the need to be aware of 'gaps' between medical concepts of menstruation and associated disease and lay women's concepts of menstruation and associated illness.

There is evidence that beliefs about menstruation tend to be acquired at an early age and generally reflect cultural stereotypes about menstruation as a negative and symptom-laden phenomenon. Such beliefs are likely to influence girls' menarcheal experience, and most apparently 'expect' to experience negative feelings and symptoms (Woods, Dery, and Most 1982). Whisnant and Zegans (1965) found that when adolescents were asked to describe their first menstrual period, they frequently used words like 'scared', 'upset', or 'ashamed'. This is consistent with studies of adult women's recollections of menarche (Shaines 1961). It has been suggested that a negative menarcheal experience may influence subsequent menstrual attitudes and symptoms. Woods, Dery and Most (1982) set out to test this hypothesis. They interviewed 179 women aged 18–35 and found that negative recollections of the first menstrual period had little effect on current menstrual experience: 'Thus, the self-fulfilling prophecy that might have been set in motion by negative menarcheal experiences seems more a myth than reality' (Woods, Dery, and Most 1982: 292). They do suggest, however, that current menstrual attitudes may well be influenced by current menstrual symptoms.

Scambler and Scambler (unpublished) asked their sample a number of questions relating to attitudes towards menstruation. They found that women tended to fall into one of three broad categories, which they entitled 'acceptance', 'fatalism' and 'antipathy'. These can be elaborated as follows:

Table 5 *Most distressing menstrual symptoms*

week before period			*during menstrual flow*			*either before or during period or both*		
	symptom	*% reporting as distressing*		*symptom*	*% reporting as distressing*		*symptom*	*% reporting as distressing*
1	irritability	38	1	irritability	29	1	irritability	49
2	swelling	24	2	pain	23	2	pain	30
3	headaches	22	3	tiredness	22	3	tiredness }	28
4	depression moods } weight gain	19	4	depression moods }	18		moods	
7	tiredness	18	5	backaches	15	5	swelling	27
8	tension	15	7	headache	14	6	headache	25
9	backache } tender breasts	14	8	swelling weight gain }	13	7	depression	24
11	pain	13	10	anxiety avoidance of social activity lowered performance }	11	8	weight gain	22
12	anxiety	11				9	backache	20
						10	lowered performance	19
						11	tension	18
						12	anxiety avoidance of social activity }	16

1   *Acceptance* (25 per cent of women)   This category contained those
    women who experienced no menstrual symptoms or who were only
    marginally affected by them. They defined their periods as 'normal'. It
    was in this category that women came nearest to displaying a
    'positive' attitude towards menstruation, some actually referring to it
    as 'healthy' or 'feminine': 'It's a normal, healthy thing; everybody has
    one.' Those who did experience menstrual symptoms thought
    nothing of them or played them down: 'Just don't take no notice of it
    really'; 'I just accept it as part of the process of life.'

2   *Fatalism* (27 per cent of women)   This category comprised those
    women who felt their periods were 'a bother', 'a nuisance', and so on.
    They always qualified their remarks, however, with statements like:
    'It's something you just live with, isn't it? They are a nuisance but I'd
    rather have them than not'; 'Well, I suppose it's a necessary evil so a
    woman can have a baby'; 'I know I've got to have them so I put up
    with them.' These women were 'resigned' to their periods.

3   *Antipathy* (48 per cent of women)   In this category were all those
    women with an unconditional dislike for menstruation. This ranged
    from negative feelings of inconvenience to downright hostility, and
    was based on perceptions of menstruation as 'unclean', 'messy',
    'unhealthy', and so on. These women would dispense with periods
    altogether if they could do so with no side-effects. Examples of
    comments include: 'I don't like them. I'd rather not have them. It's
    messy and I don't like mess'; 'I don't like it. I hate it – especially in the
    summer with the heat if you've got to wear a pad'; 'I don't bloody like
    them. I think it's because I have so much trouble with them – all the
    backaches and the stomach aches and the heavy bleeding. I've had so
    many problems with it ever since I started.'

An overall menstrual distress score was calculated in the following
way. A woman scored one point for each of the thirty-four symptoms she
defined as strong or acute during the seven days prior to menstruation.
When totalled, these gave her a pre-menstrual distress score. The same
procedure was adopted for symptoms defined as strong or acute during
the menstrual flow. When totalled, these gave her a menstrual flow
distress score. A combined or overall menstrual distress score was
created by adding these two scores together. This meant that a woman
who experienced a level of distress on an individual symptom both
before *and* during the menstrual flow had her overall menstrual distress
score automatically weighted to allow for both intensity of distress *and*
discomfort over time. Any woman with an overall menstrual distress
score of four or more was said to have a 'high' level of symptom distress.

Not surprisingly perhaps, a higher proportion of women showing
antipathy towards their periods were experiencing a high level of

symptom distress (76 per cent) than was the case with women showing either fatalism (45 per cent) or acceptance (40 per cent). This is consistent with the suggestion of Woods, Dery, and Most (1982) that current menstrual attitudes may reflect current menstrual symptoms. Both antipathy towards menstruation and high level of symptom distress were associated with the utilization of general practitioner services for menstrual symptoms in the year prior to interview. However, these associations were not statistically significant and, as Hannay found when he examined self-referral for all types of symptoms, 'incongruous' referral behaviour was by no means uncommon. To reiterate an earlier point: self-referral is not simply a function of how people perceive and evaluate their symptoms.

A TYPOLOGY OF NON-CONSULTERS FOR MENSTRUAL SYMPTOMS

Concentrating on those women who had not consulted their doctor for menstrual symptoms for over a year (63 per cent of the sample), Scambler and Scambler developed a typology of non-consulters. Four types were delineated:

1 The *unaffected* (35 per cent of non-consulters) This group neither experienced symptom distress nor saw menstruation as a health problem. None felt periods had any effect on the quality of their lives and most of them displayed attitudes of acceptance, although a few were fatalists. It might be argued that these women would need to re-define menstruation as problematic should they experience distress in the future.

2 The *alienated* (33 per cent of non-consulters) This group experienced high symptom distress levels, with a mean overall menstrual distress score of 11 per woman, and regarded menstruation as a health problem. Almost all felt the quality of their lives to have been affected, and most held antipathetic attitudes towards menstruation. Eighty per cent of these women had consulted a doctor about menstrual distress in the past (i.e. more than a year before interview). Women from social classes four and five were over-represented in this group. These women tended to feel disillusioned with medicine. A number had long-term symptoms which they had learned to 'put up with': 'I don't consult – I haven't bothered again – I don't feel they understand the problem and it's so hard to explain.' Some women felt either 'let down' by their doctor or convinced that medicine could offer them no relief. Another sub-group were so used to their symptoms that they felt they could cope adequately through self-medication. Yet another reason for not consulting was a dislike of medical examinations. Some women clearly used 'delaying tactics', despite frequent attempts at 'sanctioning' by relatives: 'I would go, but only when it was really

necessary – men [i.e. her general practitioner] haven't been through it, so they can't know all about it.'

3   The *realists* (17 per cent of non-consulters)   This group did not experience symptom distress but did see periods as potential health problems. They did not define periods as affecting the quality of their lives, but tended to be fatalists rather than acceptors in their attitudes. These women may perhaps be predisposed to consult a doctor in the event of future symptom distress.

4   The *marginals* (15 per cent of non-consulters)   This group experienced high symptom distress levels, but lower than the alienated (with a mean overall menstrual distress score of five per woman). Unlike the alienated, they did not define menstruation as a health problem. They were almost equally split between those who accepted their periods and felt the quality of their lives to have been unaffected, and those who were antipathetic and felt the quality of their lives to have been affected. Less than half had had a menstrual consultation in the past, and these averaged more than five years before interview. Almost all had one or more of the following attitudes: they didn't like medicine, doctors or examinations; they preferred women doctors; they felt they had had bad experiences with doctors in the past. It may be that these women had some unmet need for consultation which was partially repressed by these reservations.

The construction of typologies like this is a common feature of social scientific studies, and it is instructive to contrast the nature and function of typologies in sociology with those in medicine. Schneider and Conrad (1981) discuss three important differences. First, sociological typologies derive from pre-existing lay typologies, the essential meanings of which must be preserved.

'Sociological analysis strives to locate those everyday typifications within a more abstract system of meanings, making 'sociological problems' out of segments of others' everyday worlds. Through this and other scientific operations, the sociologist aims to understand and explain, rather than solve, practical problems.'

(Schneider and Conrad 1981: 213)

Medical typologies such as diagnostic classifications, on the other hand, do not derive from lay typologies; indeed, from the medical perspective the clinician (or medical scientist) is the sole arbiter of meaning and he or she need not be concerned with any 'lack of fit' with lay typologies patients might present. Second, sociological typologies rarely enter the experience of those under study, while medical diagnoses 'are "realities" with which people so designated must contend, independently of the physiological aspects of their conditions' (Schneider and Conrad

1981: 213). And third, sociological typologies generally invite critical reflection, while medical typologies are pragmatic and likely to become taken-for-granted aspects of routine medical practice.

In their discussion of epilepsy, Schneider and Conrad argue that the official dominance of medical typologies has resulted in a 'one-sided, incomplete understanding of epilepsy for both medical personnel and, to the extent that these medical types are popularly known, the larger society' (1981: 214). For epilepsy one might of course substitute problems of the menstruum. The value of sociological typologies of the kind developed by Scambler and Scambler (unpublished) then, is that they complement medical understanding and challenge doctors and other health workers to take full account of lay or patient perceptions and evaluations of illness when asked for advice or help.

Conclusions

In this chapter, the extent and relevance of the so-called illness iceberg have been discussed, and some of the ways social scientists have linked the experience of illness with the seeking of medical help selectively reviewed. Examples were given of psychologically and sociologically oriented models of illness behaviour and both were subjected to criticism. Special attention was devoted to recent studies prompted by Freidson's notion of lay referral systems. Finally, aspects of an unpublished study of women's experiences of menstruation were reported, tracing links between perceptions and evaluations of symptoms, attitudes towards periods and illness and consulting behaviour. This study was examined in some detail because of the authors' belief that it is highly focused work of this kind that will pay the highest dividends in the exploration of illness behaviour. It is also believed that no doctor or other health worker can afford to neglect such exploration if he or she is to engage patients' trust and confidence. Indeed, in many circumstances it would seem to be a precondition of effective treatment.

4   Social class, ethnicity, and illness

Ray Fitzpatrick
and Graham Scambler

Introduction

In everyday life it is commonplace to categorize people into a particular
social class or ethnic group. We generally entertain a complex series of
assumptions about a person's attitudes and behaviour once we have
placed the individual into a social category. This may be of enormous
value in social interaction as the two characteristics point to major social
differences in our society. Yet the ease with which such terms are used in
social life is of course deceptive. Stereotypes of particular classes or
ethnic groups may prove inappropriate and misleading in any particular
encounter. In social life therefore, social categories are double edged,
sometimes useful, sometimes misleading.

There are parallels in the more formal use in the behavioural sciences
of these two social concepts as means of understanding differences
between individuals or groups in their actions in response to illness.
Social class and ethnicity are important potential means of understanding social and cultural differences and they are increasingly being
incorporated into studies of health care. Yet, as this chapter seeks to
indicate, it is insufficient to include such characteristics in the investigation of behaviour without also giving critical attention to the meaning
attributed to them (Suchman 1967: 109). One needs constantly to ask

which specific aspects of social background or experience are involved in any particular piece of research where social class or ethnic identity appear to be implicated.

A full explanation of what sociologists call 'stratification', the 'arrangement of society into layers' (Reid 1981: 4), in the form of social hierarchies of class, ethnicity, and other qualities, is beyond the scope of this book. The disadvantages that attend a lower position in society are, of course, crucial to an understanding of health and illness. This chapter attempts critically to review the ways in which two major indicators of social background and social resources have been used as explanations of differences in behaviour with regard to illness.

Social class

THE MEANING OF SOCIAL CLASS

There are sharply differing views held as to the meaning of social class. People variously emphasize status and prestige, level of income or power and authority when pressed to state the basis of social distinctions in British society. Opinions differ also with regard to where the fundamental dividing lines occur in society and how many classes there are. Sociological debate inevitably reflects such differences and offers a variety of conceptions of class. The Black Report (1980), a recent enquiry into inequalities in health published by the British government, offers one definition which appears useful in its brevity and clarity: 'segments of the population sharing broadly similar types and levels of resources, with broadly similar styles of living and (for some sociologists) some shared perception of their collective condition' (Townsend and Davidson 1982: 47). In practice, the social classes have been most commonly conceived as groupings of occupations which share similar social status and the classes so formed constitute a hierarchy of relative prestige. The Registrar General's classification of occupations into five social classes is the most familiar schema for Great Britain. The five classes are listed in *Table 6*, together with some examples of occupations in each category and an approximate proportion of the population that falls into each class. Also provided in the table are the adult standardized mortality ratios (SMR) for each class.

This measure provides a summary expression of the extent to which the death rates of any group, such as a social class, differ from their expected death rate, which is the rate that prevails for the whole population. The SMR takes account of the different age structures of groups. It is apparent from the table that there is a deteriorating gradient of SMRs from social class one to social class five. Similar social inequalities are to be found in surveys of reported illness.

Table 6 *Registrar General's social class classification and standardized mortality ratios*

social class	descriptive definition	examples of occupations	proportion in populations	adult mortality		standardized ratio (15–64)	
				male		*female*	
I	professional	doctor, lawyer	4	77		82	
II	intermediate	sales manager, teacher	18	81		87	
III	skilled non-manual	clerical worker, shop assistant	21	99		92	
III (M)	skilled manual	bricklayer, electrician	28	106		115	
IV	partly skilled	farm worker, bus conductor	21	114		119	
V	unskilled	office cleaner, railway porter	8	137		135	

Sources: Le Grand (1982); OPCS (1978a).

The Black Report generated intense discussion regarding the explanation for such differences. The view taken by that document is that class inequalities in health reflect differences in the material and economic circumstances of different social groups in Britain. The evidence that they review points to the influence of such factors as income, diet, housing conditions, and employment status. The role of the health service in this analysis is of less importance in influencing inequalities. Nevertheless, one important section of the Black Report considers inequalities in health service provision that might also be implicated in differences in health between social classes. Again the evidence that they assemble suggests that there are major regional and local differences in the quantity and quality of health services which seriously disadvantage occupational classes four and five. The report also discusses differences between social groups in their use of health services. It is the evidence regarding this suggestion that is of importance for the present discussion.

PROBLEMS IN THE CONCEPT OF SOCIAL CLASS

Before the use of health services is considered, however, there needs to be some recognition of the fact that there are advantages and disadvantages attached to the use of the Registrar General's classification of social class. Its advantages are that it is widely used in official statistics, has a quite long history of use and is relatively simple. Also it is a reasonable assumption that occupation is a sensitive indicator of many aspects of life-style. On the other hand, one major purpose of research into social class differences in, for example, use of health services, is to arrive at more specific explanations of such differences. For that purpose there is a need for more specific social indicators such as income, housing conditions, and educational level to explore more precisely the meaning of differences and the researcher may be frustrated by the limitations of conventional social measures.

There are other cautionary points to be made about social class as a means of explaining behaviour in relation to health. First, Illsley (1980: 19) reminds us that classes are not static 'things' but are summary expressions of complex changes in the economy and division of labour and in the social movement of individuals over time. Thus the size, composition, and stability of classes constantly change. Second, one needs to be wary of the divisions and distinctions commonly used in health services research: to take a simple example, the middle class–working class distinction may imply very different assumptions about the processes at work producing differences from a poor–non poor distinction. Yet all too frequently the results of surveys conducted in terms of the former distinction may be explained in terms more appropriate to the latter and vice versa. The very familiarity of the distinctions can lead to uncritical interpretations of differences.

Research into class differences in the use of health services has drawn upon a number of different theories or perspectives to explain results. The theories attempt to state more clearly how differences in behaviour between classes occur. It is important to recognize that finding a relationship between social class and any particular variable is the beginning and not the end of a social explanation. Moreover, the alternative interpretations of class differences have in principle quite different implications. For the sake of simplicity, interpretations of social class differences in this field can be divided between, on the one hand, those explanations concerned with the use of health services and, on the other hand, explanations of class differences arising in interaction with the doctor.

THEORIES OF SOCIAL CLASS AND THE USE OF HEALTH SERVICES

The culture of poverty thesis

One view of class differences in relation to illness that has at times been influential is the 'culture of poverty' thesis (e.g. Rosenstock 1975). According to this view, communities that experience poverty and low status develop, in response to their situation, a culture central to which is a sense of powerlessness, passivity, and fatalism. In some versions of this thesis, the culture of poverty may be so pervasive in a community as to dominate individuals' views of the world even when their economic circumstances improve. The culture of poverty includes acceptance of low levels of health, mistrust of modern medicine, and is particularly incompatible with a future-oriented, preventive view of health. It has been applied most frequently as an explanation of the survival of distinctive values and attitudes in particularly poor communities in North and Central America.

The middle class–working class division

The first approach sharply contrasts the cultural values of the poor with the majority of society. There is an alternative conception of society often reflected in the social investigation of differences in the use of health services (e.g. Tuckett 1976: ch. 4). This would draw a more fundamental dividing line between middle-class and working-class groups. This is probably one of the most frequently used of distinctions employed in research into social differences in Britain. It is employed in such disparate fields as political attitudes, leisure activities, educational achievement, or whatever. The distinction derives from various socio-logical traditions which view non-manual occupations as enjoying fundamental advantages over manual occupations with regard to power, status, and income. Differences in rewards and experience at the work place parallel two sharply distinctive life-styles and sets of attitudes characteristic of middle-class and working-class communities. However, complex changes in the economy have resulted in considerable differences of rewards and prestige *within* both the non-manual and manual sectors (Parkin 1979) that might lead to a questioning of the value of such dichotomies. It continues to be the working assumption of much survey research that there are two broadly different life-styles and sets of values. Unfortunately, the meaning of class in this tradition is often too all-embracing yet ill-defined that almost any part of the broadly delineated stereotype of, for example 'working-class' can be invoked to make sense of attitudes or behaviour identified in surveys.

The cost-benefit approach

Although the two approaches so far identified differ in how they conceive divisions in society, they are similar in placing most emphasis, in their explanations of social differences, upon cultural beliefs, attitudes, and life-styles. A third approach to explaining social differences in the use of health services would stress the different costs and benefits involved in their use, as perceived by individuals of differing social backgrounds (e.g. Le Grand 1982). The costs are particularly of time: those who are dependent on public transport, have further to travel for health care facilities, and are more likely to lose wages for time taken to go to the doctor, incur greater costs which are a disincentive to consulting the doctor. If, also, the benefits of consulting are less, either because certain groups have less health knowledge to understand benefits, or because they actually derive less benefits, this will also decrease the likelihood of consulting. This cost-benefit approach is simple but potentially a 'powerful tool' (Le Grand 1982: 32) for understanding differential use of services and is favoured by the Black Report:

> 'It is hard to resist the conclusion that this pattern of unequal use is explicable not in terms of non-rational response to sickness by working class people but of a rational weighting of the perceived costs and benefits . . . These costs and benefits differ between the social classes.
>
> (Townsend and Davidson 1982: 89)

THEORIES OF SOCIAL CLASS AND INTERACTION WITH HEALTH WORKERS

Cultural compatibility

There are a number of different theories to explain differences of experience that appear to occur between patients of varying back-grounds when they consult a doctor. One view (e.g. Freidson 1970) stresses the varying cultural backgrounds which shape patients' views about illness and treatment. In this approach, middle-class patients' ideas are more likely to be compatible with the scientific medical approach of the doctor. Thus various problems of communication are more likely to occur with working-class patients whose views, drawing on more traditional or folk medical principles, most contrast with the medical model.

Social skills

A somewhat different theory would emphasize the variability in social skills and confidence amongst patients (e.g. Bochner 1983). Middle-class patients are more likely to be confident in meeting middle-class doctors and hence more likely to be successful in achieving their objectives from the consultation. Common to both approaches is the implied prediction that the greater the social distance (whether assessed by social status or education) between patient and doctor, the less likely it is that there will be empathy and understanding between the two parties. The two approaches differ in that the first places emphasis upon the cognitive aspect of consultations, the ideas and explanations each party holds about illness; whereas the second perspective would regard the differing styles of behaviour and social skills of patients as ultimately influencing the pattern of consultations.

The influence of the health worker

Both approaches focus primarily on the patient. An alternative perspec-tive (e.g. Hooper *et al.* 1982) would argue that equally important are the differing perceptions and stereotypes in terms of which doctors and other health workers relate to patients. It may be that doctors' implicit assumptions about patients of different social backgrounds are a major influence over the outcomes of consultations.

It is important to stress that, although clearly there are points of overlap between approaches, it is essential that effort is made to assess their relative merits. The implications of theories vary: to take an extreme contrast, if the costs of access to health care most satisfactorily explain different levels of use then different solutions would be required than if cultural beliefs about acceptable levels of health were the more powerful explanation. In simple terms, the former interpretation would imply reducing financial costs and barriers to health care; the latter interpreta-tion might point to educational changes.

EVIDENCE REGARDING SOCIAL CLASS AND USE OF HEALTH SERVICES

The first question that needs to be asked is whether there are social class differences in the use of health services. Owing to the type of data available in the United Kingdom, much more evidence has accumulated about the use of general practice than other parts of the National Health Service. The General Household Survey (GHS), which questions a large sample of respondents in the United Kingdom annually, has recently included items about health status and the use of health services. For several years, the survey has found that lower social classes are more likely to have attended general practice in the study period. However, the survey has also found that the same groups report much more illness. Thus the question that really needs to be considered is whether there are significant differences between social groups in their use of general practitioner services in relation to differing levels of illness. Brotherston (1976) examined this question by means of GHS data for England and Wales, 1972. For each social group, from professionals to unskilled workers, the numbers of general practitioner consultations reported in the two weeks covered by the GHS were calculated. At the same time, the number of days in which activity was restricted by illness was calculated for the same groups. The first calculation gave an expression of the level of use of services; the second an expression of the level of 'need' for services in each of the social groups. The two sets of figures were then combined to provide a simple 'use in relation to need' ratio for each group. The ratio of use in relation to need was highest for professionals (133) and declined steadily to the lowest use–need ratio (57) for unskilled workers. Townsend and Davidson (1982) repeated the exercise for GHS data for the period 1974–76 and obtained the same pattern of greater use of services in relation to given levels of sickness by higher social groups.

Townsend and Davidson (1982: 78) acknowledge that there may be limitations to such calculations: for example, people with illness severe enough to restrict activity may be using hospital rather than general practice facilities. Collins and Klein (1980) point out that in the calculation of use–need ratios, it is not necessarily the same individuals who are reporting illness as are reporting consultations with their doctor. They offer a more rigorous analysis of GHS data for 1976 in which they examine the use of services of individuals linked to their health status. They examine separately the rates of use of general practice of the acutely sick, the chronically sick with and without restricted activity and those reporting no illness.

Amongst the acutely sick and the chronically sick without restrictions, particularly for men, it is the lowest social groups who are more likely to have attended general practice. Amongst the chronically sick with restricted activity, there appear to be no significant social class differences. Generally their results therefore go against the patterns established in other studies by finding equitable use of general practice by the different social classes. Various limitations have been suggested with regard to the study. Townsend and Davidson (1982: 24) argue that it only takes one year into account and examines only the numbers of users of general practice rather than how frequently services are used by different social groups. The study does not consider the degree of severity of illness in class differences in use. Both considerations, they argue, would restore the trend of lower use in relation to need by working classes. Le Grand (1982: 30) suggests that no account is taken of the purpose of visits to the doctor: the working class rates of use may be high because of more frequent needs to obtain sickness absence certification from the doctor. Until research takes account of such issues it is premature to say that there is equitable use of general practice. The other sources of evidence are mainly specific studies of particular health services. Cartwright and O'Brien (1976) and Townsend and Davidson (1982) argue that the clearest evidence that there are social differences in the use of health services appears in the field of preventative care. Here the evidence should in principle be less difficult to assess since rates of use are less complicated by varying levels of need which have to be considered in interpreting rates of consultation for illness. The evidence that they assemble shows increased levels of use of services such as antenatal care, immunization for children, and screening for cervical cancer by the higher social classes. These gradients of increased use are the reverse of patterns found for cigarette smoking in which the higher social classes are less likely to smoke. Such data are sometimes taken together to give support to a cultural explanation in which lower social classes are less oriented to the future with regard to their health and hence less likely to take appropriate preventative action. However, the evidence needs careful interpretation. Several of the studies of social class and preventative services are quite dated and need to be repeated. Given the problematic state of evidence regarding class differences in the use of services for illness, it may not be justified to infer that class differences in behaviour are so much greater in preventative compared with acute services. This inference is especially dangerous since with it tends to be invoked the all too readily available explanation that the greater differences in preventative services are due to fundamental cultural attitudes such as fatalism in working-class communities which inhibit the use of preventative services. The ever present risk is of creating over-simplified stereotypes to explain differences. Little evidence is available to support such class-typical forms of explanation.

SOCIAL CLASS AND THE MEANING OF ILLNESS
Surveys of the kind that have been discussed so far can provide evidence as to the extent of class differences in use of services but little

understanding of the meaning of differences. A few studies have recently attempted more intensively to examine class-related attitudes and beliefs in relation to illness. Blaxter and Paterson (1982) examined, by intensive interviewing, the perspectives of two generations of mothers in Aberdeen from unskilled and semi-skilled occupational backgrounds. The women accepted as normal quite considerable levels of symptoms, sometimes for example viewing as essentially healthy, children who were suffering recurrent ear infections and coughs. Health appeared for many to be judged in functional terms such as the ability to continue going to work. There was little evidence of a positive sense of health that the individual could actively promote. The women of both generations had become mothers or grandmothers at an early age and accepted the degree of physical decline that attended their premature ageing as normal since the same thing happened to most of the people that they knew in similar circumstances. There were differences between the two generations in readiness to seek help for medical problems: a fatalistic reluctance to seek medical help being more common among the older women. The younger generation reported a wider range of attitudes: on the one hand a demanding readiness to seek medical advice, especially for those illnesses in their children which evoked fears from their families' histories of such diseases as tuberculosis; on the other hand not consulting for a variety of symptoms defined as normal in their relatively low expectations of health. Generally however, the extreme set of fatalistic attitudes portrayed in the culture of poverty were uncommon in the younger women and it was difficult to identify any single characteristic orientation among the views expressed.

The sample studied by Blaxter and Paterson was working class in composition and although the values reported appear different from those associated with the middle classes, no comparative material is provided in the study. Another study of health beliefs in an Aberdeen community (Williams 1983), conducted amongst elderly respondents, appeared to find no significant social class differences in attitudes to health. Blaxter and Paterson's study presents an important point with regard to class and one which is similar to the findings of a study by Pill and Stott (1982) who investigated the health beliefs of a sample of working-class mothers in Cardiff. Both studies find important *intra-class* differences in beliefs. Blaxter and Paterson distinguished, within their sample, between two groups of more and less disadvantaged by means of an assessment of their housing and economic circumstances and of their social stability (taking account of such factors as the quality of their marriages). All of the small group who were rated as apathetic and pessimistic about health had also been rated as more socially disadvantaged. Moreover, the more disadvantaged group were less likely to have consulted a doctor or dentist for their children in a six-month period. In

Pill and Stott's fairly homogeneous sample of mothers of a semi-skilled occupational background, living in one estate, they found significant differences in health beliefs between home owners and those who rented their homes from the council. The home owners were more likely to view a variety of diseases such as heart disease and cancer as caused in part by aspects of individual behaviour such as diet, mental attitude to work, and life-style generally. The authors viewed home-ownership as part of a cluster of social attitudes which emphasized the individual's control over life as opposed to notions of fatalism. Both studies show how variations in specific social and material conditions within class categories need to be considered in understanding attitudes to health.

These two studies focus primarily on cultural and social factors involved in response to illness. A few studies have directly examined the possible role of costs and benefits in class differences in use of health services. Cartwright (1964) surveyed a sample of people who had been hospitalized. Whereas over half of the working-class respondents had felt some financial strains, largely through loss of wages during hospitalization, this was true of less than 10 per cent of middle-class respondents whose salaries were normally not affected. Le Grand (1982) points to evidence that semi-skilled and unskilled workers are less likely to own cars and have further to travel to health care facilities. In a study of children in Welsh hospitals (Earthrowl and Stacey 1977) the financial costs and practical difficulties of travelling to visit their children were much more frequently cited as a problem by working-class respondents. The discussion of the benefits of care to different social classes partly turns on the studies of consultations and their outcomes considered later in the chapter, as well as on evidence of social inequalities in provision, of the kind discussed in Le Grand (1978).

SOCIAL CLASS AND USE OF HEALTH SERVICES IN THE UNITED STATES

One limitation of the investigation of class differences in the United Kingdom is the lack of research that considers together the role of social, cultural, and economic factors in explaining the use of services. American research has made more progress in the use of survey methods to explore such issues.

Many direct financial barriers to health care for the poor were removed with the passage of Medicare and Medicaid legislation. The differences in the numbers of visits to the doctor between the poor and non-poor have subsequently disappeared (Rogers, Blendon, and Moloney 1982). There is some evidence that lowest rates in use of health services now occur amongst middle-income families (Rundall and Wheeler 1979). However, as in British studies, the highest levels of morbidity occur in low-income families. In a study of Medicare benefits for the elderly,

Davis (1979) reports that, if the health status of respondents is standardized, low income is associated with fewer visits to the doctor at every level of health. Crandall and Duncan (1981) in a sample of low-income Chicago families, examined the influence upon visits to the doctor of economic factors such as the individual's level of insurance cover and travel time to the doctor's office and of social attitudes such as the level of belief in the effectiveness of medicine. They found that the two sets of variables interacted to influence patterns of use. It was amongst respondents with fewer financial barriers to health care that beliefs in the effectiveness of medicine were most positively associated with visits to the doctor.

Rundall and Wheeler (1979) examined the use of preventative care of a large sample of Michigan households. They found that lower-income households were less likely to visit their doctor for check-ups. Most of the association between income and use could be explained by two other variables. Low-income families were less likely to perceive themselves as susceptible to such disorders as heart disease, stroke and blood pressure. This view about their health was less likely to be associated with regular visits for check-ups. The authors see this link as consistent with the culture of poverty thesis and support for the view that even if financial barriers are reduced, health may be less salient for some groups. Their second finding is that higher-income households were more likely to have a regular doctor and that this led to more frequent visits. Poorer households were more likely to use public hospital out-patient clinics or accident and emergency departments which provided more impersonal care. This also resulted in less frequent attendance for check-ups. The influence of both cultural variables and aspects of the health care system on use is supported by Dutton (1978) who examined the use of services of a mainly black sample in Washington. The more frequent use of preventative services by those with higher incomes was explained by more positive cultural beliefs in the value of medicine and of prevention: whereas more frequent use of the doctor for illness by households with higher incomes was explained by the fact that they were more likely to be able to attend doctors in group practices rather than hospital accident and emergency departments.

Thus the direction of such American research is towards supporting modified versions of a culture of poverty approach: that is that associated with very low incomes are attitudes regarding health which make the use of health services less likely, particularly in discretionary instances. In addition, the quality of the health care facilities to which low-income groups have access acts as a separate disincentive to more regular use of facilities. This research shows the value of simultaneous consideration of cultural, economic, and health system factors in understanding patterns of use of services. Clearly the results should not be uncritically applied to

Britain, where it is arguable that there is less variability in the type of health care facility available to different sections of society and fewer direct financial barriers to care even if indirect costs remain important.

SOCIAL CLASS AND MEDICAL CONSULTATIONS

Earlier, various cultural and social psychological perspectives were reviewed which suggested that the social status of the patient might influence interaction in medical consultations. Again the question has received most attention in relation to general practice. Perhaps the simplest and most consistent evidence is on the length of consultations received by patients of differing social backgrounds. Buchan and Richardson (1973), in a study of over 2,000 consultations, found a clear gradient in the length of consultations from an average of 6.1 minutes for patients in social class one to 4.4 minutes for those in social class five. Cartwright and O'Brien (1976) report a study of elderly patients' consultations in which middle-class patients' consultations lasted for 6.2 minutes on average compared with 4.7 minutes for working-class patients. Bochner reports a study by himself and Pendleton of seventy-nine general practice consultations which were videotaped (Bochner 1983; Pendleton and Bochner 1980). They classified the patients into three groups according to socio-economic status. The average lengths of consultation for the low, medium, and high status groups were 5.8, 6.3 and 7.3 minutes respectively. In this study, the possibility was considered that the differing lengths of time were due to varying degrees of complexity in the problems presented which would require different amounts of time. When the doctors' diagnoses were used to classify patients' problems as simple or complex, no difference was found in the proportion of complex problems presented by each of the three social groups, suggesting that other, more social factors determined the length of consultations.

The content of consultations also differs according to the social background of the patient. Bain, a GP, (1976) recorded and analysed 480 consultations in his health centre. He found that more explanations were given to patients of social classes one and two than to patients of social classes four and five. In Pendleton and Bochner's study the doctor volunteered more information and explanations, the higher the social status of the patient. One possible explanation for such differences is simply that middle-class patients ask more questions of the doctor and thereby elicit more information. Both Bain and Cartwright and O'Brien showed that middle-class patients do ask more questions, although Bain points out that questioning generally was not common by patients of whatever status. These two studies do not indicate whether it is the more frequent questioning by middle-class patients that leads directly to them obtaining more information. Pendleton and Bochner, although they do not report on differences in the amount of patients' questioning, nevertheless show that high and middle status patients' questions were more likely to elicit explanations and information than those of low social class patients. The implications of this would be that class differences in experience are due more to doctors' decisions about how to respond to different kinds of patients rather than to the different degrees of influence that patients have in consultations through questioning the doctor. However, Bochner (1983) reports of the same study that there was little evidence that the doctors involved assumed their working-class patients to be less curious about their problems. Generally, the evidence is not yet sufficient to sustain an exact explanation of social class differences. The tendency of research has been to resort to some kind of social skills theory. Thus Bochner concludes that 'the medical consultation, like any stylized social encounter has a set of rules and assumptions, a culture. These rules are better known by some groups than by others' (Bochner 1983: 137).

The influence of cognitive cultural factors such as the degree of compatibility between patients' and doctors' concepts of illness upon consultations is discussed in other chapters. Few studies have directly investigated the possibility that social class differences in concepts might be important in consultations. One often cited hypothesis that warrants attention is that 'a tendency to express emotional distress and discomfort in bodily terms is stronger among people of less education and lower socio-economic position' (Barsky and Klerman 1983: 280). The potential impact of such a tendency upon the outcomes of consultations could be immense (Kleinman 1980). However, for understanding class differences, more attention has been given to the style and manner of patients' presentations than to their content (Boulton 1983).

SOCIAL CLASS AND THE OUTCOMES OF CARE

Another aspect of the consultation that merits attention is the broad issue of outcomes. To what extent are there significant differences in benefits for patients of different social backgrounds? Bain (1976) and Pendleton and Bochner (1980) demonstrate one outcome that differs – the amount of information obtained. Indeed, Bain (1977) followed up some of his patients and assessed, by means of a simple questionnaire, understanding of information given and found much more misunderstanding in social classes four and five. Blaxter (1983b) also provides evidence to suggest that, amongst older men and women, higher social classes are more likely to obtain referrals to specialist out-patient clinics. The issue of outcomes is not only of importance in terms of the principle of equity but also plays a part in one form of explanation for class differences in rates of use, that is the view that there are differential costs and benefits. Although there is suggestive evidence of differences in the content of consultations between social groups, the extent to which there are differential benefits, obtained, or perceived, still needs examination.

COMMENTS

The role that social class membership plays in influencing responses to illness is by no means simple. No single perspective can be said to have greater explanatory power in relation to differences. A variety of cultural, social, and economic factors mediate between class position and be-haviour. One problem is the paucity of studies that incorporate social class as a focus (Hauser 1981: 108). Much of the evidence regarding the use of services has been collected for a wide variety of other purposes and has only limited potential for resolving the issues discussed in this chapter. In particular, more work is needed that combines the intensive attention to the meaning of illness shown in research, such as that of Blaxter and Paterson, with quantitative evidence on patterns of be-haviour in the use of services or consultations.

It is now commonplace to remark upon the limitations of conventional classsification of class for understanding social factors in health (Collins and Klein 1980: 115; Illsley 1980: 16; Townsend and Davidson 1982: 48). Several studies in this chapter made important contributions by investi-gating the influence of social and material variation within social class. This is not to argue for the abandonment of social class as an explanatory variable but to recognize the urgent need for greater specification of the social factors operating in the health field. Overdependence upon the dichotomies of social classification in terms of which much data are gathered or interpreted may not do justice to the complex social processes involved, may perpetuate misleading class-typifications, and may limit the potential contribution of research to bringing about more equitable health care.

Ethnicity

ETHNICITY AND HEALTH STATUS

The literature linking ethnicity with health and health care is marked more by anecdote than scholarship. There remains a dearth of reliable studies, both quantitative and qualitative. Although, for example, ethnicity has often been associated with health inequalities, commen-tators have tended to rely on extrapolations from social class-related health inequalities rather than cite any 'direct' evidence of association. A typical argument runs: as immigrants to Britain from the New Common-wealth and Pakistan (NCWP) – whose ethnic identity is apparent from their skin colour – are known to experience social and economic disadvantage, it can be assumed that they have higher than average rates of mortality and morbidity. The Black Report (DHSS 1980) highlights the difficulties of testing this hypothesis. Its authors also note that the age standardized mortality ratios of immigrant males compare favourably with those of their British-born equivalents in social classes four and five (if less so in social classes one and two). They speculate that this favourable comparison may reflect a tendency for migrants to select themselves on the grounds of health and fitness. They then call for further research on ethnicity and health inequalities, especially in relation to second and third generation immigrants.

Some writers have also claimed associations between ethnicity and inequalities in the provision and use of health care services, again largely inferring as much from data on social class-related inequalities. The authors of the Black Report acknowledge there is 'a clear lack of adequate facilities in some of the areas in which (immigrants) have been obliged to concentrate' (Townsend and Davidson 1980: 115) but sound a note of caution concerning claims about ethnicity and the under-utilization of these facilities by stressing once more the sparseness of information.

The ensuing discussion will concentrate on ethnicity and 'the experience of illness', on the various ways in which the concept of ethnicity has been used to analyse and account for differences in people's perceptions of illness; their knowledge, impressions and use of health care services; and their interactions with health workers.

THE CONCEPT OF ETHNICITY

Introducing his *Ethnic Minorities in Britain*, Krausz (1972: 10) writes: 'The label "minority" applies here broadly to all those groups which, by virtue of ethnic differences – i.e. racial, religious, national, linguistic and other cultural factors – are singled out for differential treatment and in consequence regard themselves as objects of collective discrimination.' Cashmore and Troyna (1983) employ a similar definition of 'ethnic groups', emphasizing that members of such groups are essentially aware of sharing a common origin or destiny. They write:

'Usually, though not always, they are descendants of immigrants who left their lands either to seek improvements elsewhere or were forcibly taken from their lands, as were African slaves. Conversely, they might be original inhabitants of lands alienated from them by invaders – like North American Indians or Australian aborigines. Whatever the circumstances, the ethnic group reveals a response of disadvantaged peoples who believe themselves to be participants in a common plight but who also feel that they can find comfort, stability and perhaps further their interests, by emphasizing the features of life, past and present, they share.'

(Cashmore and Troyna 1983: 161–62)

Banton (1977) has distinguished between ethnicity and race, 'so that the former reflects the positive tendencies of identification and inclusion where the latter reflects the negative tendencies of dissociation and exclusion' (Banton 1977: 136).

Cashmore and Troyna (1983) make the point that it is impossible to be more precise than this in defining ethnicity because the forms it takes are so varied. Key ethnic minorities in Britain include: West Indian or Guyanese, Indian, Pakistani, Bangladeshi, Chinese, African, and Arab. After discussing the various 'push' and 'pull' factors which led to the

Table 7   *Ethnic groups—people in employment: by sex and socio-economic group, 1981*

| | Great Britain | | |
| | ethnic group | | |
	white	West Indian or Guyanese	Indian/ Pakistani/ Bangladeshi
males (percentages)			
professional	6	2	8
employers and managers	16	4	12
intermediate and junior non-manual	18	7	14
skilled manual and own account non-professional	38	49	35
semi-skilled manual and personal service	16	27	25
unskilled manual	5	11	6
armed forces and inadequately described	1	1	—
all males aged 16 and over in employment (= 100%) (thousands)	13,325	120	243
females (percentages)			
professional	1	—	3
employers and managers	7	2	4
intermediate and junior non-manual	53	50	41
skilled manual and own account non-professional	7	4	13
semi-skilled manual and personal service	23	34	35
unskilled manual	8	8	3
armed forces and inadequately described	—	1	—
all females aged 16 and over in employment (= 100%) (thousands)	8,945	107	104

Source: Central Statistical Office (1983).

migration of such groups to Britain, Krausz (1972) stresses the absence of any comprehensive statistics. In the 1971 census, information was collected for the first time on the country of birth of individuals and of their parents, but attempts to extend the data on ethnicity and race to be obtained by the 1981 census were thwarted when the matter became politically contentious (White 1979). Much of the literature on ethnic minorities in Britain is based therefore on *ad hoc* surveys and small-scale studies.

Before turning to ethnicity and the experience of illness, it is worth briefly commenting on the nature of the association between ethnicity and social class, at least as far as minorities from the NCWP are concerned. It has already been implied that these minorities are over-represented in the manual or working classes. *Table 7*, deriving from the 1981 Labour Force Survey (Central Statistical Office 1983), shows that this is indeed the case, especially for those of West Indian or Guyanese origin. Data from the same surveys also show extremely high rates of unemployment for minorities from the NCWP, again most notably for those of West Indian or Guyanese origin (CSO 1983). No fewer than 21 per cent of men of West Indian or Guyanese origin aged 16–64 were unemployed in 1981, and this percentage rises to 38 for those aged 16–24. There are differing interpretations of such statistics, but most social scientists would broadly agree with the following: that post-war expansion in Britain created gaps in the labour market which only came to be filled with the help of immigrants from the NCWP. These immigrants, first from the Caribbean and later from South Asia, tended to occupy jobs either not wanted or not needed by native workers; Glasgow (1980) calls them 'cellar jobs'. Persistent racialism reinforced their subordinate position in the labour market, while their position in the reserve army of labour made them especially vulnerable when the economic situation deteriorated.

If the high levels of unemployment of the early 1980s continue, it is quite probable that 'whites' will increasingly come to see 'blacks' and Asians as competitors for jobs to which they believe they, historically, have the better claim. In the light of this, Banton (1983) lists four possible future scenarios:

1   A 'class unity process', whereby members of ethnic groups come to be absorbed into the classes of the native social structure and to define their major problems as class issues;
2   'ethnic organization', whereby the different ethnic groups organize politically as independent units;
3   a 'black unity process', whereby all non-whites combine together to form a co-operating group;
4   a situation in which, instead of their being absorbed into the native

working class, ethnic groups remain as an underclass, a reserve army of labour of the type envisaged by those who write of internal colonialism.

(Banton 1983: 325–26)

Banton suggests that a number of different combinations of these scenarios could come to pass. Rex and Tomlinson (1979) argue that for both West Indians and Asians 'the question of the absorption of immigrant minorities into the working class has been settled against absorption', with the native working class uniting with other indigenous classes against them. On the basis of their work in the Handsworth area of Birmingham, they contend that both minorities, still constituting an underclass, have resorted to what Banton calls 'ethnic organization':

'In the Asian communities it takes the form of defensive organization within which individuals may aim at capital accumulation and social mobility; in the West Indian community it may take the form of withdrawal from competition altogether with emphasis upon the formation of a black identity, even though a small minority might achieve, and a larger continue to aspire towards, assimilation.'

(Rex and Tomlinson 1979: 276)

THE PERCEPTION OF ILLNESS AND THE USE OF HEALTH SERVICES

Cultural differences

While there have been several theories linking social class membership with experiences of illness and health care utilization, there have been few attempts to generate equivalent theories around the concept of ethnicity. It is possible, however, to discern a number of interlocking 'themes' in the research and discursive literature. Most emphasis has undoubtedly been placed on aspects of cultural differences between ethnic minorities and the majority population. The clearest manifestations of such differences are those modes of comprehending and responding to illness which are far removed from western medical paradigms. Eisenbruch's (1983) recent case-study of Mrs Xuyen, a 46-year-old mother of six who settled in Britain after leaving Vietnam, illustrates the point well. Called in to see Mrs Xuyen's 17-year-old son, who was reported to be suffering from severe depression at school, Eisenbruch noticed that during each of his visits Mrs Xuyen herself was withdrawn and unresponsive and formed the impression that she was clinically depressed. Her family referred to her bad 'headaches' over many years and to other bodily pains. These headaches became particularly severe with the trauma of resettlement; but Mrs Xuyen had no faith in western medicine and only agreed to see a general practitioner as a result of increasing pressure from the younger members of her family. The general practitioner diagnosed tension headache and pre-scribed a course of self-relaxation. Mrs Xuyen was confused and disappointed: 'despite the help of an interpreter, she had understood nothing of what had occurred and could see no possible connection between her headaches and the prescribed exercise' (Eisenbruch 1983: 323).

Over a period of time Mrs Xuyen made passing references to 'wind'. Eisenbruch discovered that the onset of her headaches dated back sixteen years, and that the initial problem was not a headache but 'something bad'. It transpired that after the birth of her third child, Mrs Xuyen had failed to observe the (Chinese) ritual of 'doing the month' (for a detailed description of this ritual, see Pillsbury 1978).

> 'Consequently, she had become poisoned and her headaches were a final manifestation of this poisoning. Mrs Xuyen explained that when she was "dirty" after having delivered the child, she had cleansed herself with a wet towel and rinsed it out in clean water. Feeling fatigued, she lay down to sleep, placing the moist towel under her head as a pillow. During her sleep, the "wind" emerged from the towel and entered her head, where it had stayed ever since'.
>
> (Eisenbruch 1983: 324)

She was suffering from 'wrong menstrual wind illness' *(lom phit duan)* caused during the first postpartum month by a breach of postpartum custom. Eisenbruch (1983: 324) continues: 'It is noteworthy that, of the entire sibship, this child, whom I was first called on to see, is the only one to have developed depressive symptoms and headaches during his childhood.' Mrs Xuyen believed that her son had contracted 'wind illness' via her breast milk. Her attitude to her own illness was fatalistic. She had tried without avail to 'right the wrong' by taking special care with the ritual of 'doing the month' after the birth of two further children. Herbal remedies had also failed. She was convinced there was nothing anyone, including western doctors, could do. (In the event, a course of acupuncture led to an improvement: her headaches diminished and she became more involved in family affairs.)

Eisenbruch raises the complex question as to whether Mrs Xuyen was the victim of 'wind illness' or somatic depression. Ethnographic and clinical research has suggested that Chinese populations commonly explain psycho-social distress, such as depression, in somatic or situational terms. Indeed, this 'somatization' of affective disorder has been cited as one reason for the under-utilization of mental health services among Chinese minorities in the United States and elsewhere. In a study involving samples of (Caucasian) American and Hong Kong Chinese students at the University of Hawaii, White (1982) set out to test the hypothesis that 'somatization' is essentially a cultural phenomenon: 'In this view, "somatization" can be seen as an interpretive process which conceptualizes particular medical problems with less reference to psychological (affective) constructs than would be expected in Western theories of illness (both popular and professional)' (White 1982: 1519). He was aware that *other* factors – such as the stigma associated with mental illness – might influence the interrelated phenomena of 'somatization' and under-utilization of mental health services among the Hong Kong Chinese and designed his study to minimize the effects of such 'social contextual factors'. He found that the American students made more use of emotive constructs in explaining several of a series of 'somatic' and 'affective-type' complaints than did the Hong Kong Chinese and judged this a 'limited' corroboration of his hypothesis.

White's reference to stigma is a reminder that factors other than the cognitive bases of cultural explanations of illness are implicated in any under-utilization of health care services by minority ethnic groups. Henley (1979) has noted that diseases like Hanson's disease, eczema, tuberculosis, asthma, epilepsy, and all forms of mental illness are profoundly stigmatizing in many Asian communities in Britain. Moreover, the stigma may affect not only the patient but all members of a family. 'Some parents will not allow their child to marry into a "diseased" family. A serious disease in one child, therefore, may ruin the marriage chances of all the others' (Henley 1979: 63). One consequence is that diagnoses may be rejected or the existence of diseases concealed. Other more obvious cultural factors functioning as barriers to health care include inability to speak English and ignorance of, or unfamiliarity with, available services. In a study of elders of the ethnic minority groups, Bhalla and Blakemore (1981) discovered that no fewer than 88 per cent of the Asian elders interviewed could not speak English. A survey undertaken by the Wandsworth Council for Community Relations found that 60 per cent of Indian and 77 per cent of Pakistani women speak English only slightly or not at all. Bhalla and Blakemore (1981) also found Asian elders to be 'pitifully lacking in knowledge about the basic services and help available to them' (Bhalla and Blakemore 1981: 27). For example, only 19 per cent had heard of home helps (compared with 94 per cent of Europeans and 83 per cent of Afro-Caribbeans) and only 13 per cent of meals on wheels (compared with 96 per cent of Europeans and 80 per cent of Afro-Caribbeans). None of the Asian elders had actually benefited from home helps and/or meals on wheels. They tended to rely much more heavily than the Europeans and Afro-Caribbeans on their extended families for help and care. Horn (1982) found that Asians of all ages made less general use of the social services in Bradford than the native population, but she notes that a comparatively high number of Asian referrals concerning children (e.g. wanting day centre places) suggests that the extended family system may be losing some cohesion in Britain. She concludes: 'This may eventually have implications for the Asian elderly of future years. Social workers should therefore cease to assume that the Asian communities will always "take care of their own" within the extended family' (Horn 1982: 61).

Henley (1979) makes the point that many Asians brought up in rural areas of the Indian subcontinent had little or no experience of hospitals before coming to Britain; for many, 'hospitals conjure up ideas of serious or fatal illnesses and are extremely frightening' (Henley 1979: 54). This is equally true of some other ethnic groups. Watson (1977) for example, found it to apply to the Hong Kong Chinese, most of whom work in the restaurant trade in London's Soho. When they are ill they tend to rely either on Chinese doctors who practise with the Public Health Service, or on a particular Cantonese-speaking Indian physician who once lived and practised in Hong Kong. Asians too sometimes seek out Asian doctors, although it should be remembered that there are frequently differences of language, 'class', and culture between Asian doctors and their patients. They also make widespread use of traditional healers or 'hakims', of whom there are several in most Asian communities in Britain; hakims combine the role of doctor with those of counsellor and pharmacist and always treat bodily ills in their social context (Davis and Aslam 1979).

Migration

A second theme concerns the implications for health of the process of migration itself. After a comprehensive review of the evidence, Hull (1979) concludes that 'in migrant studies there is not a reliable, direct relationship between change and illness' (Hull 1979: 35). Nevertheless, the 'common-sense' assumption that migrants coming from rural parts of India or Jamaica to settle in urban Britain were likely to experience high rates of psychiatric illness while they sought to adjust to a radically different and sometimes hostile social environment seemed to receive some support from several small studies published in the 1960s. Most of these studies, however, have since been criticized because of their small sample size and because too little attention was paid to variables like age, sex, and social class. More recently, some larger-scale surveys of psychiatric hospital admissions have been conducted. *Table 8*, composed by Rack (1982), summarizes the results. It can be seen that the rates for West Indians are about one and a half times the rates for the indigenous population, and that the rates for women are a little higher than those for men. The figures for Asian patients are simply inconsistent. Rack counsels extreme caution in interpreting *all* such data, adding: 'At present it is probably fair to say that no consistent trends can be detected, and such differences as exist cannot be explained by any simple

Table 8 *Summary of admissions data*

country of birth	England and Wales 1971 (Cochrane 1977) all admissions		Bradford 1968–70 (Hitch 1975)		Manchester 1973–75 (Carpenter and Brockington 1980) first admissions only		South-east England 1976 (Dean et al. 1981)	
	male	*female*	*male*	*female*	*male*	*female*	*male*	*female*
Britain (base rate)	100	100	100	100	100	100	100	100
West Indies	103	113	72a	22a }	156d	185d*	136*	156*
Africa			88	59a			121b	129b
India	85	79	134	191* }	236c*	325c*	149*	123*
Pakistan	68	68					59*	55

Notes: There are substantial differences in the rates quoted by different authors for the British-born patients in their series. Presumably these reflect differences in the organization and utilization of psychiatric services in different areas. To obtain rough comparability therefore the rates for each immigrant group have been converted to a percentage of the rates given for British-born patients in the same sample.
* indicates statistically significant difference from British-born rate (p < 0.01) calculated by the authors in each case.
a Hitch comments that the numbers in these categories were too small for any important conclusions to be drawn.
b includes ethnic Africans and ethnic Indians (refugees from Kenya and Uganda).
c all Asians amalgamated, including Bangla Deshis.
d includes 'negroes from sub-Saharan Africa' (13 per cent of sample).
Source: Rack (1982).

generalization' (Rack 1982: 162). Studies are badly needed which control not only for variables like age, sex, and social class, but also for the number of beds in particular areas, the legal and administrative procedures for admission, the distance of hospitals from the community, discharge policies, the availability of out-patient, private, and community facilities, and, most obviously, how particular ethnic minorities perceive and cope with mental illness (Littlewood and Lipsedge 1982). A review by Cochrane (1983) of some of the most recent studies of migration, ethnicity, and mental health highlights the difficulty of interpreting very limited data in this area. Although, for example, it has often been suggested that immigrants may experience relatively high rates of psychiatric illness prior to assimilation, Cochrane counters that there may actually be a negative association between assimilation and mental health. He writes: 'It is quite possible that the groups which are the most isolated from the host community, both because of prejudice and because of a desire on the part of the ethnic minority to maintain their separate traditions, are the least vulnerable to psychological disorder' (Cochrane 1983: 105). Advocates of both of these plausible but seemingly contradictory views claim a measure of support from the research literature. It is clear, however, that until a lot more is known about perceptions of mental illness and coping strategies in different ethnic groups, all views of this type must be regarded as essentially speculative (see Chapter 3).

Social and material disadvantages

Another theme focuses on social and material disadvantages. It is known that members of ethnic minorities, especially from the NCWP, are over-represented in manual or working-class occupations, and that they share many of the socio-economic disadvantages experienced by the indigenous poor. In its evidence to the Royal Commission on the National Health Service, the Community Relations Commission reported that

'the 1971 Census shows that nearly three-quarters of the ethnic minority population is concentrated in one-tenth of the census enumeration districts, in which they constitute over a fifth of the total population. When these 10 per cent of enumeration districts are compared with others on indicators of deprivation, it is found that they contain nearly three times the mean for Great Britain of households who share or lack hot water, twice as many who share or lack a bath, nearly three times as many living at a density of over 1.5 persons per room (the statutory over-crowding level) and nearly four times as many households lacking exclusive use of all basic amenities.'
(CRC 1977)

These socio-economic deprivations are of course associated with poor health. Wallis (1981) illustrates this by means of graphic case-studies in her report on Bengali families in Camden, London. Adelstein, Davies and Weatherall (1980) found that in 1977 the infant mortality rate for children of women born in Pakistan and living in Britain was 50 per cent higher than the rate for women born in the United Kingdom. Having suggested that this rate may well be associated with 'poverty' amongst the Pakistani community in Britain, Blaxter makes the point that 'there is no collection of information or major programme of research on the health, service use, or needs of racial minorities' (1983b: 1144). The CRC conclusion that because of social and material disadvantage, ethnic minorities are likely to be 'over-represented among those seeking help from the health services' is entirely speculative (and, given cultural barriers to help-seeking, rather unlikely).

Special needs

A fourth theme is that ethnic minorities have special needs relating to health. For example, it has been found that Asian babies in Britain have low birth weights and, as has already been seen, high levels of perinatal and infant mortality in comparison with the indigenous population. The CRC complained that this problem has never been properly investigated and expressed anxiety at Asian under-utilization of antenatal and postnatal care services. Certain dietary deficiences have also been identified among Asians – for example, iron deficiency or vitamin B12 deficiency causing anaemia. A relatively high incidence of rickets and osteomalacia has been reported among infants, adolescents and preg-nant Asian women. A recent study comparing hospital morbidity in Asians and non-Asians found that Asian patients in certain age groups were more likely than non-Asians to be diagnosed as having asthma; leukaemia; diabetes mellitus; blood, thyroid, and eye disorders; certain forms of heart disease; and spontaneous and other types of abortion (excluding therapeutic abortion). The recognized excess of cases of tuberculosis among Asians was also confirmed (Donaldson and Taylor 1983). Other ethnic groups also show 'special needs'. Sickle cell anaemia affects the West Indian community and thalassemia affects Cypriot babies; both conditions are much rarer in the indigenous population and few facilities exist to deal with them.

Some racially motivated commentators in the 1960s argued that the utilization of maternity beds by mothers of NCWP origin constituted a special 'burden' on the welfare state. The Runnymede Trust and Radical Statistics Group retort that, even if it were true that maternity beds were used disproportionately by mothers of NCWP origin, it would not follow that people from the NCWP therefore make more or excessive use of the health services.

'Such a conclusion can only be drawn if evidence is available which compares use and non-use of *all* NHS facilities. For instance, greater use of NHS maternity beds may be "offset" by lower use of geriatric beds. In sum, one must distinguish between "special needs" which are particular and specific and overall demand or use which is general.'
(The Runnymede Trust and Radical Statistics Group 1980: 108)

Racism

The final theme is racism. There is ample evidence of racial prejudice and discrimination in many spheres of life activity in Britain, especially employment (Smith 1977). In relation to employment in the NHS, the Royal Commission on the National Health Service (1979: 219) noted that: 'Posts in the NHS are normally competed for, and on the whole overseas born graduates compete less successfully than UK trained doctors. As a result, they tend to get pushed into the 'unpopular' specialties such as geriatrics and to get left with the less attractive posts.' In a study of 2,000 British-born and overseas doctors, Smith (1980) reports that 20 per cent of the 'black' doctors he interviewed said they had 'experienced' racial discrimination of some kind when applying for hospital jobs; he refers to some consultants taking pride in keeping their departments 'white'.

A recent edition of *Issues in Race and Education* contains the following assertion:

'In a racist society, society's response to the health problems of minority group members is likely to be racist. There are differences of degree of course. The National Front use health issues in an overtly aggressive and propagandist way. The state, in patrolling its borders at Heathrow, uses health as a means of intimidating new arrivals and banning entry to Britain. The medical profession makes erroneous and damaging assumptions based on notions of cultural superiority and ignorance: less vindictive in motivation, perhaps, but not necessarily less damaging in effect on the victim.'

(1983: 1)

Leaving aside the crudities of the National Front, what evidence is there that either the state or the medical profession act as agents of racism? Not surprisingly it is piecemeal and highly contentious. The Manchester Law Centre makes the point that people can be prevented from coming to Britain on health grounds; in other words, that health is used for purposes of immigration control. 'As a result of this', they write, 'there has developed a whole paraphernalia of health officers and immigration officers whose job is to keep black people out of this country' (Manchester Law Centre 1982: 14). The Centre claims that the Conservative government's new Nationality Act (1983) and their new health regulations – 'Charges to Overseas Visitors' (1982) – together form a pattern of second-class citizenship. The health regulations require the sick to prove they are 'ordinarily resident' in the United Kingdom before being entitled to free treatment. Despite government assurances to the contrary, a letter in the national press from six general practitioners at a London health centre still insisted that

> 'this scheme will subject non-white or foreign-sounding citizens to further harassment and suspicion, continually putting upon them the onus of proving their identity and eligibility – thus reinforcing their position as second-class citizens. They will feel discouraged from seeking health care and will suffer delays in receiving it if sought.'
>
> (Manchester Law Centre 1982: 5–6)

The Manchester Law Centre Report claims, with supporting case-studies, that the new health regulations have in fact legitimized what has been common practice in some localities for twenty years. MacCormack (1980) argues that members of ethnic minorities are often frightened of government/medical bureaucracy, afraid that jobs in the 'black economy' or immigrant status might be uncovered; she suggests they may be increasingly turning to private treatment with allopathic doctors from their own ethnic groups.

It has also been contended, by the Black Health Workers and Patients' Group for example, that the concept of ethnicity itself has racist connotations. Policies of 'multiculturalism' have been attacked in this connection: such policies, it is said, 'on the one hand, objectify black culture and lifestyles and, on the other, try to divide the black community into separate and competing ethnic groups' (Black Health Workers and Patients Group 1983: 50). Divisions between ethnic groups have been replicated in welfare agencies and even self-help groups, so that black organizations – segregated off as Asian, Afro-Caribbean, and so on – compete for resources. In terms of Banton's scenarios cited earlier, 'ethnic organization' is being fostered by the state at the expense of a much more threatening 'black unity process'. Research on multiculturalism of the kind frequently referred to above may be used directly for surveillance or be stored to help justify future policies.

The fragmentary and conjectural nature of a lot of the work linking ethnicity with the perception of illness and use of health services is readily apparent. It is equally apparent that all such work has political overtones. Complexity of concept and phenomenon and paucity of statistical and research material has led to a largely atheoretical literature. Although it seems reasonable to suppose, on the one hand, that factors like migration, social and material disadvantage, and special needs serve to increase the general *need* for health care, and, on the other hand, that factors like cultural difference and racism serve to depress the general level of *demand* for health care, there is a dearth of published studies considering the combined effect of such factors. As Blaxter and others suggest, remarkably little is known about the illness behaviour of members of ethnic minorities which is not merely anecdotal.

INTERACTIONS WITH HEALTH WORKERS

It is axiomatic that many of those cultural factors which constitute barriers to help-seeking also inhibit doctor–patient communication and interaction when help is sought. Henley recounts, for example, how cultural differences restricting Asian attendance at antenatal classes can also create apprehension and fear on entry to maternity hospitals.

'Instead of being in her own bed surrounded by the women of her family in the privacy of her home, the woman delivers her baby in a technology-filled room attended by strangers, often men. At some stages she may even be left alone. She has no idea what will be done to her next, or what she should do, and she cannot ask. Her fears can make things difficult for the delivery team, and any frustration and irritation they may show will make things worse.'

(Henley 1979: 78)

If appropriate religious ceremonies are not permitted after birth, the relationships between mother and child or husband and wife may be more or less permanently affected. The Asian mother may find separation from her baby – still common in many British hospitals except for feeds and, sometimes, bathing – cruel and unnatural. She may nevertheless show reluctance to return home too soon after birth, believing that a long period of rest is essential for her own health.

Poor communication as a result of cultural difference is perhaps most obviously damaging in the area of mental health. Rack (1982) argues that 'a reliable psychiatric diagnosis cannot be made unless the patient is interviewed in his own language by someone who knows what to look for'. He points out that although junior doctors coming to Britain from India or Pakistan for postgraduate training have been invaluable in this context, 'it would be an unusual Asian doctor who was equally fluent in Hindi, Urdu, Punjabi, Pushtu, Bengali and Gujerati (to name only the six commonest languages), let alone their regional dialect variations' (Rack 1982: 198). Nor, of course, are cultural differences between Asians purely linguistic (Henley 1979).

Despite the general lack of systematic investigation in this field, there is some evidence that poor communication based on inter- and intra-ethnic difference can lead to non-compliance, and hence affect the outcome of treatment (Steffenson and Colker 1982). Unterhalter (1979) studied compliance among a group of 150 black ambulatory patients attending various out-patient clinics at a large urban hospital for blacks in Soweto, Johannesburg. Three categories of patient were seen: children with upper respiratory tract infection, adults with diabetes and adults with hypertension. In unannounced follow-up interviews from three to fourteen days after attendance at the clinics, non-compliance was found to be highest among the hypertensive patients, closely followed by those with diabetes; compliance was highest in the children with acute infections. Unterhalter argues that while the 'overwhelming majority' of the parents of the children with upper respiratory tract infection knew what was wrong, only a third of the diabetic patients and a quarter of the hypertensives understood the nature of their problems despite having regularly attended specialist clinics. Non-compliance, he suggests, can be related to this lack of comprehension, which is rooted in 'the absence of knowledge of diseases such as hypertension and diabetes in the Black indigenous culture' and exacerbated by factors like crowded clinics, lack of continuity of care and failure to provide health education; also mentioned are barriers of language and race and the authoritarianism of predominantly white doctors. Unterhalter ends by suggesting that non-compliance by black patients in South Africa may be one way they can preserve their integrity.

Some writers have argued that a 'transcultural view' is a prerequisite to inter-ethnic or inter-cultural communication in medicine. In Weidman's terms, this approach demands an ability to 'adopt a degree of perceptual distance from any two health cultural traditions involved in specific health-related interactions ... Under the circumstances of assuming a transcultural posture, the health professional becomes sufficiently free to become a cultural negotiator' (Weidman 1979: 86). Hurdles to be cleared include a largely pre-conscious or unconscious ethnocentrism among health professionals, and a similarly unreflecting commitment to what has often been termed the 'biomedical model'. Good and Good (1981) say of this model:

> 'When symptoms are treated as biological indicators rather than meaningful realities, when "disease" is treated to the exclusion of the personal experience of suffering, the physician loses a very fundamental and primitive healing function. Such problems are inherent in the interpretative strategy of empiricist clinical models and are grounded in the epistemology of contemporary medicine.'
>
> (Good and Good 1981: 192)

Weidman (1979) notes that while the doctor may be responding to the same set of symptoms as the patient, his efforts at treatment and re-assurance may have no meaning for his patient. 'Such instances begin to border on an unintended but very real intolerance and possibly contempt for the patient's cognitive system' (Weidman 1979: 86).

It is not always easy to distinguish between ethnocentrism and racism. Brent Community Health Council (1981) has written of the existence of institutional or 'camouflaged' racism in NHS hospitals (i.e. racism which is not open and visible but concealed in the routine practices of hospitals). Writing on psychiatry, Littlewood and Lipsedge (1982) contend that overt racial discrimination is rare, perhaps because of the large numbers of psychiatrists and psychiatric nurses who themselves belong to ethnic minority groups. However, they note that West Indian men are more likely to be admitted to psychiatric hospitals than British-born men; that psychotic black patients are twice as likely as British-born and white immigrants to be detained involuntarily in hospital, 'sectioned' under the Mental Health Act (section 136 is known in some black circles as 'the Mental Health Sus Law' (Black Health Workers and Patients Group 1983)); that Asian-born patients in Britain are also more likely to be involuntary patients in psychiatric hospitals and less likely to refer themselves; that black patients – when differences in diagnosis are allowed for – are still more likely to receive phenothiazine drugs and electro-convulsive therapy; and that black patients are less likely to get the more 'attractive' types of psychiatric care like individual or group therapy (Littlewood and Lipsedge 1982: 65).

Research into ethnicity and doctor–patient interaction is scarce and *ad hoc*. Although, for example, poor communication due to cultural difference has obvious and important implications for quality of care, both social scientific studies and policy innovations to improve the situation are in extremely short supply. The relative importance of cultural difference, ethnocentrism and racism is unknown. If more flexible and sophisticated research is needed on social class and the experience of illness, the same need is even more obvious in relation to dimensions of ethnicity and the experience of illness.

Conclusions

It is apparent that careful thought is required when using the concepts of social class and ethnicity in a psycho-social perspective of illness experience. Both concepts draw attention to a complex array of social, economic, and cultural differences in society. Their familiarity as concepts may result in incautious and over-simplified arguments as to their role in explanations of behaviour. There are as many dangers in perpetuating simplistic social stereotypes as in neglecting the importance of social differences in behaviour. This chapter has argued in particular that vigilance is needed with regard to the conceptualization of the basic social divisions of society in terms of which explanations of behaviour are couched. Moreoever, the variety of alternative social processes which may link individuals' social position and how they respond to illness, needs to be recognized.

A complete picture is not yet possible. The insights into the nature of social class differences provided by such data sources as attendance rates in general practice cannot be matched for ethnicity. There is considerable sensitivity about the recording of information on ethnic origin. Much less research has been conducted which could contribute to clarifying the nature and extent of ethnic differences in the experience of illness and treatment. An uneven emphasis has resulted in current discussions of inequalities in health. The extent and nature of social differences in behaviour and in benefits in relation to health care remains an urgent issue for the behavioural sciences.

Part 2
The experience of treatment

5   Communicating with patients

James Thompson

Introduction

The interview is the one thing which distinguishes medicine from
veterinary surgery. Despite being the cornerstone of medical practice, it
is often seen as a tiresome interface between the doctor and the disease,
yet it may determine the form and content of the information provided, and may totally determine whether the advice given is heeded.
Relatively little attention is paid by medical curricula to interviewing
skills, the assumption being that such abilities come naturally with
unsupervised practice. Yet dissatisfaction with medical communications
remains the most prominent of patient complaints and a major factor in
the move to alternative medicine, with its focus on good and reassuring
communications and the patient as an informed participant in treatment.
Patients prefer to be able to give an account of their problems in their
own terms, yet these expectations of communication are often unmet.
This chapter will outline the perspective which social psychology brings
to the study of social interactions. It will then discuss some of the
problems which have arisen in communicating with patients, will
consider the interview process as a decision-making task and will then

go on to study the training methods which have been employed to improve communication skills.

A social-psychology perspective on communication

THE CONSULTATION AS A PERSONAL ENCOUNTER

Important as the interview is to the practice of medicine, it is only one of the many social interactions which people must negotiate in everyday life, and is best understood in the context of the social psychology of personal encounters.

The consultation interview is a relatively formal means of communication and remains the most common means of interacting with the health service for most patients. Once patients are hospitalized they are open to a wider range of communications with other health professionals. Other members of staff will talk to them, instruct them and attempt to reassure them. Nurses and others will also communicate informally by the extent of attention they pay the patient or his complaints, suggesting that they see some problems and some patients as more important than others. Tones of voice, facial expression and failures to look the patient in the eye may communicate more to the patient about his condition than words could ever do. Although these factors are present in out-patient interviews, their effects are even stronger when the patient is in the dependent position of the hospital bed.

Social encounters are preceded by working assumptions about the purpose of the meeting and the status and role of the participants. Most medical encounters are initiated by patients, whose needs impel them to the consultation. The purpose of the meeting from the patient's point of view will be to seek relief from pain, to recover lost function or well-being, to gain professional validation of incapacity through illness, or to receive reassurance about a health concern. The purpose of the meeting as seen by the health professional may be to reach an accurate diagnosis, prescribe appropriate treatment, and then turn promptly to the needs of the next patient. Whereas the patient may be concerned about a pressing fear the doctor may be concerned only with verifiable physical signs and may give reassurance a lower priority. Consultation is therefore a special type of encounter, which Goffman (1961) has described as a focused interaction in which both parties try to sustain a single focus of attention. Stimson and Webb (1975) list three features which distinguish consultation with the doctor from other social interactions. First, consultations take place at restricted appointed times and specific places; second, there is a specific reason for the interaction and third, there is a competence gap between the advice seeker and advice giver. They found that patients prepared their stories as best they could before going in to see the doctor, nearly two-thirds expected that they would be given a prescription, and altogether 83 per cent of patients had a fairly clear expectation of what would happen when they saw the doctor. Faced with the prospect of a fairly predictable interaction, patients tried to raise the issues which concerned them but were not always able to do so and were easily put off during the consultation.

Status differences may restrict the ease of communication in cultures which lay a lot of stress on occupational stratification. Where the status of doctors is high relative to their patients, the transmission of information is likely to be halting and imperfect. Freidson (1961) argues that there is always a conflict between the separate worlds of the layman and the professional. Vocabularies may differ considerably, and the value placed on health and long-term prevention may also differ in ways not initially obvious to the participants. Assumptions about the role or function of the participants can strongly determine the nature of the interaction. If only the health professional is seen as being capable of opening up lines of enquiry and determining what is considered a legitimate subject for discussion, then one-sided interactions may result. Pritchard (1983) has given an account of the steps which have been taken by patient participation groups to increase the contribution made by patients to the nature of the interview.

SOCIAL SKILLS

Speech is the main channel of human communication but non-verbal communication may often transmit emotions and attitudes which would rarely be spoken about out loud. Argyle (1972) has argued that such signals work most powerfully on important but unvoiced inter-personal issues, so that affection and affiliation are more likely to be demonstrated by eye gaze than by words in the formative stages of relationships. Putting an emotion into words may over-commit the actor and render him vulnerable to rejection. A glance is more ambiguous and can be used in order to test out another's feelings without too much danger. Successful interactions depend on the social skills of the participants, who must find a means of regulating their separate needs if the interaction is to proceed at all. As with most skills, training and practice proceed by observation, imitation, and informal tuition (Argyle 1981). The unpredictable nature of unknown human beings is reduced by rituals which constrain the interaction in its early stages and make it more manageable. Greeting rituals reduce the threat values of strangers and ritual talk on neutral and impersonal subjects allows the participants to learn about and adjust to each other before revealing themselves in a more vulnerable fashion. These are precisely the rituals which are often jettisoned from medical consultations, where they are seen as non-functional distractions from the task of doctor-defined diagnosis and treatment. In addition, these rituals embody cultural rules which govern the nature and extent of bodily contact. Jourard (1966) studied body accessibility and found clear restrictions as to which part of the body could be touched by different people. As one would expect, touching in genital areas was done by friends of the opposite sex but these friends touched more in other areas as well. Within families, mothers touched their children more than fathers did and many of these student-age subjects were touched by their fathers only in the region of the hands. Medical examinations break all these restrictions and cross private boundaries.

STEREOTYPES

In the opening stages of meetings, the superficial characteristics of the participants will often determine the working stereotype which allows each actor to make preliminary guesses about the appropriate approach to the other actor. Hooper *et al.* (1982) argue that stereotypes held by doctors about social class lead to implicit assumptions which influence the outcome of consultations. Age, race, perceived social class, will all encourage the selection of particular approaches, which may in turn determine the subsequent course of the meeting. Although each participant regards the behaviour of the other as revealing their intentions and character, the behaviour is largely determined by the nature of the interaction itself.

Social behaviour is a two-way process. The behaviour which a person exhibits is often determined by the lead or focus which the other person provides. Kelley (1950) was able to show the power of bias by telling one half of a class that the next lecturer was a warm person and separately informing the other half that he was a cold person. The lecturer then addressed the entire class and answered questions in a discussion at the end. When the students were asked to evaluate him at the end of the session, they maintained their earlier acquired bias about him, and significantly, those who had been told he was a warm person participated more in the discussion than those who were told that he was cold. Interviewers can also be biased in more specific ways. For example, they may form an impression during a respondent's answer of what he means to say, and then interrupt or ignore anything which does not fit in with this preconception (Kahn and Cannell 1957). When interviewers are authoritatively given incorrect data about a person before interviewing him, they often persist in reporting these falsehoods even when the person denies them at interview (Stanton and Baker 1942).

BODY POSITIONING

In the early stages of a meeting location, distance, and posture can transmit important cues about power and attitude. Face to face '180 degrees' across the table meetings are perceived as more competitive and potentially confrontational than seating configurations which are closer to the co-operative '90 degrees' across the corner of the table meetings (Cook 1970). Most participants like to maintain a comfortable distance between them. Too close suggests intrusion of body space with consequent threat, while too far suggests coolness and dislike. Cultural differences about correct distances can cause considerable misperceptions. For example, American diplomats taught to accept the closer body distances preferred by Arabs were then rated as friendlier than those who maintained their own preferred distance (Hall 1966). Posture can reveal perceived status and attitudes. Goffman (1961) has described how, in psychiatric hospital ward meetings the highest status staff adopted relaxed postures and sat at the front of the room, while lowlier staff sat more stiffly at the back. LaCrosse (1975) found that non-verbal behaviours such as leaning slightly forwards, gestures, and head nods make patients see the doctor as warmer and more attractive. Larsen and Smith (1981) found that higher patient satisfaction was associated with doctors' forward lean and body posture.

A lack of attentive orientation and posture in an interviewer can make the interviewee feel unimportant and disregarded, which inhibits full disclosure of important material and makes it unlikely that the interviewee will feel able to ask questions and participate fully in the interaction.

EYE CONTACT

Normal social conversations are generally preceded by a period of eye contact. Once the conversations are under way the participants look each other in the region of the eyes with intermittent glances of varying but generally short durations between 1 and 10 seconds, partly to continue to establish contact and partly to monitor agreement, surprise, protest, and the wish to interrupt. Kendon (1967) found that in two-people conversations the speaker looks up at the end of, or just before the end of, long utterances, which is the point at which they need feedback. The person listening gives longer glances than the person talking and tends to look considerably more. If eye contact is broken or severely reduced then the nature of the conversation is likely to change, becoming more formal, impersonal, and brief. If people are placed very close together then they are likely to reduce the amount of eye contact, so as to try to maintain social distance (Argyle and Dean 1965). Measuring this in experimental circumstances presents methodological difficulties but a general trend towards decreased eye contact with increasing proximity is observed. Further, when conversation in an interview turns to intimate topics then eye contact is likely to diminish. Some clinicians will deliberately reduce eye contact by busying themselves with some minor task to assist the process of disclosure. Others have found that patients will often disclose personal matters when the doctor's attention and eye contact are taken up with a physical examination.

Social interactions are normally terminated by a well-signalled departure ritual which allows both parties to complete the conversation and finish by consent. Failure to do this is generally seen as rude and unfeeling, communicating that the person left in this manner and the conversation were of little value.

Problems of medical communication

INTERVIEW STYLES

Byrne and Long (1976) in a study of over 2,000 tape-recorded general practice consultations revealed that three-quarters of the interviews were 'doctor-centred' in the sense that the doctor concentrated on closed questions about the first complaint the patient had presented, often brushing aside or ignoring verbal leads about other problems, thus quickly achieving an 'organic' diagnosis and terminating the interaction with a prescription. The remaining quarter were more 'patient-centred', with the doctor taking a less controlling role and letting the patient give his own account of symptoms, fears, and stresses. Such doctors were more apt to ask open questions which did not restrict or determine the nature of the possible answers. Closed questions can reduce patients to monosyllabic responses, whereas an open question such as: 'How did you feel after treatment finished?' gives the patient the option to introduce new facts and not merely confirm or deny a hypothesis held privately by the doctor. Byrne and Long (1976) found that the doctors they studied tended to have consistent interview styles regardless of what sort of patients they were seeing. It appears that they develop a set of interview behaviours, and use these stock patterns whatever problem is presented to them. Verby, Holden, and Davis (1979) in a study of video-taped interviews found that length of experience in general practice did not correlate with interviewing skill. This suggests that doctors develop a coping style early on in their careers and subsequent experience does not materially alter their behaviour. Lloyd (1974) found that some doctors' consultation styles were authoritarian and out of keeping with community needs. Gough (1977) investigated the factors which made doctors characterize patient complaints as trivial and found that this tended to be done by those who had been older than average at medical school, better prepared at pre-medical subjects, more able at science, unconventional in obtained academic goals, and somewhat intuitive by nature. The characterization of a complaint as trivial is an indication of a complete mismatch in doctor and patient perceptions. Without specific training the majority of practitioners are below standard as interviewers and are likely to remain so.

Seven interviewing styles were described on the patient-centred to doctor-centred dimension, though such discriminations are more a matter of qualitative than quantitative judgement. In essence these styles vary from those in which patients can express their fears, hidden problems and expectations in the presence of an understanding doctor to those in which the doctor determines the course of questioning once the patient has presented the initial problem.

THE BALANCE OF POWER

In power terms each participant has an agenda which he would prefer to follow and attempts to run the meeting with that in mind. Only if shifts of power are possible within the interview will there be a chance of the separate lists of items being covered to the satisfaction of both parties. Katon and Kleinman (1981) regard this as a process of negotiation which goes through several stages. The first step is to elicit the patient's explanatory model of his illness, which involves assumed causes, course of illness and treatment expectations. Stimson and Webb (1975) have shown that patients, anticipating the limited time available, rehearse a brief coherent account which they attempt to provide in the first few moments before the doctor takes over the agenda. Lazare *et al.* (1978) found that although 99 per cent of patients expressed at least one request regarding treatment on a standard written form, only 37 per cent expressed them spontaneously to the physician and a further 26 per cent did so only when prompted. This suggests that, unless carefully encouraged, patients may withold requirements and then leave the consultation dissatisfied with the advice they have been given. Roter (1979) has reported an experimental study in which some poor, black women patients attending an out-patient department in Baltimore were given a preparatory tutorial in order to make them more active as patients. The 15-minute session identified questions the patient wanted to ask and gave her rehearsal in asking them. The interactions with the doctor were recorded and compared with a control group who had had a session about available hospital services. The prepared patients asked more questions, took a more assertive line and were more efficient in that their sessions took no longer than the more passive control patients. They also improved slightly in their appointment keeping. Doctors judged the prepared patients as more angry and anxious and it seems that both parties were disconcerted by the more active participation obtained by this means, since established roles and styles of interaction were being challenged.

The next step in a successful interview is to elicit illness problems as seen by the patient, as distinct from disease problems as seen by the doctor. Stiles *et al.* (1979) point out that patients appreciate an opportunity to tell their story in their own terms but are often constrained by their sense of inferior role from taking a more active part in the consultation.

Patients' problems may involve family or financial difficulties or major changes in identity and status brought about by being ill. Inappropriate resort to the sick-role may further complicate the effects of illness. When bargaining itself begins in order to reach an agreement about treatment then, as Katon and Kleinman (1981) point out, each party begins from a different power base. The physician has high social status, perceived power and competence, while the patient generally has lower status, no special relevant competence and presents himself as a petitioner in a time of need. Zola (1981) has graphically described how a standard medical history can serve to make the patient feel foolish as he struggles to remember childhood illnesses and details of medication given to him in the past. After examination he may be told not to worry, thus communicating not so much reassurance as a guilty feeling of having wasted time by being over-anxious. Even then, the precise circumstances which would have warranted consultation are rarely given, so the patient only learns that he should be more cautious about coming to see the doctor.

Another feature of the power balance is that the physician has strong and established legal support, while the patient has a weaker, though growing, defensive legislation to protect his rights. Principled medical negotiation develops trust, establishes expertise, explains treatment options fully and encourages health behaviour. It involves a therapeutic alliance in which conflicts are openly discussed and resolved by considering proposals from both parties. Although Katon and Kleinman (1981) champion the cause of the therapeutic alliance and give case histories, they do not present detailed findings on how the outcome of this approach compares with other consulting styles.

DETAILED STUDIES OF THE DOCTOR–PATIENT INTERACTION:
THE LOS ANGELES STUDIES

Problems of medical communication are well illustrated by the work of Francis, Korsch, and Morris (1969) and Freeman *et al.* (1971), Korsch, Gozzi, and Francis (1968) who have conducted extensive studies of doctor–patient interaction at the Children's Hospital of Los Angeles. They point out that the quality of medical care depends on the interaction of the patient and the doctor and that over half a physician's working time is spent on problems involving primarily psychological factors, and the need is for communication rather than technical knowledge. The prevailing ideology is that medical practice should be a series of short-term specialized technological encounters centred on functional biological needs and not a long-term relationship based on personal rapport. To such doctors the 'bedside manner' seems a concession to salesmanship unbefitting a medical scientist.

The method of investigation used was to tape-record 800 successive consultations between doctors and mothers who had brought their children to a walk-in clinic for acute disorders. In this way the complicating factors of previous knowledge of the patient could be excluded. The visits tended to be short and led to a specific recommendation from the doctor to the parent. The doctors were full-time, young, well-trained paediatricians and because most of the interaction was with the mother of the child, she was designated the patient. Mothers were interviewed immediately after they came out from seeing the doctor concerning what they had expected from the visit and what they felt about it and they were then followed up within fourteen days to see if they had complied with the advice they had been given. The rationale of the study was to investigate the one-off consultation as carefully as possible, avoiding the long-term repeated consultative process with its many uncontrollable variables. Previous knowledge of the patient can naturally influence the doctor in his interviewing and prescribing behaviour. Previous knowledge of the doctor can influence the patient in his interviewing and compliance behaviour and may determine whether he bothers to consult in the first place.

The investigators were concerned lest the presence of the tape-recorder affect the nature of the interaction and so, as a control, omitted it from 300 of the consultations, yet found that neither doctors' performances nor patients' reactions showed any effects. The presence of recording apparatus seems to have less effect on interactions than that of an observer in the room, since it tends to be quickly ignored and forgotten.

Immediately after the mother came out of the consulting room she was questioned by the interviewers to find out how she felt about her child's illness, what she had expected of the doctor and how satisfied she was with his performance. Seventy-six per cent of them were more or less satisfied with the doctor's performance during this brief encounter but this figure looks less reassuring when their specific reactions are considered. Nearly a fifth felt that they had not received a clear statement of what was wrong with their baby and almost half of the sample were left wondering what had caused their child's illness. This failure of explanation is particularly worrying, since 38 per cent of the mothers felt that they were to blame. A failure to understand and reassure on this count leaves the child's main care provider in doubt and confused about her role, with poor consequences for co-operation with instructions. Within the next fortnight the mothers were visited at home and the extent of their compliance was assessed by interview, pill counts, and pharmacy checks. Forty-two per cent had complied as advised, 38 per cent only partially, and 11 per cent not at all, the rest having received no instructions.

One of the strongest determinants of compliance was satisfaction with the consultation. Patients who had had a satisfactory interview were three times as likely to have followed instructions as those whose interaction with the doctor had been unsatisfactory. This result shows very clearly that good communications can have major practical consequences.

A common complaint of doctors is that they do not have the time to communicate as they would wish with their patients. As a consequence, it would be expected that the longer interviews would lead to greater patient satisfaction. However, there was no significant correlation between the length of the session and either the patient's satisfaction or the clarity of the diagnosis of the child's illness. Inspection of the transcripts revealed that some of the longer sessions were taken up with the time-consuming sorting out of misunderstandings and did not lead to better or more detailed explanations.

The severest and most common complaint from the dissatisfied mothers was that their anxiety about their child had not aroused much sympathy. They had the clear expectation that when they told the doctor about their worries he would be sympathetic and supportive but this was rarely the case. The tape-recordings showed that less than 6 per cent of the doctor's conversation was friendly, though this rose to 46 per cent of his communications with the child. The doctor's perception must have been that the mother did not need his support, whereas the child sometimes did. In most of the consultations the doctor paid no attention to the mother's feelings and devoted himself solely to a technical discussion of the child's condition. This constitutes a major misperception of the medical role. These physicians perceived their responsibility as the identification and treatment of the disease, not the treatment of the patient. In some sense they must have felt their responsibilities at an end when they had solved the diagnostic puzzle and announced their solution. However, for the patient treatment had yet to begin and until they could see the connection between the worries which brought them to the doctor and the advice given, they were unlikely to follow instructions.

Patients also experienced difficulties in getting the doctors to understand the real nature of their worries. One mother was understandably concerned that her child's febrile convulsions might permanently damage his brain but was unable to get her doctor to pay attention to her concern. Other mothers were subjected to lines of questioning which did not seem to be related to the presenting symptom. The doctor had a clear idea of the hypothesis he was testing but his failure to explain that his enquiry related to the worrying symptom, left the mother bewildered and dissatisfied. A full 26 per cent of mothers said that they had not revealed their greatest concern to the doctor, either because he hadn't asked them to or they hadn't been given an opportunity to do so. This frequently resulted in a complete breakdown of communications. The doctor was attempting to solve a puzzle along lines which he understood, while the mother was so involved in her pressing worry that she could not concentrate on what she was being asked.

The experience of illness typically involves a narrowing of concerns and a major change in the usual priorities of life. A failure to go into these worries means that the doctor and his patient are driven by different priorities and real communication is unlikely. Among the mothers who felt that their main concerns had not been understood, 68 per cent expressed dissatisfaction with the doctor's performance, whereas among those who felt that they had been understood, a full 83 per cent expressed satisfaction with the interview. This massive change in evaluations hinges on the simple fact of understanding motivation, which should be the key concern of any physician who wishes to be an effective practitioner.

The tasks which face the interviewer may well diminish his capacity to monitor his own performance. Most of them felt they had been friendly but only half of the patients felt this and the evaluators of the tapes noted a considerable imbalance between the emotional tone directed to mother and to child. The successful doctors in this study were those who established a good and friendly relationship with the parent and questioned them about their worries and expectations early on in the interview. Such doctors did not condemn as irrational fears that did not fit in with their system of medical knowledge. They had the capacity to listen and to reassure once they had understood the basis of their patient's fears. A further feature of these doctors was that they expressed continuing concern about the welfare of their patients and made it clear that they could contact them should they wish to at a later date.

When the interactions were studied in detail, the nature of the power relationship between doctor and patient was made apparent. Patients were diffident, did not open lines of enquiry, even when they very much wanted to, and the doctors maintained a social distance which, far from impressing patients into meek compliance, made them politely rebel once they had left the surgery and heed their own counsel rather than follow the doctor's advice. In the consulting room, patients rarely expressed open dissent but stated that they were worried and tense (such remarks accounting for 10 per cent of utterances). Doctors rarely responded with reassurance. Patients who were tense and diffident when in the role of petitioner then exercised their freedom, once they had left the consulting room, to tend their children as they thought best. The failure to understand that poor communication is as serious a problem as mistaken diagnosis results in a major deficiency in health care, which is the more regrettable for being avoidable.

PATIENT COMMUNICATION AND THE MEDICAL HIERARCHY

The task of communication in medicine is not restricted to doctors. Nurses spent more time with hospital patients than physicians and surgeons and as such have more opportunity to interact with their clients. Patients are often too diffident to interrupt apparently busy staff with an account of their concerns and this suggests that the rate of disclosure should be inversely proportional to perceived status. This would suggest that communication is worst with senior doctors and best with junior nurses. Johnston (1976) asked surgical patients to complete a hospital adjustment inventory to describe their worries and simultaneously a nurse filled in a similar form to evaluate how much she had been able to pick up from the patient about their worries. The two accounts showed very little concordance, revealing that communication on these issues had been poor. Without such basic knowledge appropriate reassurance will not be possible.

Johnston (1980) showed that surgical patients still experienced high levels of anxiety long after they had been discharged from hospital after surgery. This suggests that reassurance has indeed failed to reach its target. In more recent work, Johnston (1982) has studied patients' disclosure of personal worries and measured the extent to which nurses and fellow patients have been aware of these. Fellow patients are naturally seen as outside the medical hierarchy and have more time on the ward to find out about each other. The patients used in this study were twenty female in-patients on a gynaecological ward, who filled in the hopital adjustment inventory which contains twenty-two items asking about the presence or absence of different worries. The patient then named the nurse and fellow patient on the ward with whom they had most contact and they were asked to fill in the inventory to indicate how they thought the patient felt. Patients admitted to an average of 3.9 items, fellow patients assumed they were experiencing 4.8 worries and nurses thought that they were experiencing 7.75 worries on average. Nurses therefore significantly overestimate the amount of worry experienced by their patients, while other patients on the ward are far closer to the mark. Nurses tended to overestimate worries about discharge from hospital, problems about work and progress in recovery. They under-estimated fears about catching diseases from other patients, feelings of being very confined on the ward and worry that they would not be liked by staff. Fellow patients were more accurate but they agreed with nurses as to which problems were more likely to be experienced overall. This suggests that nurses are responding to some 'average patient' they may have been taught about, rather than the individuals in the beds in front of them. The patients themselves are of roughly equal perceived status and are sharing common experiences, which gives them a better basis for real communication. Although nurses know what subjects are likely to cause worry, they do not know who is being worried by what, so that most of their attempts at reassurance are misapplied.

The technique of asking both patient and nurses and fellow patients to fill in simple inventories offers a useful method of measuring communication efficiency. Rather than relying on indirect measures such as satisfaction, a direct measure of communicated knowledge can be obtained. The measure cannot be considered perfect, since the items on the list may not cover all of the possible topics on which communication has taken place. For example, the omission of uncommon fears from the list would artificially improve communication scores, while the inclusion of important but subtle messages would provide a harsher test of communication. It is not sufficient simply to add up the number of points on which both patient and nurse agree. Account must also be taken of false positives – items which the nurse assumes are causing worry but which the patient does not confirm. The usual way to do this is by calculating an overall sensitivity measure using signal detection theory. Johnston found that such a measure tentatively confirmed that fellow patients were more accurate than nurses but the small sample size mitigated against a more confident conclusion. However, this is a promising technique which could be used more widely to bring common standards of measurement to a research field which would otherwise lack any consistent method of evaluation.

Consultation as a decision-making task

In conducting a medical interview a doctor is faced with a variety of tasks which compete for his attention. Stated very simply, he must:

1 Get the patient to talk. She/he must provide a starting point and encourage the patient to give an account of his complaint.
2 Control the relevance of what is said. She/he must guide the patient with appropriate questions and selective encouragement so as to provide the necessary factual information.
3 Record the answers. She/he must either write them down or hold them in her/his memory during the consultation.

4 Think of what to say next. She/he must have in mind a series of appropriate questions depending on what she/he has just been told.
5 Achieve a diagnosis. She/he must come to a decision as to which of the hypotheses she/he held during his questioning is best supported by the answers she/he received. She/he may need to perform physical examinations and carry out further investigations before she/he can reach an answer and some uncertainty may always remain.
6 Decide on treatment. She/he must remember what sort of treatment is appropriate and must decide what to do if no effective treatment is available.
7 Communicate her/his findings to the patient. She/he must do this in a clear and convincing manner, since her/his effectiveness here will largely determine the success of the consultation.
8 Present her/himself throughout as a credible health resource. Her/his competence and credibility are being evaluated by the patient during the entire consultation and she/he must maintain a high rating if she/he is to continue to get patients.

The patient also has tasks to perform in consulting the doctor, though she/he may often appear to take a passive role. He or she must:

1 Prepare some rationale for having consulted the doctor. She/he may have to justify having requested a consultation and will probably have rehearsed her/his account of her/his problem to ready her/himself for questioning.
2 Answer questions appropriately. She/he may have to do this even if their purpose and meaning are unclear and may have to recall facts which did not appear important to her/him at the time.
3 Remember to tell the doctor all the important points. She/he must judge what needs to be communicated and be sure that she/he does so even if the questions do not lead to it.
4 Understand and remember the instructions given. She/he must be clear what is required of her/him and recall it when she/he comes to follow treatment instructions and advice.
5 Remember to ask the questions which are important to her/him. She/he must obtain answers to her/his anxieties and queries about her/his illness and its treatment.

The task demands on the doctor have predictably gained more attention. A physician conducting an interview has a limited amount of attention which he must direct according to an inner sense of priorities and a perception of signs, circumstances, and requirements. For information to be processed it must be noted, coded, and stored while decisions are made. Patterns must be recognized and compared with past memories, or they will simply pass through the short-term memory buffer store and be lost (Baddeley 1976). Repeated exposure can establish a pattern which lowers the recognition threshold. For example, most people are sensitized to and easily recognize their own name. A foreign language, on the other hand, will be far more difficult to note and remember, because there are no long-term patterns of memory to give meaning to what is heard. According to the training and priorities of the doctor, some of what he is presented with by the patient will be perceived as meaningful, some dismissed as irrelevant, and some not consciously perceived at all. Students in training, whose attention is largely taken up by the tasks of recording data, may not note or pay attention to non-verbal cues.

Hunt and MacLeod (1979) use the concept of 'attention budget' to describe how a doctor apportions his information processing energies. They use the analogy of a policeman directing traffic to explain that although there are a multitude of stimuli such as passing cars and traffic lights impingeing on the senses, only a few key stimuli are used to carry out the basic task. In the same way, an interviewer must focus his attention on what he believes to be the crucial cues.

The patient operates under the same constraint. He must select from a wide variety of experiences those which he believes to be relevant to the initial presentation of his case. Some important facts will not have been noted. Others will be recalled if an effort is made and the physician directs memorization to certain key events and experiences.

One of the main attentional demands on the physician will be the need to generate and prove a hypothesis about the patient's illness. Once the physician forms a hypothesis his bias will be, like most hypothesis-testers, to ask questions which confirm it, rather than the more logical process of asking key disconfirming questions which may lead to fresh hypotheses. The tendency, described by Wason and Johnson-Laird (1972) can lead to a premature focus that can then close off important lines of enquiry. Although it is not usual at present, expert systems using artificial intelligence concepts may provide a more effective means of assisting physicians to explore hypothetical diagnoses. Davis, Buchanan, and Shortliffe (1977) have reported on MYCIN, an artificial intelligence program for evaluating systemic infections. This program asks for patient data, explains its decision logic if asked and puts forward its diagnostic hypotheses. It can fairly easily be taught new knowledge so as to extend its scope of application. Other programs cover internal medicine and other aspects of patient care. All require an expert to make explicit his clinical decision-making processes.

Elstein, Shulman, and Sprafka (1978) found that clinicians were more influenced in hypothesis generation by disease frequency than disease seriousness and that knowledge of underlying pathophysiological processes was rarely used. They also found that the most common error in hypothesis testing was to assign positive importance to non-contributory findings. Barrows *et al.* (1977) report that physicians actively search out data to confirm hypotheses rather than rule them out and Wallsten (1978) showed that data collected in the later half of interviews was systematically distorted to support prior opinions. Elstein and Bordage (1979) have outlined the various inferential and decision-making processes which may be utilized to improve clinical reasoning. However, it remains the case that a lot of clinical communication is directed to an inefficient and error-prone hypothesis testing procedure. While this remains so, opportunities for real communication will be lost.

Training in communication skills

It has long been usual in medical education to assume that interviewing is a skill which any student can pick up with repeated unsupervised practice. The material to be elicited in a history taking interview is generally listed on written forms, though these will vary from speciality to speciality. The student then finds a patient on the ward, who will probably have been interviewed several times before, and proceeds to fill in his 'shopping list' of questions. He then brings back an account, of varying plausibility, of what he has found out about his patient, which is then compared with other previous accounts or a subsequent interview with a senior doctor that the student observes. This method at least allows the student to compare the answers he has obtained with those elicited by other people. If the doctor he observes is a good interviewer he may pick up some good habits as a communicator. On the negative side, the shortcoming of this approach is that there is no observation of the interview itself. The impact on the patient of the student's manner is rarely considered. Errors in questioning can become ingrained and deficiencies in the interview can sometimes be glossed over in the subsequent presentation of the case. Worst of all, the interview is inevitably seen as a data extraction process in which inter-personal issues count for very little.

However, if this process produced good communicators there would be little objection to the potential shortcomings of the system. Both the evidence of studies that have directly monitored student performance and the reports of patients suggest that the traditional method has failed to achieve a satisfactory standard. A particular difficulty experienced by students is a reluctance to question the patient on 'personal' issues, however relevant to their problems and an insensitivity to those verbal and non-verbal cues whereby patients can lead an observant listener to their real problem. At a more mundane level, students are often unable to keep patients to the point and to find out the precise details of their complaints (Anderson *et al.* 1970; Tapia 1972). Practice does not appear to improve matters. Helfer (1970) found that senior medical students were more cursory on psychological and social aspects of their patients and tended to question them in a way that gave them little opportunity to explain the real nature of their disorder. The interest junior students showed in their patients as people had diminished through exposure to the limited range of the medical interview.

Maguire and Rutter (1976) conducted an evaluation of fifty students' history taking skills during a psychiatry clerkship, at which stage they had had extensive interviewing experience in the major medical specialities and were within fifteen months of their final examinations. They were asked to interview a psychiatric patient whom they didn't know and to find out his or her present problems within fifteen minutes. They were told that they must prepare a report on the patient at the end of the interview and that they should assume that the patients did not know what was expected of them. The preparation for the task was intended to ensure that students gave of their best and fully understood that their skills were being evaluated.

Patients were only selected when they were very willing to co-operate and were able to give a coherent history in the time available about their problems, which always involved affective disorders or anxiety states.

The interviews were video-recorded and then rated by independent assessors for a variety of previously determined behaviours. The student write-ups were compared with the medical notes and rated for the number of accurate and relevant facts they contained. A median value of fourteen facts were obtained, slightly less than one a minute and only one-third of the number readily available from the patients. Virtually nothing about the impact of the psychological problem on the life of the patient was obtained. This omission and the low rate of fact-finding came as a surprise to the students, who had the impression that they had collected a lot of information.

Analysis of the tapes revealed very clearly the hidden assumptions which these medical students brought to the interaction. Only 16 per cent bothered to explain about the video-recording and check that this was acceptable, only 8 per cent bothered to explain the purpose of the interview and a mere 4 per cent checked that the patient was at ease, understood that there was a time constraint, and was willing to have his or her answers written down. Coupled with the finding that 30 per cent did not introduce themselves by name and 44 per cent did not mention their status as students, the assumption of a passive relatively unimportant role for the patient is obvious. The message seemed to be that because the interviewers knew who they were and what they were doing no further explanation was necessary. Contrast this behaviour with that shown by the students at vivas and job interviews and the assumed power relationship is seen. Failing to mention the time restriction and the purpose of the interview maintains power firmly in the hands of the questioner, who can work to a plan while the respondent remains baffled by the purpose of the questions.

Apart from avoiding personal issues, students tended to accept many descriptions and explanations at face value and were thus often misled about the true nature and intensity of patient complaints. The interviewers frequently accepted inconsistent and unclear accounts without further enquiry and failed to press for precise answers when given hazy descriptions of drug dosages and past treatments. Only 4 per cent were able to consistently pick up verbal leads and three-quarters only registered a fraction of those emitted by respondents. Patients give verbal leads when they are unsure about a matter of concern to them and a lack of response will cause most to retreat into frustrated non-co-operation.

Over half the students lacked the ability to control their respondents when they talked on about irrelevant matters, though those who asked patients to return to the point found them happy to do so. This lack of control partly stems from the failure to inform the patient about the purpose of the interview and the restricted time in which it must be carried out. Such an explanation would allow the patient to structure his account into the required format and would establish a co-operative role in which both could participate. Although most students were able to get their interviewees to talk, a third found it difficult to facilitate the flow of the conversation and paid more attention to their notes than their patients. This may stem from the restrictions on attention brought about by trying to remember what to ask next, but is more likely to relate to unease with the interaction.

A third asked questions in a way which determined the form of the answers. The most common in the experience of this author is the assumption when questioning about effects of treatment that the outcome will have been positive. One-quarter asked questions which were so complex that patients could not give a clear answer.

A more cognitive type of failure on the part of the questioners was premature focus: the incorrect assumption that the first problem presented was the main or only problem. Students were particularly apt to believe that problems of one type precluded patients from experiencing problems which fell into another category and their questions reflected this restricted vision. Naturally such restrictions in the collection of data can then contribute to the stereotype that patients or disorders fall into mutually exclusive categories.

Ninety per cent of students had not finished their task when the time was up.

Maguire and Rutter were able to show by conducting interviews with audio rather than video-recording that the findings were not an artefact of the television cameras, since the same problems came up in the auditory recordings and these were identical with the problems which students had admitted to in conversation with the investigators.

In order to overcome these problems Rutter and Maguire (1976) devised a training programme which has since served as a model for many subsequent investigators. A consecutive sample of twenty-four medical students were randomly allocated, half to a training group and half to a no-training control group. Each student conducted a fifteen-minute interview with a patient, wrote up their account of the information they had obtained and then a week later repeated the exercise with another patient. As before, the students were told that the patient had an affective disorder, that the interview would be videotaped, that they must end the interview on time and write up the findings as fully as possible afterwards. The patients were suffering from clearly diagnosed affective disorders and each took part in only one interview.

Students in the no-training control condition completed their first interview and were then sent away without comment and told to return for their second interview the following week. Students in the training condition attended a tutorial, at which they were first given a standard, structured scheme for taking histories that they discussed in detail with their tutors. The scheme drew attention both to the information that should be obtained and to the techniques that should be used. Then the videotape of the interview was played and was interrupted and re-run at any point of interest so that the performance of the student could be analysed in detail. At the end of the hour-long tutorial the trainer would emphasize the need to study all the points raised in the handout.

The effects of training were assessed by comparing all the student write-ups with an abstract of the facts derived from the patient's notes. Any fact in the write-up also in the notes was credited and if the student provided information not denied by anything in the notes he was given the benefit of the doubt. The scoring was done 'blind' by one of the authors who did not know whether the student was in the training group or not. In total the trained students reported 35.5 accurate and relevant facts, compared with 13.5 for the untrained group, a highly significant difference. Five of the nine categories of information showed this significant effect of training. Symptoms, the course of the disorder, effects on adjustment, details of treatment, and previous episodes of the disorder. The effects of a one-hour tutorial are that trained students report almost three times as much information as those who have not received any specific guidance.

In order to establish the relative contributions of the handout and the videotape playback Rutter and Maguire conducted a further experiment in which twenty-eight students were randomly allocated to either a full training group as above, or a partial training group. In this latter group students did everything as before but did not see and discuss the videotape, confining themselves to a discussion of the handout. Fully trained students obtained 25.5 relevant and accurate items, while the partially trained obtained 21.5 items. This difference, though statistically significant is small in practical terms and shows up significantly only in the details of treatment category of information. Rutter and Maguire conclude that videotape playback is not the most important feature in training data collection. The measure of interview is not restricted to data collection. The playback of the videotape may well have helped with those features not assessed in this study, such as the extent of rapport and the patient's level of satisfaction with the interview. It was this observation which led Thompson and Anderson (1982) to extend the analysis to include patient preferences and more detailed analysis of interview performance. The authors accepted the findings that training improved interview performance and that the major factor in this improvement was discussion of the handout. They therefore distributed and discussed the list of topics to be covered with all students before any training began. They argued that if performance is judged by the extent of coverage of a set of topics, then there is the danger of circularity or self-fulfilling prophecy if this set is revealed halfway through training. Improvements may then be due not to real advances in interviewing skill but to fitting the questioning to the measuring device. To overcome this they made sure that every student knew what topics they should cover before they met the patient.

In order to ensure that the training technique had wider applicability than affective disorders, they used surgical patients, with a variety of conditions, chosen only because they were available on the day and were well enough and willing to participate. As in the Rutter and Maguire model, students were given fifteen minutes with the patient, told to get as clear a picture as possible of the patient's main problems and how they had affected the patient's life, and to write up their findings. They then attended a tutorial in which they were given the part of the handout which related to suggestions about interviewing technique and went through the videotape in the usual fashion, before going on to interview another patient the following week. However, each patient was interviewed by three students in turn and was thus able to state their preferences and to rate each student on some simple scales. Each patient was asked by a researcher after the interview: 'If you had to choose one of those students to be the doctor looking after you which one would it be?' Then the patient was asked to choose between the two remaining students so that a preference order could be obtained.

In order to get a more detailed understanding of the interview than would be gained by a fact count, the videotapes were randomized and rated blind by an independent assessor using a detailed rating scale derived from Maguire and Rutter's work. There were forty-three interview videotapes in all.

Although post-training improvements were not the main purpose of the study, analysis of the videotapes revealed that after their tutorial, students were significantly better at introducing themselves, preparing the patient for the interview proper, asking clear, open, simple questions, giving explanations, and terminating the interview in an appropriate manner. Their overall interview performance had improved by about 20 per cent on the assessor's rating scales, a significant improvement. Thus, even though the list of topics to be covered had been given to the students prior to training, the tutorial itself made a significant contribution to interview competence.

Turning to the more interesting question of what features of an interview make for good communication, students were categorized by the rankings ascribed to them by patients. As expected, the preferred students got the highest ratings on the scales which patients filled in on each student at the completion of each interview. Preferred students were on average seen as easier to talk to, more sympathetic, less irritating, warmer, and easier to confide in about personal problems, though all these differences fell short of statistical significance. The sole patient evaluation that significantly differed between rankings was competence, which was perceived as highest in the preferred students. The sensitivity of the patient scales was somewhat diminished by a grateful diffidence and unwillingness to be critical, even when the videotapes revealed examples of clumsy enquiry. More extended debriefing later in the evening often produced accounts of criticism and reservations which had not been apparent on the scales, together with understanding, for those students seen as not having coped adequately with the task they had been set.

Analysis of the videotapes allowed Thompson and Anderson to have a better understanding of the characteristics of preferred interviewers. These turned out to be linked to avoiding repetition, being aware of verbal leads, being good facilitators by giving appropriate encouragement, controlling the interview well, being precise in questioning, and being self-assured in presentation. To repeat a line of questioning is damaging to rapport, since it transmits the unintended message that the interviewer has not been listening, or did not consider what he was told accurate or relevant. Precision in questioning is often comforting to patients, who may feel that a cursory questioning will fail to elicit important facts whose exclusion will diminish the success of their treatment. The independent assessor's ratings of competence were also significantly different, indicating that both assessor and patients noted differences in the students' interview styles.

In order to determine which aspects of behaviour led to a patient ascribing competence to a student, the detailed features of the interview were compared to the competence ratings. The first finding to emerge was that 'competence' correlated with more aspects of the interview than any other of the patients' ratings. It related to the more technical aspects of interviewing such as a proper introduction, clarification of statements, handling of emotional material, avoidance of repetition, precision of questioning, and empathy. It also correlated highly with a measure of how well the key complaints were elicited and with finding out about disruption. Patient and assessor ratings of competence were significantly correlated. It emerges from this analysis that the concept of 'competence' used by the patients goes beyond any circumscribed notion of brisk, insensitive data collection. Appropriate enquiry about personal matters was seen as a token of concern and thoroughness and was welcomed by these patients.

This study reveals that the ingredients of the interview which result in patient satisfaction are capable of being taught and that there remains considerable scope for improving interviewing skills. Increasing attention is being paid in medical curricula to interview training but such skills still occupy too small a place in medical education.

Conclusions

Many factors determine the nature and extent of communication in social interactions and all these come to bear on the more focused and delimited interaction of the medical consultation. The expectations and social roles the participants bring to the meeting can establish powerful restrictions on what can be communicated between the two parties. Within the meeting itself communication styles and beliefs about health and treatment can further determine what is communicated. Most medical consultations must negotiate conflicting needs, with the balance of power tilted in favour of the practitioner and the patient largely restricted to negative and non-participatory reactions when his or her needs are not met. The responsibility of having to come to the decision regarding diagnosis can often severely limit the subjects covered in the consultation and the mood of the interaction. Failure to notice cues is unfortunately common and many meetings result in miscommunication and dissatisfaction. With training many of these problems can be overcome but essential limitations remain while the patient is restricted to a subordinate role as a communicator.

6   *Compliance*

James Thompson

> 'It is so hard that one cannot really have
> confidence in doctors and yet cannot do
> without them.'
>
> *Goethe*

Introduction

Being ill can bring in its train anxiety, dependency, frustration, and depression. It can forcibly reduce an independent individual to the level of a helpless petitioner. Being ill does not mean that all capacity for critical judgement is lost but that this capacity must be brought to bear on a matter of considerable personal importance at a time when the processes of illness may make judgement difficult.

Consultations do not take place in a social vacuum. Ideas about the correct role of the patient, family and peer pressures, treatment fashions, and commercial drug advertising can all have their effects. Nor is the process of consultation static. Decisions as to the best form of treatment can fluctuate as the illness itself varies, a process the doctor may see as the necessary search for the best therapy and the patient may perceive as prevarication or uncertainty. This same process of adapting treatment to the apparent course of the illness, if carried out by the patient, may be seen by the doctor as vacillation and a failure to follow advice. Therefore, the consultation process can be as much about perceptions as about the 'facts' of illness.

'Compliance' is the term used to describe health behaviour on the part of the patient that follows medical advice. Other terms that have been used are obedience, adherence, co-operation, collaboration, and therapeutic alliance, each representing a different point on the authoritarian–democratic dimension, with consequent ideological assumptions as to how patients and doctors are expected to behave. Compliance carries the unfortunate implication that patients are either passively obedient or wilfully disobedient in the face of medical wisdom, which tells us more about the inherent assumptions behind medical practice than it does about the process of consultation. Despite these connotations the term is in common usage, figures extensively in the research literature, and will be retained here. However, it will be argued that it is more fruitful to use the term 'compliance' to describe the extent to which the doctor's perception of the correct form of treatment is shared by the patient. This way of describing patient behaviour underlines the fact that both patient and doctor have their own ways of interpreting the facts and unless these are in substantial agreement successful treatment is unlikely.

In order to set this topic in context, the first step will be to describe the extent of 'the problem of non-compliance'. The second section will look in closer detail at the factors which determine the success of consultations and the last section will suggest remediation.

The problem of non-compliance

Data on non-compliance have been obtained from three main areas of study:

1 Attendance rates at clinics.
2 Medication and advice uptake.
3 Medication and advice uptake when a person is looking after another dependent person.

ATTENDANCE RATES

The most basic form of non-compliance is not to turn up as instructed when an appointment has been made. Sackett and Snow (1979) reviewed fifteen studies and found that attendance rates were only about 50 per cent when appointments had been initiated by health professionals, rising to about 75 per cent when initiated by the patient. Data analysed by the author on attendance rates covering 19,400 appointments at the out-patient department of a teaching hospital revealed higher rates. First attenders were slightly more likely to turn up than re-attenders, the figures being 87.4 per cent and 83.8 per cent respectively. A slightly bigger effect was found for time of year with February showing 88.5 per cent and June 81.0 per cent, suggesting that holidays and other summer pursuits may have had a competitive pull on patients' time. In terms of specialities, ante-natal obstetrics and adult psychiatry were well attended, with failure rates below 6 per cent while general medicine at 20 per cent and geriatrics at 25 per cent were far less well attended.

Berrigan and Garfield (1981) studied the non-attendance and drop-out rates of patients receiving psychotherapy and found a very strong effect of social class on the uptake of these services. None of those in the highest socio-economic class dropped out of therapy, 12 per cent of class two, 27 per cent of class three, 32 per cent of class four and 50 per cent of class five. The highest three social classes had a failed appointment rate of around 18 per cent, while for class four it was 50 per cent and for class five it was 70 per cent. Because of the special nature of psychotherapy, with its stress on verbal discussion of feelings, it would be unwise to generalize from this finding to other forms of treatment.

Attendance rates at three NHS clinical psychology clinics have been studied by Weighill, Hodge, and Peck (1983) over a six-month period, during which there were 929 consultations. There were 12.4 per cent broken without notice, 8.4 per cent were cancelled, and in 6.4 per cent patients were late – a total failure rate of 27.1 per cent. The strongest determinant of broken appointments was lower social class, followed by lack of a private car and having children aged between eleven and fifteen years. Social class was also a determinant of premature termination of treatment. Some comfort can be drawn from the fact that once a patient had kept the first appointment, non-compliance was halved at the second appointment. The authors note the finding of Hochstadt and Trybula (1980) that a reminder letter or phone call may produce a substantial improvement in appointment keeping.

MEDICATION AND ADVICE UPTAKE

Estimating the extent to which those patients who do attend have carried out their instructions depends on the nature of the advice. Pill taking is easier to monitor than more general changes in life-style, so compliance studies tend to concentrate on medicine taking in the short term. Within this compass people are more apt to credit themselves with compliance than can be confirmed when the pills are counted, and this estimate in turn generally has to be revised downwards when blood samples or urine is analysed to determine drug levels. Feinstein *et al.* (1959) found that while interviews suggested that 73 per cent of patients were good compliers, with only 19 per cent in the questionable category, on a pill count basis only 55 per cent could be confirmed as good compliers, with 35 per cent in the questionable category. Other studies (Park and Lipman 1964; Rickels and Briscoe 1970) note that much of this discrepancy is due to small disparities between prescribed and actual pill taking and patients were more likely to admit non-compliance when they had encountered real difficulties and when the disparities were large. In the Park and Lipman (1964) study of psychiatric out-patients on imipramine therapy 100 patients were compliers as judged by interview but only 57 by pill count and of the 14 who were non-compliers by pill count, only 7 had admitted as much at interview.

Gordis (1979) points out that both pill counts and urine tests have their error terms, since pills may be discarded and the rate at which drugs are excreted from the body can vary considerably from one subject to another. The classification of a patient as a non-complier can be problematic, since although this should be done on the precise basis of failure to achieve the level of dose required to achieve a therapeutic response such data are rarely available. The more common procedure is to select an arbitrary level and then calculate a percentage compliance level. Such figures hide considerable differences in the pattern of response, failing to distinguish between the patient who adheres faithfully to the regime and then gives up halfway for some important but unknown reason, and the patient who is erratically semi-compliant throughout because they try to follow instructions but cannot remember to take their tablets consistently.

MEDICINE AND ADVICE UPTAKE WHEN CARING FOR OTHERS

It has been usual in compliance research to pool together results from the person as patient and the person as carer for another dependent patient (Francis, Korsch, and Morris 1969). However, some caution is necessary, since the monitoring of the illness process may be better in the second case and since those caring for others may feel a sense of responsibility they would not feel in dealing with their own ailments. Gordis, Markowitz, and Lilienfield (1969) found that mothers being interviewed about their children's taking of penicillin tended to overstate compliance as measured by urine tests of penicillin excretion. Children's statements also overstated adherence. This led the author to suggest that interview reports are not to be trusted, but DiMatteo and DiNicola (1982) point out that such conclusions prematurely curtail crucial lines of enquiry. Interviewing techniques may be poor, face to face meetings may make the admission of failure very stressful, patients may simply have forgotten some of their difficulties, or have adapted the treatment regime for reasons they feel they cannot discuss unless specifically encouraged to do so. It is interesting that in the study reported by Francis, Korsch and Morris (1969) a mere 8.5 per cent of mothers were found to be discrepant in their self-reports of compliance with medication prescribed for their children, as compared to pill counts done at the same time. The reason for this may lie in the fact that the follow-up interviews were conducted not by the prescribing physicians but by specially trained interviewers, who took pains to avoid the practitioner's perspective and understand the patient's point of view. For example, their question to mothers about compliance was: 'When did you feel able to stop giving him the tablets?', which allowed the patient to explain the symptomatic changes or side-effects which may have caused them to depart from the treatment regime for their child. Stone (1979b) suggests that the error lies in assuming that compliance is a quality of the patient rather than the shared responsibility of expert and client. This error, in his view, results in non-compliance being seen as the moral culpability of the patient, which he is thus unlikely to confess should it occur. In addition, episodes of non-compliance can be forgotten in the constrained setting of the medical interview. These are not isolated memory failures. Marquis (1970) reports that 12–17 per cent of hospital admissions, 23–36 per cent of medical consultations, and 50 per cent of documented health problems are not reported by patients in health interviews. Health interviews can yield important findings but considerable care must be taken to ensure that patients are given encouragement fully to reveal their concerns and suitably prompted to remember the important facts about their condition.

POOLED RESULTS OF COMPLIANCE STUDIES

Pooling together the results of disparate studies inevitably combines different criteria and different circumstances but allows a rough overall view that can lead to an understanding of the extent of the problem.

Ley (1982) has summarized three reviews of non-compliance and it will be seen in *Table 9* that over 40 per cent of patients fail to take their medicine. Dietary and other advice are not followed by roughly 50 per cent of patients (Ley 1976; 1978), so it is clear that medical consultations often fail to convince patients of the wisdom of the proposed treatment.

The traditional approach has been to view this as a regrettable state of affairs that must be countered by more effective persuasion. Attempts

Table 9   *Patient non-compliance*

type of medication	Ley (1976)	FDA (1979)	Barofsky (1980)
antibiotics	49	48	52
psychiatric	39	42	42
anti-hypertensive	—	43	61
anti-tuberculosis	38	42	43
other medications	48	54	46

Source: Ley (1982): table 2.

have been made to determine the deleterious consequences of not following advice. Ausburn (1981) estimated the proportion of hospitalized patients whose admission could be attributed to non-compliance as a probable 20 per cent. This estimate should in fairness be compared with the proportion of patients whose hospitalization could be attributed to the side-effects of drugs. Further, many disorders are self-limiting and should not be medicated in the first place, so non-compliance is the correct response to inappropriate prescription. Many minor disorders such as coughs and colds will resolve themselves of their own accord and prescriptions of drugs which are supposed to accelerate this process are unnecessary. Some doctors over-prescribe and patients are quite right to exercise their own judgement where their own health is concerned.

The economic consequences of non-compliance are considerable, including as they do the direct costs of drugs and medical wages and the indirect costs of wasted time on the part of the patient. It is not only the patient who exercises judgement when deciding whether to follow advice. Ley (1981) reported that health care professionals do not always follow the best available recommendations when treating patients (an 80 per cent non-compliance rate) and that on 65 per cent of occasions the medication and advice they give is not appropriate. Many of these findings were obtained by sending pseudo-patients to pharmacies and then checking the appropriateness of the advice they were given. Gordis, Desi, and Schmerler (1976) studied physicians' management of acute sore throats by investigating their self-reported procedures by questionnaire. Of the general physicians 76 per cent did not use cultures to reach a diagnosis, or did not use the results when deciding on treatment. Paediatricians performed better, with 21 per cent in this category. When a judgement was made on the percentage who used appropriate antibiotics, at an adequate dosage for an adequate duration, then 88 per cent of the paediatricians were up to standard, compared with only 41 per cent of the general physicians. Even here the appropriateness of using antibiotics at all might be called into question, since the condition is self-limiting. However, these variations in the quality of therapeutic advice are not entirely unknown to patients, who note that individual doctors differ in their treatments, that fashions change in medicine, and that not all treatments have beneficial effects on all patients.

A final point that should be noted is that non-compliance is not restricted to medicine. Not every bit of advice given by solicitors, architects, business consultants, and other professionals is followed by those who have sought their services. Clients exercise their judgement, as is their right, when presented with professional advice even though they may not have the expertise claimed by their advisers. They are capable of healthy scepticism, of balancing advice from different sources, and of requiring supportive evidence. Clients' failure to follow advice may have serious consequences, yet these professions tend to see this independence as part of clients' rights and if they study non-compliance at all, do not do so in terms of client deficiency but in terms of necessary improvements in the services they offer.

Factors that determine the success of consultations

The criterion of a successful consultation has generally been seen as the short-term assessment of the degree to which the patient has co-operated with the advised treatment. This criterion implies that the patient has given informed consent and has been free from pressures that might restrict his freedom of choice of treatments, and has fully participated in deciding which of the options in treatment are likely to benefit them most. For example, a woman's participation in the treatment of her breast cancer will involve decisions that go further than the purely medical.

Sackett (1976) has stated the preconditions for ethical compliance thus: the diagnosis must be correct, the therapy must do more good than harm, and the patient must be an informed willing partner. The whole trouble from the patient's point of view is that he must make a judgement on all these matters without the specialized knowledge which would give him a truly independent perspective. He must trust but also doubt, accept but also question if he is ever to achieve informed consent. Being a patient is hard work, since he must make up his mind on a matter of considerable personal importance without much outside guidance and place himself trustingly in a position of dependence.

The variables most often mentioned as probable factors in non-compliance do not show reliable strong effects. Davis (1966) found that roughly 60 per cent of doctors and medical students believed that patient's 'unco-operative personality' was the main cause of non-compliance and were far less likely to implicate legitimate difficulties for which they as doctors bore some responsibility. The personality of the non-compliant patient shows no consistent pattern when measured with the usual personality inventories, though it may be argued that subtle differences exist which the tests cannot easily identify. Also, there are very many personality characteristics that might conceivably be related to compliance, and not all of these have been studied in medical contexts. Social class is not a factor, nor are the characteristics of the doctor, nor the duration and severity of the illness (Ley 1976).

The following factors have been shown to influence the effectiveness of consultations:

STANDARD OF SERVICE

Patients cannot be expected to comply with advice perfectly if the process is made difficult and unrewarding. Finnerty *et al.* (1973a, b) investigated the reasons for non-attendance at an out-patient clinic. They found a 42 per cent drop-out rate, which was associated with long waiting times, lack of twenty-four-hour availability and lack of continuity in the staff seen on different visits. By attending to these factors so that patients were seen more promptly by the same staff the drop-out rate fell to 8 per cent. In a study of 1,300 patients' views on the service offered by general practitioners (Consumer's Association 1983) it was found that the most common problem was getting to see the doctor in the first place. Long waits at the surgery were cited by 26 per cent, difficulty in getting an appointment by 20 per cent, lack of confidence in the general practitioner by 14 per cent, and then at 12 per cent inconvenient surgery hours, problems with receptionists, feeling rushed when with the doctor, and not having things fully explained. Fixed appointment times were preferred over a queuing system, though they were not always available. These findings show that the standard of services offered can have important effects on attendance rates and the choice of health care resources. It is unwise to assume that illness will be of such overriding personal concern that patients will see the convenience or otherwise of the services offered as irrelevant. Aside from the unconscious casualty, most patients retain preferences as to how they should be treated and will avoid inconvenient and unfriendly services wherever possible.

DOCTORS' LACK OF AWARENESS

Many doctors assume without further enquiry that their recommendations are followed faithfully. Davis (1966) found that only 11 per cent of the doctors seeing patients in a general medical clinic correctly estimated that only half the patients were actually complying with advice. Forty-seven per cent estimated that three-quarters were compliant and an astounding 42 per cent claimed that almost all their patients adhered to the advice they were given. This distorted perception of reality on the part of the doctor may result from ego involvement, the feeling that no patient is likely to diminish excellent advice by ignoring it. Possibly this sense of personal importance, coupled with an assumption that people value preventative health measures, leads doctors to avoid checking up on what their patients are actually doing. Caron and Roth (1968, 1971) found that even when patients had been in a ward for three to four weeks the majority of physicians significantly overestimated the extent to which their gastrointestinal patients took antacid medication. Though they had definite ideas about their patients' adherence, they were unable to spot the non-compliers.

One simple reason for this state of ignorance is that many doctors do not question their patients on this issue. Svarstad (1976) found that when physicians checked with patients about their compliance, patients were more likely on follow-up to have been found to comply. The more extensive the monitoring of adherence, the more accurate the feedback, the more honest the answers, and the more likely that problems with co-operation would be admitted. These problems, once admitted, elicited friendly concern and support from most of the practitioners. Conversely, those physicians who did not explicitly question their patients did not get these admissions about difficulties. Their failure to question meant that there was no forum for the patient to put forward his own views about treatment. Their patients were apt to conceal their non-compliance and adherence was poor, possibly because the lack of questioning erroneously transmitted the impression that the doctor thought the treatment unimportant or unlikely to work. Patients are often very diffident and this passive response when faced with the doctor may be mistaken for acceptance of the advice given (Stimson 1974).

PERSUASION

Surprisingly, techniques of persuasion have rarely been used. The professional ethic favours a 'soft sell' and many doctors regard their duty as completed once they have reached a diagnosis and prescribed treatment. Persuasion seems to be a pursuit tainted with salesmanship and therefore not to be countenanced. Yet major advances in health can only be achieved by persuasion, since so many hazards are self-inflicted. Such work as has been done has largely been concerned with studying the effects of fear-arousing messages as a prompt to health action. Dabbs and Leventhal (1966) studied the effects of fear arousal in a series of messages intended to encourage subjects to get themselves inoculated against tetanus. The authors point out that much of the work in this area has been simplistic, since it has often failed to distinguish between changes in attitude and changes in actual behaviour, and has often ignored the fact that a health behaviour may be perceived as ineffective or painful. A group of 182 university students were given a ten-page pamphlet about tetanus inoculation and then a check was made as to whether they eventually went to get inoculated. Pamphlets were systematically varied so that there were three levels of fear about the disease, two levels of effectiveness of the procedure, and two levels of pain involved in the injections. At the end of each were specific instructions as to how to get vaccinated at the university health department. Neither effectiveness nor pain were influential. Only fear led to an increased intention and to actual vaccination. None of the personality measures correlated with vaccination taking, except for self-esteem. Subjects who had a poor opinion of themselves were persuaded even by low fear conditions, whereas those with higher self-esteem complied most in the high fear condition. Possibly these subjects feel that they can cope with most dangers on their own and only comply with advice when self-sufficiency is shown to be inappropriate. Judgements of this sort are part of rational decision-making, yet can be interpreted by others as being foolhardiness. This study also highlights the necessity of giving subjects clear instructions as to what they have to do. There is little purpose in scaring people unless they are given detailed communications as to where and how they can take appropriate health action.

Fear can be a powerful motivator, though the direction in which it influences behaviour can be determined by many factors. Knowledge that cigarette smoking may lead to lung cancer does not of itself lead to the majority of smokers giving up their habit. This is partly because the feared consequences can be seen as delayed and unlikely and partly because this generalized fear needs specific assistance if it is to be translated into action. Raw (1981) has shown that compliance with advice about giving up smoking depends upon the provision of both a supportive social group and a temporary nicotine gum to substitute for the physiological effects of tobacco. Fear of cancer seems only to be effective when it is too late and the patient has been diagnosed. Therefore, it would appear that fear assists compliance only when clear guidance and appropriate support is given to the desired health action.

ATTRIBUTION

One way to get a person to behave in a particular fashion is to let them know that you expect them to do so. You credit them with the characteristic of sensible obedience and then let them sensibly obey. This attribution technique is often used by doctors in an informal way when they say, 'I'm sure a sensible person like you will agree to this course of treatment.' Some evidence that attribution can be more effective than persuasion as a means of modifying behaviour is provided by Miller, Brickman, and Bolen (1975) who found that children's tidiness and clearing up after others and performance in mathematics was most improved by appropriate attributions. Children who were repeatedly told that they were cleaner and tidier than other children, or better at mathematics, improved more on objective criteria than those who had been urged to improve their behaviour. The authors suggest that persuasion often suffers because it involves a negative attribution (a person has faults which he ought to overcome), while attribution generally succeeds because it disguises a persuasive intent behind a compliment.

DEGREE OF SATISFACTION

As discussed in Chapter 8, satisfaction has been described and measured in a number of ways, yet it is consistently associated with compliance. Although a cluster of variables probably contribute to a patient being satisfied with a consultation, once a state of satisfaction is achieved then major changes occur in patients' health behaviour. To a certain extent the patient believes in the power of the doctor, which can lead to dependency, uncritical acceptance, and exaggerated respect in some cases. Satisfaction with the consultation (Francis, Korsch, and Morris 1969; Korsch, Gozzi, and Francis 1968), with communications (Kincey, Bradshaw, and Ley 1975; Ley 1976, 1979a) and in general with medical care received (Haynes, Taylor, and Sackett 1979) are all correlated with patient compliance.

Korsch, Gozzi, and Francis (1968) conducted a detailed study of 800 consultations in which mothers brought their children to a well-staffed walk-in clinic for acute disorders. Consultations were recorded, patients interviewed as they came out from seeing the doctor and then visited at home a fortnight later. As an exercise in communication, many of the consultations left a lot to be desired. Doctor's language was often full of jargon and whilst this impressed some patients, it left most baffled as to what was wrong with their child and what they were supposed to do about it. Although 76 per cent of the mothers said they were more or less satisfied with the doctor's performance in their brief encounter, their specific reactions were less favourable. Nearly a fifth of the mothers felt that they were given no clear indication as to what was wrong with their child and almost half left the surgery still wondering what had caused the child's condition. This last finding is particularly worrying since many mothers would be left blaming themselves for their child's condition. Patient's stated satisfaction on emerging from the interview was the most powerful determinant of compliance as measured on the home visit a fortnight later. Satisfied mothers were three times as likely to have followed instructions as those who were dissatisfied. The rates were 53 per cent compliance for the highly satisfied and 17 per cent for the highly dissatisfied.

When the mothers were interviewed and the recordings studied several factors emerged as contributing to satisfaction. If the doctor indulged in friendly talk not directly concerned with the illness, then satisfaction was increased. The doctors studied were often friendly with the child but distant with the mother, though they had the impression that they had been friendly. The doctors also had the impression that the patients had done most of the talking, yet the recordings showed that the true position was the reverse, and when there was a rough balance between the parties in amount of talking, satisfaction increased. If the patient had a chance to express their concerns and the doctor registered these and dealt with them appropriately, then this feeling of having been understood on an important matter was strongly associated with satisfaction. Also, if patients had strong expectations about the form of treatment they should receive, then these had to be discussed and catered for if treatment was to be successful. For example, one patient expected that her child's persistent cough would be dealt with by some cough mixture and was mystified when an unknown type of nose drops were prescribed. The doctor did not bother to explain that a drip from the nose was inflaming the back of the throat and that the drops would deal with this. On follow-up it emerged that she had spurned the prescription and bought a proprietary cough mixture. Compliance with instructions showed no relation to the length of the interview and if anything, some of the longer interviews were those in which communication and compliance were poorest.

PATIENT COMPREHENSION OF MEDICAL INSTRUCTIONS

Medical and lay vocabularies differ in content and extent. A typical finding is that doctors know two to three times as many words as the average patient, though education is the major factor in this difference. Medical education is largely concerned with the identification and classification of biological processes and inevitably this requires specialized vocabularies. In addition, this vocabulary can be used in an exaggerated and unnecessary form to impress and occasionally confuse patients. Jargon is an ingredient of the maintenance of professional identity and can demarcate medical territory and preserve dominance over the most educated and enquiring of patients. Samora, Saunders, and Larson (1961) took fifty words which physicians judged to be suitable for use with patients, embedded them in context sentences and got 125 largely working-class patients to say what they meant. The average number correctly defined of these supposedly easy words was twenty-nine and a quarter of the patients knew only twenty or fewer words. Among the most commonly misunderstood words were: malignant, secretions, cardiac, respiratory, tendon, terminal, and nerve. Segall and Roberts (1980) suggest, in a more recent replication, that these professional–lay differences have decreased.

Whatever the cause, the result is that much of what doctors say is not understood by their patients. When patients are asked to report whether they have understood the doctor's instructions then 7–53 per cent admit that they do not (Ley 1980). This method is likely to be an underestimate, since it will not pick up those who have misunderstood what was required of them but do not realize it. However, the harsher behavioural tests of comprehension, which imply even lower rates of understanding, in the range of 53–89 per cent, are subject to some of the other factors which reduce compliance. Unless specific care is taken to ensure that what is said can be understood by the patient then the effectiveness of medical advice is considerably reduced.

RECALL OF MEDICAL INFORMATION

Even if a message is understood, it must be remembered if it is to be acted upon. Since the typical procedure is for the doctor to give oral instructions, with only some basic dosage advice being printed on the label of the medication, the usual method of investigation has been to ask patients how much they can recall of what they were told at varying times after the consultation. Ley and Spelman (1965, 1967) found that immediately after the consultation roughly 40 per cent of what had been said by the doctor had already been forgotten. Recall of instructions at 44 per cent was poorer than recall of statements giving information about the illness at 56 per cent and diagnostic statements were recalled best of all at 87 per cent. From the practical point of view the essential facts to be remembered were the instructions but the patients and also the doctors did not appear to perceive the consultation in this way. The general finding has been that the amount forgotten increases with the number of statements made, though this relationship is not always a simple linear one. Even though forgetting is proportionately greater when the doctor has made many statements, patients still recall more in absolute terms. Therefore, if it is essential that the patient remember something, then only two statements should be made in a consultation. Even so, only 82 per cent remembered them both in Ley and Spelman's study. If it is necessary to give the patient a general understanding of his illness and treatment, then up to six statements can be made but only three or four are likely to be remembered by the average patient. In general doctors appear to tell their patients more than they can hope to remember without writing down the instructions. Getting patients to write down what they are told itself marginally improves unprompted recall and naturally ensures that the patient has a record to refresh his memory later.

Age does not consistently influence the recall of personal medical information. The general finding has been of no association (Anderson 1979; Brody 1980; Joyce *et al.* 1969; Ley 1979c), with the work of Ley and Spelman (1965) perhaps surprisingly showing better recall for older patients in one study but no difference in the other studies and more recent work (Anderson 1979; Ley *et al.* 1976) suggesting that patients over sixty-five years of age may forget more, which would be in line with psychometric findings for verbal recall.

In their original work Ley and Spelman found no association between intelligence and recall. Intelligence as inferred from higher educational levels was associated with better recall in the work of Bertakis (1977) and Anderson *et al.* (1979), which may in part be due to better knowledge about medical matters. The extent of medical knowledge is influential in that those who, as judged by a medical knowledge questionnaire, can understand medical terms find it easier to remember them. Greater ease of recall for meaningful material is a well-established finding in memory research.

The other influential factor in recall is the patient's level of anxiety during the consultation. Early work in this field suggested that those who are moderately anxious remember more than both those who are too relaxed to bother to pay attention and those so anxious that they are unable to do so. In general it has been found that some moderate level of anxiety, neither too high nor too low, is necessary for the best performance at tasks. This curvilinear association between recall and anxiety prompted Ley and Spelman (1967) to suggest that putting people at their ease could be an important prerequisite for successful communication. On occasion it would also be necessary to underline the seriousness of a problem in order to obtain their attention. However, Anderson (1979) found in a study of rheumatology patients that those with highest levels of anxiety showed the best recall of what was said to them. It is interesting to note that a similar move from the curvilinear to the simple linear association has now occurred in the study of anxiety and post-operative recovery. It may be that assessments of anxiety have changed, or that there is an interaction effect with the generally improved levels of public knowledge about medical matters. Whatever the precise nature of the association, anxiety remains strongly implicated as a factor in patient recall.

Most of the research studies have concentrated on memory for a single consultation, which is naturally easier to study than the more usual and complicated pattern of building up communication over successive consultations. Hulka *et al.* (1975a,b) found that with prolonged and repeated contact recall rates were in the range of 67–88 per cent, which is better than single contacts though still short of optimal levels.

PROVISION OF WRITTEN INSTRUCTIONS

Written information seems to be an effective means of improving compliance in the short term. Morris and Halperin (1979) found that six out of seven studies reviewed showed greater compliance for those who had received written instructions but in the case of long-term treatment only six out of eleven studies showed this improvement. This suggests that such instruction is capable of dealing with one of the components of non-compliance, immediate understanding, but has less effect on the long-term perceived utility of treatment.

However, written instructions can only improve compliance if they can easily be read by the people to whom they are directed. In the same way that doctors in spoken instructions often use words that patients cannot understand, in written instructions both the vocabulary and the construction can reduce understanding. One attempt to measure the extent of this difficulty is to use readability measures, which, by counting the number and length in syllables of the words in the sentence, give a rough estimate of the percentage of the population which could be expected to understand them. Ley (1973, 1977) found that the longer the words and the longer the sentences the smaller the number of people who could make sense of the pamphlet. However, in later work (Ley 1980) he warns that while a poor score on the readability test indicates that the material is difficult to understand, an apparently good score may still let through difficult material.

Despite this, use of any of the readability formulas will improve the understandability of written information, which many investigations have revealed to be regrettably low. Non-prescription drug leaflets would on nine occasions out of ten be misunderstood by 60 per cent of the population (Pyrczak and Roth 1976); opticians' leaflets on twenty-seven out of thirty-eight examples be misunderstood by the same proportion; and even in the case of health education leaflets eight out of fifteen would equally be misunderstood by 60 per cent of the population. In a summary of these findings over seven separate studies Ley (1982) found that a staggering 69 per cent of these written communications would be misunderstood by 60 per cent of the population and that only 20 per cent could be expected to gain the understanding of three-quarters of the population. The likely explanation is that the writers do not bother to test comprehension adequately and simply assume that their attempts at explanation will be successful. This may be part of the larger bureaucratic tradition in which the public is communicated with little, if at all, but in those who purport to be encouraging their patients to understand and co-operate in treatment, these findings are highly regrettable. It is clear that considerable gains can be made in patient comprehension by paying careful attention to the ways in which medical communications are written.

IMPROVING RECALL OF MEDICAL INFORMATION

Ley (1982) has summarized the effects on recall of memory improving techniques and has shown general improvements can be achieved, though no single technique can always guarantee success. Ley and Spelman (1967) had originally found that patient recall was best for statements about diagnosis, which tended to come early in the interview, and worst for instructions, which were generally left to the end of the consultation. Recall was also better for those portions of the interview patients perceived to be most important and because of the emphasis doctors laid on the topic, this was another reason for the diagnosis being seen as the fact worth remembering. Work on improving recall has thus concentrated on the systematic manipulation of these factors, as well as making the different types of information more apparent to the patient by explicitly organizing what is said into separate categories.

The results of different studies can be simplified by giving the average percentage improvement in recall according to the main technique used. Naturally this will pool different patients in different circumstances and can serve only as a rough indication of the sorts of results that might be expected from particular procedures. Analogue studies, in which volunteers recall medical information, are included because the results closely mirror those found in real-life studies, suggesting that as far as recall goes, the major factors are general cognitive memory limitations rather than personal specific responses.

These results must be interpreted with caution. For example, the apparently outstanding effects of specific statements have been evaluated only in the field of slimming advice, which, while it offers the objective measure of weight loss as a criterion of success, does not cover all contexts of patient compliance. However, it does suggest that it is easier to remember that one must lose a specific amount of weight than to comply with generalized advice about slimming. Furthermore, inspection of *Table 10* reveals that substantial improvements are possible using simple readily available techniques to improve patient recall of medical information.

Table 10   *Improvement in recall from various techniques of giving information*

technique used	number of studies	percentage improvement (%)
specific statements	3	242
primacy	2	46
stressed importance	1	38
simplification	6	32
explicit categorization	2	28
repetition	4	26
mixture of techniques	5	19
adjunct questions	1	−20

Source: Ley (1982): adapted from table 5.

Achieving patient compliance

PATIENT'S BELIEFS

If a patient has given informed consent to competent medical advice, then techniques that achieve compliance are to the benefit of both patient and doctor. Achieving this requires an understanding of the social psychology of personal interaction. No single technique on its own will achieve success.

DiMatteo and DiNicola (1982) have reviewed theories and findings in the field of compliance and their conceptualization is based on Ajzen and Fishbein's (1980) 'Theory of Reasoned Action'. This states that action is a reasoned outcome of cognitive beliefs and emotional attitudes, conditioned by group subjective norms. They propose that for there to be a change in behaviour there must be a change in beliefs. Although there are many theoretical formulations of compliance behaviour, most research attention has been given to one that emphasizes the belief compqnent in rational decisions and serves as a convenient framework in which to place the results of further research.

The Health Belief Model (Becker 1974; Rosenstock 1966) proposes that for people to seek out and comply with health advice they must:

1   Possess some basic knowledge about health and the motivation to achieve it so as to provide a cue to action.
2   Believe themselves to be vulnerable to illness.
3   Believe that the illness has significant consequences.
4   Believe that treatment will work.
5   Believe that this can be attained at acceptable cost, in its broadest sense.

The basic tenets of the model are similar to those proposed for other forms of decision-making under uncertainty. This model had been complicated by the addition of 'modifying and enabling factors' which include evaluation of the doctor, the standards of service, the nature of the interaction with health advisers, financial cost, accessibility, and prior experience of treatment. Cues to action now include the perception of symptoms, media coverage of illnesses, and the facilitatory effects of encouragement from loved ones (Becker and Maiman 1975). The sorry truth is that each bold conceptualization flounders on the complicated reality of compliance research and must then be elaborated to fit the findings. The health belief model serves to order the countless variables into simpler categories but is still very far from being able to predict compliance behaviour. It does give patient perceptions a key part to play, which offers a productive approach to the topic.

FACTORS RELATED TO COMPLIANCE

Basic health motivation   This has been shown to be related to compliance. Becker *et al.* (1977) found that mothers with an active preventative orientation were more likely to bring their children for check-ups than those with a fatalistic orientation, who were more likely only to bring their children when they had had an accident or were already ill. Radius *et al.* (1978) showed that maternal health motivation correlated with compliance in the treatment of children's asthma and children's obesity and Kirscht *et al.* (1978) further showed that such motivation was positively related to obese children's weight loss at follow-up. However, as DiMatteo and DiNicola (1982) point out, these encouraging findings are not a pure measure of motivation, since belief in the efficacy of treatment is also involved.

Vulnerability to illness   This factor is correlated with health behaviour over a wide range of disorders, including screening for cancer (Fink, Shapiro, and Roester 1972; Haefner and Kirscht 1970; Kegeles 1969); for tuberculosis and for heart disease (Haefner and Kirscht 1970). Belief in vulnerability also correlates with obtaining immunization (Leventhal, Hochbaum, and Rosenstock 1960; Ogionwo 1973) and other preventative measures (Becker *et al.* 1977). Vulnerability seems to be an important factor in compliance, as the rational model and common sense would predict. Naturally, perceptions of vulnerability may change through experience and propaganda.

Consequences of the illness   These are not related to compliance, unless the patient's perception of severity matches the reality. Whenever a condition is believed to be serious, regardless of medical estimates of severity, then compliance is increased. This has been shown for dental care (Tash, O'Shea, and Cohen 1969), accident prevention (Suchman 1967) and seeking treatment for a variety of conditions (Battistella 1971). A mediating factor in estimates of vulnerability and severity may be anxiety, which is a strong motivator of behaviour.

Effectiveness of treatment   This is always hard for doctors to judge till proper random controlled trials have been carried out and must be judged by patients on the basis of public media and the reports of people known to them. Compliance is higher when treatments are perceived as effective (Becker, Drachman, and Kirscht 1972; Feinstein 1976; Hartman and Becker 1978; Kirscht and Rosenstock 1977). Subjective assessments of effectiveness are influenced by the subject's view as to how much his illness is under control.

Locus of control   Rotter (1954) proposed that a person's potential for carrying out a behaviour is determined by his expectancy that it will lead to a particular outcome and the value he places on that outcome. People who have a generalized expectation that reinforcement is under their individual control are said to have 'internal locus of control'. They would be likely to agree with the sentiments that 'life is what you make it' and 'rewards in life go to those who work for them'. People who have a generalized expectation that reinforcement is under the control of outside forces such as fate or chance are said to have 'external locus of control'. They would be likely to agree with the sentiments 'life depends on luck' and 'rewards in life go to those who are offered the best chances'.

When these propensities are measured on Rotter's (1966) scale, they are shown to be moderately associated with compliance. Internal locus of control subjects are more likely than externals to be non-smokers (James, Woodruff, and Werner 1965; Straits and Sechrest 1963); to give up or reduce smoking (Steffy, Meichenbaum, and Best 1970); to use contraception (Lundy 1972; Phares 1976); to be of normal weight (Manno and Marston 1972); to use seat-belts more often (Williams 1972); to have a more inquisitive attitude about their illnesses (Seeman and Evans 1962); and even to have shorter but more painful labours in childbirth and shorter menstrual periods (Scott-Palmer and Skevington 1981). This moderate association would probably be higher if it were combined with a measure of the value the subject gives to health and the social norms and pressures on him. Wallston, Wallston, and DeVellis (1978) have developed a multidimensional health locus of control scale, which distinguished between personal control of health, professional control, and chance factors but this has yet to prove itself as a valid and useful measure. Winefield (1982) factor-analysed the results of 153 medical students, 52 healthy middle-aged men, and 53 male patients recovering from myocardial infarction on this scale and found that the internal control of health sub-scale was reliable over seven months, as was the professional control sub-scale though this rose with age, lower social class, and acute illness. The chance sub-scale showed little stability over time. Unfortunately, no predictive relationships were found between these sub-scale scores and later health or compliance. It seems more helpful to tailor advice to the general internal-external characteristics of the recipients. Cromwell *et al.* (1977) found that internals who were offered active participation and externals who were offered little participation fared better in their treatment of myocardial infarction than those who were in 'incongruent' conditions, in which the offered level of participation was contrary to their inherent preferences. Saltzer (1978) looked at the factors which influenced subjects in slimming and found that internals followed personal attitudes to weight while externals were guided more by social norms. In an unpublished pilot study of smoking reduction using individually tailored cognitive and behavioural techniques the author found that the most effective cognitive reinforcers were those derived from repertory grid analysis that focused on the issue of personal control. Externals responded best to encouragement from the group, while internals were motivated by the suggestion that they should not allow themselves to be exploited by cigarette manufacturers.

Effective communication The health belief model provides a useful framework for interpreting health behaviour and underlines the fact that the key to behavioural compliance lies in the changing of beliefs and attitudes. The accepted basic requirements for a communication-engendered change of attitude are that the person attend to the message, understand it, accept the arguments, and remember them. Aspects of the communicator, the message, and the audience affect all these factors.

An effective communicator is able to persuade by virtue of credibility, likeability, enthusiasm, and trustworthiness. Credibility is achieved by showing relevant knowledge and status. Medical jargon and a white coat are the superficial features of expertness but these lose their impact when the audience is well informed and able to require more adequate proofs of the efficacy of treatments. Liking a person is a powerful inducement to agree with their views and measures of warmth and friendliness have been found to be important in psychotherapy and compliance (Korsch, Gozzi, and Francis 1968). Enthusiasm and confidence are important, because they transmit the fact that the communicator appears to believe his own message. These 'meta-communications' probably account for the greater reported effectiveness of drugs which are prescribed by doctors who 'believe' in them and communicate this therapeutic expectation to their patients. It has also been found that when staff are told that a particular drug is in fact a placebo then the reported effectiveness decreases considerably as their lack of confidence is picked up by the patients. Trustworthiness is established by consistency and disinterestedness. A health professional's change of tack may be perceived as inconsistency and thereby destroy trust and compliance. Equally, if a physician is seen as serving his own interest then the aura of unbiased objective advice is shattered and the patient will rightly recoil from being manipulated.

All of these four characteristics can be developed in communicators by sufficient appropriate training. They are as necessary for the practice of effective medicine as training in basic medical knowledge. The characteristics of the message which make for persuasiveness are more complex. One-sided messages of the sort which are popular in medical pep talks are likely to be effective only with poorly educated subjects. Those who are able to develop counter-arguments are likely to find the one-sided approach unconvincing. They are more likely to respond to a message that mentions counter-arguments but which gives valid grounds for rejecting them (Hovland, Lumsdaine, and Sheffield 1949). The best approach is for the communicator to hear the subject's objection and then to work together with him to dispose of it. Active involvement of this sort is the best protection against any outside attack on new beliefs. Fear-arousing communications are only effective when the fear presents a credible and manageable threat with clear pointers as to what the subject must do in order to protect himself. Fears which destroy the subject's belief that he can cope are more likely to lead to anxiety and helplessness than health behaviour.

Audience characteristics strongly determine whether a message succeeds in persuading subjects to change their behaviour. An anti-smoking campaign which stresses health implications may not succeed in influencing younger people, for whom the threat of eventual illness seems distant and psychologically improbable. They may be more affected by suggestions that smoking is unattractive or unfashionable and unless this is recognized messages may miss their targets.

Ideally, messages should be complex enough to engage the audience and make them fill in the missing pieces themselves, thus generating their own reasons for accepting the argument and leading to attitude changes that are more long-lasting (Berkowitz 1980). Naturally, the messages cannot be over-complex and they must be repeated frequently for their full effect to be realized. The effect of repetition is extremely strong and is well known to all advertisers and politicians. Familiarity breeds affection and acceptance and the persistently repeated message eventually becomes internalized, thus ceasing to be perceived as a message and becoming an always-accepted received truth. For this effect to take place messages must be designed to avoid arousing immediate antagonism and should mix sentiments with which the subject is likely to agree with new material. Many medical exhortations are crudely stated and baldly repeated, making it probable that many in the potential audience will reject the advice and dislike the source in future. A more gradual approach, which recognizes the difficulties subjects experience in changing their life-styles, has more chance of eventual acceptance. Attitude change is a gradual long-term process that achieves its effects by small adjustments, many of which may be barely noticed by the subject. Eventually social changes occur that give further support to the new attitudes. Something of this sort seems to have occurred with smoking, which now, twenty years after first publication of the findings on health hazards, is increasingly seen as a regrettable, unfashionable, and unwise habit. In bringing about actual changes in behaviour, price increases can have as important effects as attitude change but attitudes must change before such legislation can be proposed and accepted.

In some individual cases persuasive messages about the need for health care may not be able to overcome the illusion of personal invulnerability. In such cases the use of role play can effect changes, by arousing in the individual the emotion he would feel if the situation were real. Mann and Janis (1968) asked smokers to role play being told that they had lung cancer and found that they were more likely to give up smoking than a control group who had heard a persuasive message. The procedure is time-consuming and requires full participation from patient and organizer but can be an effective technique and is a useful exercise for anti-smoking groups. Russell *et al.* (1979) found that when general practitioners advised patients to give up smoking there was a modest but beneficial effect, such that about twenty-five patients per general practitioner would give up permanently each year because of the advice they had received.

Changes in public attitudes to health   Medical communicators often despair of getting their subjects to comply with health instructions. In part this stems from over-reliance on the brief face to face interview as virtually the sole agent of change. The doctor's admonitions are only one factor in health behaviour and unless the subject perceives himself to be vulnerable to serious illness, immediate behavioural change is unlikely. However, some physicians are discouraged by this lack of response and easily accept the notion that their responsibility ends there. The other factors which impinge on individual behaviour are social pressures which are more easily changed by public advertising campaigns. Even here, public health campaigns tend to be under-financed, short-lived and all too often misconceived. Yet at the same time major changes are taking place in health behaviour as a consequence of social forces. The jogging movement grew out of a popular wish for healthy exercise in a form that avoided the competitive, performance-orientated official sports world. A minority was able to spread its message by personal example and private conversation. Dietary changes are notoriously difficult to bring about and it is said that of twenty heavily promoted new snacks or foods, nineteen are quickly rejected by the public. Yet commercial interests backed by advertising have succeeded in massively increasing sales of butter substitutes by referring to supposed health advantages. The original message about polyunsaturated fats was a complicated one, yet it has been transmitted and has led to changes in eating behaviour. The increases in bran and fibre consumption are other examples of changes which go beyond mere food fads and which alter national patterns of consumption in a long-term way.

The moral of these findings is that the health behaviour of the public can be changed in the long term by sustained and extensive campaigns which recruit subjects as participators in health maintaining activities. Results do not occur immediately, nor do all people change as intended but nonetheless considerable changes occur. The increased interest in alternative medicine has many causes but a prominent reason is that these approaches give subjects tasks to do which make them participators in treatment, whereas technological medicine often seems to require them to passively donate their bodies to pharmacological experimentation.

Conclusions

Being ill causes anxiety and treatment regimes can serve as a coping response. Patients must exercise their judgement at a time when they are in a dependent position and their beliefs about treatment influence their willingness to comply with specific instructions. Part of the reason for following advice is a perception on the part of patients that their actions can have an influence on their condition and that even if that influence is small the act itself is comforting. Every approach to health that gives the subject something to do and a rationale for doing it encourages adherence to advice.

An unproductive approach to the problem of non-compliance is based on an unrealistic view of human subjects and ascribes personal failings to those who are merely exercising their right to be sceptical and cautious with their own lives. A more productive approach to compliance lies in understanding all the barriers which may prevent a patient working with his advisers to improve his health. A fuller understanding of attitude change is required if the generally poor record of medical advisers is to be improved.

7   *Anxiety, hospitalization, and surgery*

Stanton Newman

Introduction

Admission to hospital for surgery is one of the many stressful events that most individuals living in an industrialized society can, or will, experience in the course of their lives. While medical staff consider certain procedures routine, from the patients' perspective any form of surgery is a cause for anxiety. This chapter considers the course of anxiety when patients are admitted to hospital for surgery, the way in which pre-surgical anxiety influences post-operative recovery, individual differences in response to the threat of surgery, and the techniques which have been developed to reduce patients' anxiety.

Studies of the relationship between anxiety, hospitalization, surgery, and recovery can be divided into four general types.

1 Studies which have examined the course of anxiety about hospitalization and surgery.
2 Those studies that have examined the course of anxiety about hospitalization and surgery but which distinguish between patients on the basis of their pre-surgical emotional state or a characteristic of personality and have studied what influence these have on recovery.

3 Other studies that have intervened with a particular psychological procedure prior to surgery and examined whether this influences the course of anxiety and recovery.
4 Studies that have investigated how an intervention technique interacts with the patient's emotional state or personality.

Instances of each of these types will be discussed below to illustrate the major research findings. The studies involve a large number of variables that need to be considered when drawing any conclusions or comparing one study with another. The most important of these are the range of surgical procedures studied and the variety of measures of anxiety and recovery.

A wide *variety of surgical procedures* have been studied. These have ranged from tonsillectomy (Ferguson 1979) through hernia repair (Andrew 1970), abdominal surgery (Egbert *et al.* 1964) to cardiac surgery (Kinney 1977). Studies have also been performed on dental patients (Auerbach *et al.* 1976; Herbertt and Innes 1979), where in some instances only a local anaesthetic was applied. Pre-surgical anxiety levels of the patient appear to be systematically influenced by the severity of the operative procedure. For instance, patients facing surgery for cancer or kidney transplant appear to have a higher level of pre-surgical anxiety than patients facing less threatening surgery. There is some suggestion that different procedures may involve different concerns which will influence the course of anxiety (see below). It is also possible that psychological intervention designed to influence anxiety may only be successful with certain procedures and not others. The net effect of this is that generalizations across different types of surgery should only be made with caution.

Pre-operative measures of anxiety have included self-ratings (Sime 1976), observer ratings (Cohen and Lazarus 1973), adjective check-lists (Wolfer and Davis 1970), treatment check-lists (Johnson, Leventhal, and Dabbs 1971), Likert-type rating scales (Johnston 1980), palmar sweating (Johnson, Dabbs, and Leventhal 1970) as well as other physiological measures such as platelet aggregation time, prolactin, and blood pressure (for more details of physiological indices see Johnston 1984a). The discussion which follows will concentrate on the psychological measures of anxiety. It is, however, worth noting that the relationship between physiological and psychological measures is not clear (Johnston 1984a). Other emotions such as depression have been assessed but the majority of studies have considered anxiety as their pre-operative measure.

A variety of *measures to assess recovery from surgery* have been used. Some studies have assessed various subjective mood states such as anxiety, pain, depression, and anger (Langer, Janis, and Wolfer 1975; Vernon and Bigelow 1974) or ratings of these mood states (Siegel and

Peterson 1980). Others have rated recovery in relation to behaviour, such as the time to achieve voicing following tonsillectomy (Visintainer and Wolfer 1975), frequency of requests for analgesics (Lindeman and Stetzer 1973), or sedatives (Langer, Janis, and Wolfer 1975). Other measures have considered the patients' physical state such as blood pressure (Langer, Janis, and Wolfer 1975), pulse rate (Schmitt and Wooldridge 1973), and post-operative complications (Lindeman and Stetzer 1973). A comprehensive measure which has also been applied is the number of days to discharge from hospital (Langer, Janis, and Wolfer 1975).

Most studies have used a number of measures of recovery and the findings have indicated that these do not always correlate. This may be accounted for by considering the variety of different influences that the measures are subjected to. For example, the number of days to discharge would be related to the policy adopted in a particular hospital making it less susceptible to alterations of a patient's psychological or physical state in comparison to subjective ratings of mood.

What is more important, these measures embrace conceptually different views of recovery. The doctor's role has been viewed as the treatment of illness, with the result that the physical measures such as blood pressure and pulse rate which are considered useful indicators of physical recovery embrace a medical concept of recovery. The patient, on the other hand, may place more emphasis on subjective feelings of discomfort, anxiety, and pain. These feelings are customarily assessed in the form of rating scales or questionnaires. They may also be reflected in measures such as the frequency of requests for analgesics. While there may be some degree of association between measures of recovery reflecting these two concepts of recovery it is unlikely, given the limited association that has been found between physiological and psychological measures, that this will always be the case.

One study examined the degree of association between different measures of recovery and produced empirical evidence to suggest that these reflect a number of separable factors (Johnston 1984b). Johnston (1984b) assessed a group of gynaecological patients on two separate occasions with sixteen measures commonly used to assess post-operative outcome. The results indicated a number of separate factors, each comprised of different measures of recovery. Three of these factors were found on both assessments. The most significant factor on both assessments was termed 'Well Being'. It included the measures of self-ratings of physical capacities such as sleep and energy, self-rating of positive mood and independent washing. The two remaining factors common to both assessments were attitudes to the hospital and a distress factor. Thus recovery in this study reflected at a minimum three separable factors. These findings confirm that the measures commonly used to assess recovery are not measuring the same phenomenon and therefore one should not expect to find all measures showing high inter-correlations. One additional interesting aspect of this study was that pain was not associated with any of the three factors and appeared as a separate factor on the second assessment. Therefore, as Johnston argues, any simple association of absence of pain with 'Well Being' is not tenable.

Before looking at studies that have contrasted patients' personality types, or examined forms of psychological intervention, or both of these together, the pattern of anxiety on hospitalization and the course that anxiety takes in surgical patients will be outlined.

Anxiety and hospitalization

Hospitalization, as distinct from surgery, is a source of stress and anxiety to patients in its own right. The hospital environment is novel to patients, and it involves a number of routines and procedures with which they are not familiar. The patients are required to meet and interact with a number of unfamiliar people and frequently have to suffer a loss of privacy. In addition they also lose a considerable degree of independence and have to endure separation from their families, friends, and work (Volicer and Bohannon 1975). Interviews to gauge the concerns of patients have found these issues to be mentioned along with fears regarding health (Wilson-Barnett 1976).

Studies have indicated that hospitalization can wield an independent effect on patients. The ease with which patients cope with the hospital environment has been found to be an important influence on the levels of anxiety they experience (De Wolfe, Barrell, and Cummings 1966). Lucente and Fleck (1972) found that the patient level of anxiety was determined to a greater extent by their personality and their view of the hospital environment, than by the severity of their condition or diagnosis.

If some of the anxiety on hospitalization derives from a lack of familiarity with the people and routines then one should expect some decrease in anxiety as the patient becomes accustomed to the hospital. Some support for this notion was found by Johnston (1980) who in one study found gynaecological patients registering their highest scores on an anxiety inventory (Spielberger, Gorsuch, and Lushene 1970) two days before surgery. This tended to coincide with the day of admission. In a further study, Johnston assessed the anxiety scores of twenty-three patients, all of whom were about to undergo a variety of forms of elective surgery that required a general anaesthetic. Anxiety was assessed on a few occasions, including six days before the operation while the patients were at home, on the morning of admission, and on the evening of admission. The highest anxiety levels were found on the morning of admission with a decrease by the evening of admission, although the difference was not statistically significant (see *Figure 1*).

While on the one hand previous periods of hospitalization may be expected to reduce anxiety by providing patients wth some familiarity and understanding of hospital routines, it may also serve to increase their anxiety because they may have a more accurate perspective on the variety of procedures and the extent of discomfort and pain they might encounter. Friedlander *et al.* (1982) found that the number of stressful events expected by a group of elective surgery patients was positively correlated with the number of previous instances of hospitalization. The information gleaned during previous hospital admissions appeared to have served an educative function leading them to expect more of a variety of stressful events while in hospital. Patients who were highly

Figure 1   Anxiety levels and admission to hospital

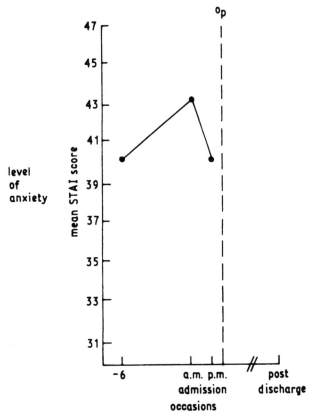

Source: Johnston (1980).

anxious tended to be those who anticipated more stressful events and perceived events to be outside their control.

If patients are asked about their concerns and worries when in hospital the concerns they express appear to be influenced by the profession of the questioner. When patients are accorded the opportunity to express what they are concerned about to an anaesthetist a large proportion of them (62 per cent) express fears about the anaesthetic and a smaller proportion (15 per cent) express concerns regarding surgery. More males than females express fears about these procedures while more females (32 per cent) than males (17 per cent) express fears regarding coma and other miscellaneous concerns (Ramsay 1972). A more diverse picture regarding patients' fears about hospital life has been found in interviews by a nurse researcher (Wilson-Barnet 1976). Two hundred medical patients were interviewed about sixty aspects of hospital life. Eight particular aspects were found to be especially disturbing to patients. These were: being away from their family, absence from work, their condition or illness, the anticipation of a painful treatment, seeing a very ill patient, barium X-rays, using a bed pan, and the night time.

Reactions to hospital are also influenced by the personality of the patient. The extent of patients' anxiety has been found to be related to the personality measure of neuroticism. Patients with high neurotic scores on the Eysenck Personality Questionnaire took longer to adjust to hospital life and were disturbed by relatively minor events (Wilson-Barnett and Carrigy 1978).

Course of anxiety

A common distinction with regard to anxiety is that made between state anxiety and trait anxiety (Spielberger, Gorsuch, and Lushene 1970). State anxiety is a transitory emotional state while trait anxiety is considered to be a relatively stable aspect of personality, reflecting an individual's propensity to anxiety. Spielberger, Gorsuch, and Lushene (1970) have developed two questionnaires to assess state and trait anxiety which have been widely used to look at levels of anxiety in surgical and hospital patients. Studies that used both of these measures before and after surgery have found little change in trait anxiety levels and fluctuations in state anxiety (Auerbach 1973; Chapman and Cox 1976; Johnson and Spielberger 1968; Spielberger *et al.* 1973). Their findings support the validity of the state–trait distinction.

The course that state anxiety measures take with surgical patients is to show a high level on admission with a gradual decline in the post-operative period (Auerbach 1973). These measures of anxiety take a considerable period of time to decline to what might be assumed to be baseline levels. Johnston (1980) examined the anxiety levels of seventy-two gynaecological patients and found that anxiety continued to decline up to fourteen days after the operation (see *Figure 2*).

It is not surprising to find that the type of operation influences the course of anxiety, in particular the rate of anxiety decline, in the post-operative period. Johnston (1980) found that orthopaedic patients maintained relatively high levels of anxiety for some four days after surgery while gynaecological patients showed a decline within the same period. Johnston (1980) attributes the continuing raised level of anxiety in orthopaedic patients to the fact that this type of patient has to wait some time until their plaster is removed before learning the results of the operation and whether the threat of disability remains. If this is so, then

Figure 2   Anxiety and surgery

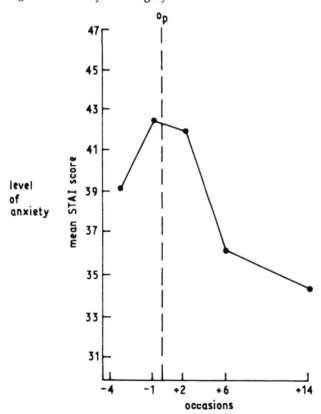

Source: Johnston (1980).

not only are patients concerned and anxious about the procedures and pain they are about to experience, but also about the result. The finding that anxiety levels remained relatively high in these orthopaedic patients, not much reduced from pre-surgical levels, suggests that either these patients switch from being anxious about the operative procedures to the results of the operation, or, that concern about the success of the operation constitutes a significant proportion of the pre-surgical levels of anxiety. Regardless of which of these proposals is correct, orthopaedic patients, and other groups for whom the result of surgery remains unclear for some time, warrant further study and comparison with patients who receive other forms of surgery.

Further evidence that different types of, and reasons for surgery influence anxiety was found in an interesting and related study which compared pain, anxiety, and depression ratings on a sample of kidney donors, kidney recipients, and general surgical patients (Chapman and Cox 1977). The results showed kidney donors to have a more volatile anxiety reaction immediately following surgery despite being least anxious prior to surgery. This study emphasizes the role that the meaning of the operation plays in determining emotions of the patient.

Relationship between pre-operative anxiety and recovery

Remaining calm at a time of threat would be considered by most individuals to be the optimum strategy for the most successful outcome. With impending surgery it might be thought that the more calm the patient, the least disturbing the procedure and the most successful the recovery. Janis (1958, 1969) however, claims that the most calm patients would show emotional disturbance in the post-operative period. He refers to this group as those who show low anticipatory fear and suggests they would remain cheerful and optimistic prior to the operation and as a result would not engage in any mental preparation of what was to follow. The effect of this would be to produce increased feelings of vulnerability and hostility directed at the hospital staff who, in the patients' eyes, would be judged to have failed to provide adequate protection. Individuals who display moderate anxiety about impending surgery would be least likely to show post-operative emotional disturbance because they would have sought out information about the surgical procedure and mentally prepared themselves for the impending threatening event. This process was termed the 'work of worrying' by Janis (1958). The high anticipatory fear group would experience constant fear about the impending surgery and would not obtain any long-lasting relief from reassurance. They would be likely to continue to be anxious after the operation. The net result of these three pre-operative attitudes to fear is that the best post-operative adjustment would be experienced by moderately anxious patients. This proposal thus results in a curvilinear relationship between pre-operative anxiety and post-operative adjustment as shown in *Figure 3a*. Janis examined these hypotheses in a retrospective study of 150 male college students who had recently undergone surgery and found support for the curvilinear relationship.

While there are certain methodological difficulties in allocating patients to the three groups proposed by Janis (see e.g. Johnston and Carpenter 1980; Sime 1976) a number of studies have attempted to examine whether this curvilinear relationship is evident in the more methodologically sound approach of prospective studies. These studies have used a variety of indices of recovery and have failed to support the curvilinear relationship, instead supporting, in the main, a small linear relationship. Those patients showing least anxiety were found to fare best post-operatively while those with high pre-operative anxiety were found to fare worst (Johnston and Carpenter 1980; Sime 1976; Wolfer and Davis 1970) (see *Figure 3b*). In addition Johnston and Carpenter (1980) examined whether low pre-operative anxiety results in anger post-operatively and failed to find a relationship, thus further refuting Janis's proposals.

One feature Janis found which distinguished the low fear from the

Figure 3a   The curvilinear hypothesis

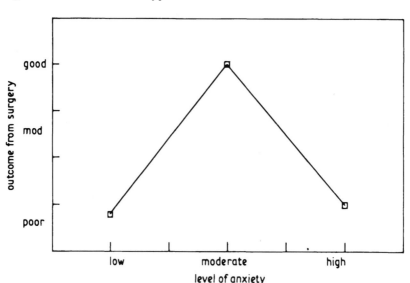

Source: Janis (1957).

moderate fear groups was the amount of information they had about the operation. The moderate fear group were found to be better informed about the operation than the low fear group. When the patients were divided into those who were well informed and those who were not, the well informed were more likely to report that they had fears in the pre-operative period and less likely to show difficulties in post-operative adjustment.

A number of mechanisms may be operating which result in the highly anxious patient making less successful recovery after surgery than less anxious patients. At the level of subjective reports of pain and discomfort the patient who is highly anxious will be more concerned about their symptoms. They would be likely to express these concerns to the medical staff and on any questionnaire or other form of enquiry into their welfare. In addition these concerns may well take the form of increased requests for sedatives or analgesics. Medical complications after surgery may result from two sources. First, highly anxious patients may be less likely to engage in the required exercises post-surgically because of concern with pain and possible effects of the exercise. Second, some researchers have suggested that in a highly anxious state, increased autonomic arousal may lead to increased levels of catecholamines and corticosteriods which may retard post-surgical healing (Mathews and Ridgeway 1981).

Figure 3b   The linear hypothesis

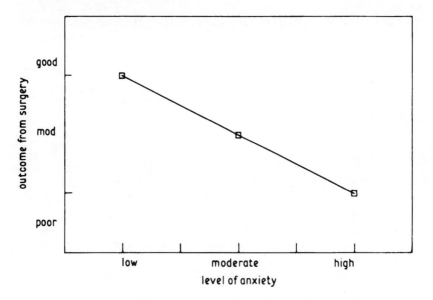

Personality variable

Persistent ways of behaving or responding which are supra-situational are considered to reflect an individual's personality. These factors can predict differences in the behaviour of individuals in a variety of situations. Within the context of anxiety and surgery a number of personality measures have been examined. These include trait anxiety, neuroticism, locus of control, and coping style.

TRAIT ANXIETY

A variety of different measures have been used to assess the propensity of individuals to experience anxiety. These measures would be expected to correlate with assessments of situational or state anxiety in the course of surgery. Studies which applied the Trait and State measure of Spielberger have found those with high trait anxiety scores tend to have high state anxiety scores (Chapman and Cox 1977; Spielberger *et al.* 1973).

The more interesting issue is whether personality differences in anxiety levels predict recovery from surgery on variables other than anxiety. The theoretical problem is to distinguish whether the effect is due to the personality measure of anxiety or the fact that situational anxiety is high, or both of these. For practical purposes, however, it would be valuable to be able to predict those patients who are liable to become anxious and thus have more difficulty in post-operative recovery.

The early studies which examined their recovery from surgery divided patients into high and low anxiety types and failed to find differences on measures of recovery (Johnson, Leventhal, and Dabbs 1971; Wolfer and Davis 1970). Later studies, however, have indicated a poorer recovery of high trait anxiety patients. In particular those with a highly anxious personality tended to experience greater pain (Chapman and Cox 1977; Martinez-Urrutia 1975).

NEUROTICISM

Measures of trait anxiety are highly correlated with neuroticism as measured by the Eysenck Personality Inventory (EPI) (Hayward 1975). This questionnaire distinguishes two dimensions of personality. The first dimension measures neuroticism, which purports to be a measure of emotionality. The second dimension measures the extent to which individuals are extrovert or introvert.

Measures of neuroticism have been found to be a relatively successful predictor of post-operative recovery (see Mathews and Ridgeway 1981). For example Parbrook, Steel, and Dalrymple (1973) found that peptic ulcer patients who had high scores of neuroticism on the EPI reported greater pain, had more injections in the first twenty-four hours, and experienced more chest complications than those with low neuroticism scores. A study with the same measures on female elective cholecystectomy patients found that high neuroticism was correlated with poorer vital capacity measure after twenty-four hours and a higher incidence of chest complications (Dalrymple, Parbrook, and Steel 1973).

LOCUS OF CONTROL

Rotter (1966) devised a scale to measure the extent to which individuals feel that events which happen to them are under their control. Those who consider they wield a strong influence on events which happen to them are termed Internal while those who feel that events are outside their control are termed External. Studies which distinguished internal from external control patients have not shown any independent correlations with indices of recovery (Johnson, Dabbs, and Leventhal 1970; Levesque and Charlebois 1977).

Those patients who have weaker internal beliefs do, however, appear to experience greater levels of state anxiety pre-surgically (Friedlander *et al.* 1982).

COPING STYLE

People appear to have a characteristic manner of coping with stressful events. This is referred to as a coping style. Typically, an avoidant and denial style of coping have been distinguished from a vigilant coping style in studies on surgical patients. The manner in which they are commonly distinguished is in relation to the patients' knowledge and inquisitiveness about impending surgery as well as their desire to discuss the surgery and feelings about the surgery. For example, Cohen and Lazarus (1973) assessed patients' current coping style by rating the patients' interview behaviour. The general characteristics of those with an avoidant coping style were that they showed 'avoidance or denial of emotional or threatening aspects of the upcoming medical experience as indicated by restriction of knowledge or awareness about the medical condition . . . the nature of the surgery, and the post-surgical outlook, and by unwillingness to discuss thoughts about the operation'. Patients with a vigilant coping style are 'overly alert to emotional or threatening aspects of the upcoming medical experience, as indicated by the seeking out of knowledge about the medical condition . . . and by the readiness to discuss thoughts about the operation'.

Cohen and Lazarus (1973) then classified patients' coping styles as Avoidant, Vigilant, and an intermediate group who were neither Avoidant nor Vigilant in style. The avoidant group experienced significantly less minor complications, and were discharged significantly earlier than the vigilant patients. Similar findings have been reported by DeLong (1970).

Two other studies have failed to find differences in recovery variables between patients with different coping styles. Andrew (1970) found no differences between avoiders and sensitizers (vigilant) and Sime (1976) also found no differences between patients classified according to their degree of information seeking.

The variability in findings in this area may be in part attributable to the various concepts and measurements of coping style used. This is supported by one study which compared three different measures of coping style. A current style based on observations of behaviour, and two more general measures as assessed by a sentence completion test and a scale which measured individuals on a repression–sensitization dimension, were examined on the same group of patients. The results indicated that the three measures showed only small inter-correlations (Cohen and Lazarus 1973).

PERSONALITY AND RECOVERY FROM SURGERY – SOME POSSIBLE MECHANISMS

The aspects of personality which have been discussed above are all seen to reflect a consistent pattern of individual behaviour which appears to have, at least in some studies, an influence on recovery. From a practical standpoint it would be an advantage to be able to predict, on the basis of a personality measure, which patients are more likely to have difficulties after surgery. To a limited extent the variables above may provide this type of predictive power. Measures of trait anxiety and neuroticism appear to be most useful in this regard.

From a theoretical standpoint it remains to be explained how these personality variables lead to poorer recovery. It may well be the case that they are all mediated through the same process. First, a number of studies have indicated correlations between the four measures discussed above. Second, they also tend to correlate with measures of anxiety. Thus, they may each offer a useful discriminator of those patients most likely to experience anxiety and all the post-operative effects may be mediated through anxiety (Mathews and Ridgeway 1981).

The one exception to this may be coping style. The avoidant and vigilant coping styles have not always shown correlations with low and high anxiety respectively (Sime 1976, but see also Cohen and Lazarus 1973). While this may reflect problems with measurement it remains possible that some individuals adopt a vigilant coping style without any concomitant increase in anxiety level. Further research is required to examine the relationship between coping style and anxiety.

Psychological intervention with surgical patients

The basis for much of the work on psychological intervention or preparation for surgery is that it may be possible to influence the patients' psychological state, which may in turn result in advantages in post-operative recovery at both the psychological and physical level. At the most obvious and simple, it may be possible to reduce anxiety by reassuring the patient. The form that preparation takes includes the provision of information about surgery and the effects of surgery, instructions about how to behave in the post-surgical period, relaxation training, hypnosis, psychotherapy, and forms of cognitive behavioural training.

A factor which should be borne in mind when considering many of the studies of psychological intervention is that some of the advantages that accrue to any group that receives intervention, may be due to the fact that they received attention from an apparently concerned member of the medical team rather than directly due to the intervention itself. This placebo effect is not easily overcome. One solution is to have as a control group patients who receive an equal amount of time with a member of the medical team who talks to them about general issues. However a problem with this approach concerns the difficulty of maintaining a conversation about non-health related issues with the control patients. The patients expect to discuss health issues with members of the medical team and may become suspicious and uncooperative if these issues are avoided and seemingly irrelevant discussions take place within the context of a busy ward (Wilson-Barnett 1984). Because of the difficulties in obtaining a group suitably controlled for the aspect of attention most of the studies have compared different forms of intervention to the normal hospital procedure.

INFORMATION

Much of the research on psychological preparation and providing information in particular stems from an early finding of Janis (1958). Janis found that those patients who were relatively well informed about surgery reported having less fears in the pre-operative period and experiencing less difficulties in the post-operative period in comparison to those who were less informed. The mechanism Janis felt was at work was that of 'emotional innoculation'. This resulted from giving patients accurate information about what they should expect together with appropriate reassurances. This would lead to mental rehearsal by the patient of the impending threats coupled with appropriate self-generated reassurances that would serve to prepare the patient for what was to follow. The provision of accurate information also serves to prevent the patient from imagining dangers and experiencing unrealistic fears.

Information provided to patients usually takes a variety of forms and is frequently dispensed by a variety of people in an unsystematic fashion. From the patients' point of view, research has tended to show fairly high levels of dissatisfaction with the information they received in hospital (Cartwright 1964; Reynolds 1978). It is important when considering this research to bear in mind that patients may not recall accurately the information that was provided (see Chapter 5).

Early research by Cartwright (1964) found that almost two-thirds of discharged hospital patients reported experiencing some difficulty in obtaining information while in hospital. The practice of providing patients with information may have changed from that time. Hospital services now place greater emphasis on providing information but it is not always successful. A later study asked hospital patients about a particular procedure, in this instance a chest X-ray. About a third did not know why it was necessary and 92 per cent received no warning that they were about to have a chest X-ray and 82 per cent were not provided with any information regarding the results of the X-ray (Reynolds 1978). As this is frequently a pre-surgical procedure the lack of provision of information may only serve to raise patients' levels of pre-operative anxiety.

At its simplest, information can be provided in the form of a booklet that either indicates details of a specific procedure or gives a more general description of surgery (see for example 'So you're going to have an operation' distributed in the Veterans Administration hospitals in the United States). Research in the United Kingdom has shown that even when booklets are supposedly routinely distributed to patients a large proportion (two-thirds) claim not to have seen it (Reynolds 1978). Almost all of those who did recall seeing the booklet, however, considered it to have been useful.

More systematic techniques of delivering information have been adopted in research studies. These have ranged from verbal information given by a nurse (Schmitt and Wooldridge 1973), a psychologist (Langer, Janis, and Wolfer 1975) and an anaesthetist (Egbert *et al.* 1964) through slides and audio information given on a tape-recorder (Weiss *et al.* 1983) to videotape or film (Andrew 1970).

The nature of the information provided to patients has varied considerably. In some studies a combination of different types of information has been used. This is well illustrated in an early study which indicated the benefits of providing patients with information (Egbert *et al*. 1964). All the patients in the study were due to have elective abdominal surgery. They were all visited by an anaesthetist who informed them about the preparation for anaesthesia, the time and approximate duration of surgery and also told them that they would wake up in the recovery room. At this point in the study the patients were randomly allocated to either a control or a special care group. The control group received no further information. The special care group were informed about the location, severity, and duration of pain they should expect and were reassured that to experience some pain after an abdominal operation was a normal occurrence. The patients then had explained to them how the pain was caused and how it was possible to experience some relief by means of muscular relaxation. Finally they were shown the use of the trapeze and where appropriate they were taught how to turn on one side by using their arms and legs while relaxing their abdominal muscles.

The follow-up of the patients into the post-operative period showed that those in the special care group required significantly less narcotics after the operation, were rated as being more comfortable and in better physical and emotional condition, and were discharged from hospital sooner than those in the control group.

While this study indicates the advantages to be gained by providing information to patients, it also serves to illustrate the variety of forms that information may take. Some of the information concerned the types of procedures patients would encounter. Egbert *et al*. (1964) provided this to both the control and the special care group when the patients were informed that they would wake up in the recovery room. Sensory information was provided to the special care group in the form of descriptions of the location and duration of pain they should expect. Information was also given to the special care group in the form of instructions on how to behave to reduce pain. In addition to these three forms of information, the patients in the special care group were given general reassurance. The positive findings in this study are thus attributable to the combined effects of a number of different forms of information and general reassurance. This study does not address the question as to whether sensory or procedural information alone are effective in assisting post-operative recovery, or even whether the effects of information are negligible in comparison with the advantages of instructing the patients to adopt certain behaviours in the post-operative period.

More recent studies have indicated that the post-operative benefits of providing procedural information alone appear to be limited. Studies which have contrasted procedural information with the customary hospital practice generally have shown either little or no post-operative benefits from providing the procedural information (see Anderson and Masur 1983; Andrew 1970; Vernon and Bigelow 1974).

One may have expected that those patients who remember the information given to them would be more likely to be the ones who show any post-operative benefits. However in a study which showed that the providing of procedural information did result in post-operative benefits, those patients who remembered the information did not show superior recovery over those who remembered little of the information. While this study needs to be confirmed, it suggests that any simple explanation on the basis of procedural information providing a reduction in uncertainty is not adequate and that the process of providing the information results in some other process that is beneficial to recovery (see below for further discussion).

Johnson, Morrisey, and Leventhal (1973) contrasted the effects of procedural and sensory information in a group of gastrointestinal endoscopy patients. They found the patients provided with sensory information moved less during the procedure. While this study involved a local examination and no general anaesthetic or surgery, later studies on surgical patients have confirmed the view that sensory information has a more significant effect on recovery than procedural information (Mathews and Ridgeway 1984). Its effects, however, are not always produced with reliability. A combination of both procedural and sensory information appear to have greater post-operative effects than either presented alone.

One assumption in many of the studies that have considered the impact of information on post-operative recovery, is that the effects will be similar on all patients. Studies that have taken into account the differences in aspects of the personalities of patients suggest that the effects of information are not uniform.

Considering the coping style adopted by patients, one might expect those with a vigilant style to welcome information about the impending surgery and the post-operative discomfort, as this would provide them with more data to consider and evaluate. Its effect would also be to allow them to base their mental preparations on accurate information, thus restricting the development of fanciful ideas. On the other hand, to provide information to those whose technique is to deny and avoid would be to attempt to force them to behave contrary to their accustomed manner, and to contemplate unwanted ideas and feelings. These views are partially supported in a study by Andrews (1970), mentioned above, who separated subjects into three coping styles: avoiders, sensitizers (vigilant), and an intermediate group. Information was found to have a beneficial effect on the post-operative recovery of the intermediate group only. They were discharged earlier and required less post-operative medication. While those with a vigilant coping style showed no advantage with information, the avoidant group had an adverse reaction to information. Those avoiders who received information required significantly more medication and although not significant, also remained in the hospital for a longer period than those avoiders who received no information (see also DeLong 1970). The implication of this study is that with certain styles of coping, information may have an adverse effect on post-operative recovery and that information should not be dispensed without regard to the patient's personality. Although the pattern of research shows a negative effect of information on those with an avoidant coping style and positive advantages for those with a vigilant coping style, not all studies have shown this trend (Wilson 1981; see also Auerbach and Kilman 1977).

Three different proposals have been made to account for the manner in which information may serve to improve recovery from surgery. Janis (1958) suggested that information encouraged patients to engage in mental rehearsal which resulted in emotional preparation for the discomfort, pain, and threat of surgery. An alternative proposal has been advanced by Johnson (1975) who claims that the function of information is to reduce uncertainty of what the patient will encounter in the post-operative period. In addition the information serves to reassure the patients that what they experience in the post-operative period is not unusual and no cause for alarm. A third proposal is based on the theory of classical conditioning. Shipley *et al.* (1978) claim that the conditioned fear response to surgery is gradually extinguished by information that acts as a desensitizer.

The three proposals are not necessarily mutually exclusive and all three operate through a reduction in anxiety. In the first case this is by mental rehearsal, in the second by a reduction in uncertainty, and in the third via classical conditioning. It remains to be seen whether it is possible to tease out which mechanism may be operating in any particular situation.

BEHAVIOURAL INSTRUCTION AND RELAXATION

It is now customary for most hospitals to provide some instruction regarding the immediate post-operative behaviour of patients. In many cases this may be limited to coughing and physical movement. When instructions regarding post-operative behaviour have been considered in research studies, they have frequently been combined with sensory and procedural information. In these instances they have largely led to an improvement in post-operative recovery in comparison to the normal hospital procedures (Egbert *et al.* 1964; Fortin and Kirouac 1976; Healey

1968; Johnson 1966). In one study where the provision of behavioural instruction without any information was compared to patients receiving the normal hospital procedure, advantages were found for the group receiving behavioural instruction on measures of physical recovery such as vital capacity as well on the number of days before hospital discharge (Lindeman and Aernam 1971).

Some studies have specifically examined whether relaxation training is an effective form of behavioural instruction for surgical patients. This training customarily involves sequential tensing and relaxing of muscle groups and may also include breathing exercises (Kaplan, Atkins, and Lenhard 1982). Wilson (1981) compared the effects of relaxation training on elective cholecystectomy and hysterectomy patients with the provision of sensory information. The patients in the relaxation group were trained in relaxation on the day before surgery and then left with a tape to engage in relaxation training whenever they wished. Those who received relaxation training scored higher than the others on an index of general recovery and also required less medication for pain. Pickett and Clum (1982) examined the effects of relaxation of patients admitted for gallbladder surgery. Two types of relaxation were applied. One took the form of direct training of the patients. This was given to those patients who exhibited an external locus of control. For those patients with an internal locus of control, the relaxation training was given in the form of instructions that emphasized self-control. The relaxation training was only administered on one occasion, on the day before surgery, and the patients were not left a tape to train themselves as in the study by Wilson (1981). No advantage was found for the patients who received either of these forms of relaxation training over the control patients. The difference in these two findings may reflect the relative frequency and availability of relaxation following the initial training. Further controlled studies are required before a reasonable evaluation can be made of the efficacy of relaxation training in promoting post-operative recovery.

COGNITIVE BEHAVIOURAL INTERVENTION

Psychological intervention techniques for patients about to undergo surgery have followed the trend of psychological therapies in general, which have come increasingly to place greater emphasis on the patient's cognitions. By intervening, it is intended to train the patients in a technique which will allow them to cope with anxieties they have regarding surgery. Two general techniques have been applied. One attempts to redirect the patient's attention away from the disturbing cognitions regarding surgery and the other encourages a re-evaluation of the threatening cognitions about surgery. Both forms of intervention have led to improved post-operative recovery.

Pickett and Clum (1982) compared the post-operative recovery of two groups who received different forms of relaxation training. A control group received the normal hospital procedure. A second group were given training in a cognitive distraction technique. This training required patients to imagine ten different surgery scenes and then to direct their thoughts away from surgery to scenes involving pleasant situations. The patients who received the cognitive distraction training had a significantly greater reduction in post-surgical anxiety than the other groups.

In a more carefully controlled study on hysterectomy patients, Ridgeway and Mathews (1982) allocated patients to one of four groups. Three of these groups received a printed manual which were all the same length. In one case the manual contained procedural and sensory information. The second group received a manual which described details of the ward and hospital routines. The manual for the third group contained a cognitive intervention. It began by suggesting that patients are able to influence how they feel about events by choosing to dwell on the more positive elements of those events. It then went on to reassure the patients by minimizing general worries about surgery. Finally it requested the patients to imagine positive elements of surgery and to reappraise the negative aspects in a positive manner. A fourth group acted as a control and received no information. The patients were visited after the manual had been distributed to ensure they had read and understood the contents. The results indicated that those in the cognitive training group took fewer oral analgesics, received fewer analgesic injections, complained of less symptoms, and became active more rapidly than the other groups.

These results considered in conjunction with other studies suggest that cognitive training methods are particularly effective in improving the recovery of surgical patients (see also Langer, Janis, and Wolfer 1975; Peterson and Shigetomi 1981). These studies also serve to emphasize the role of cognitions in determining both the meaning attached to sensations and the behaviour consequent upon a sensation.

MODELLING

The viewing of a model undergoing a fearful event has been shown to reduce fears in an observer. A consequence of this finding has been the wide use of this technique in psychological treatment of anxiety, especially phobias (Bandura 1977; Marks 1981). Modelling techniques have been widely applied to children about to receive dental treatment with relatively favourable outcomes with regard to both the child's co-operativeness and the subjective level of fear of the child (Melamed *et al.* 1975a,b; 1978). Only a few studies have applied this technique to surgical patients. One study by Melamed and Siegel (1975) examined the effects of modelling on children about to undergo tonsillectomy, hernia repairs, or operations for urinary tract infections. One-half of the children viewed a film which depicted a child successfully coping with hernia surgery. The remaining children viewed a film which was totally unrelated to surgery. The group who watched the model successfully coping with surgery were found to have fewer concerns regarding surgery, lower subjective levels of anxiety, to display less anxiety-related behaviour, and to receive better post-operative behaviour ratings from their parents.

Given the impressive effects that watching a filmed model coping with surgery has on children, it is surprising that the technique has not been well studied on adults. The few studies that have been conducted have concerned investigative procedures which have not required a general anaesthetic (Shipley *et al.* 1978, 1979). One reason for the limited research on adults may reflect the fact that the filmed model procedure appears to have been introduced specifically to overcome the difficulties that children would have with the other forms of intervention and also to attempt to hold their attention to the message that was to be conveyed.

Showing a film of the surgery with a model does generally contain both sensory and procedural information as well as exhibiting a particular coping style. Research is required to examine the relative contribution made by these factors. A variable unique to this form of intervention is the relationship between the personal characteristics of the patient viewing the film and the model displayed in the film. It may be the case that variables such as the sex and age of the model influence the efficacy of the film.

PSYCHOTHERAPY AND HYPNOSIS

Brief psychotherapy has been suggested as a valuable technique in allaying patients' fears regarding surgery and offering emotional support and reassurance. Few studies have however, evaluated the effects of psychotherapy. In those studies which have been performed it is difficult to distinguish whether any particular contribution has been made by psychotherapy over and above information and general reassurance (see e.g. Dumas and Johnson 1972).

Hypnosis has also been advocated as a valuable intervention technique. The hypnotic sessions that have been applied in studies have focused on pain reduction, a reduction in discomfort, and relaxation. Some positive advantages have been found for hypnosis in a variety of surgical procedures as well as debridement following severe burns (Bonilla, Quigly, and Bowers 1961; Doberneck *et al.* 1959; Wakeman and Kaplan 1978). Unfortunately these studies suffer from a number of methodological flaws which restrict any conclusion regarding the efficacy of hypnosis until well-controlled studies have been performed.

Conclusion

The studies discussed above have demonstrated the range of factors which influence the course of anxiety of surgical patients and the variety of psychological techniques developed to reduce anxiety levels. A number of these techniques have been shown to produce improved post-operative recovery. Firm conclusions on the relative merits of one form of intervention over another and the general applicability of a technique to all surgical patients must be tempered by the various methodological problems in many studies, as well as the difficulty in making comparisons across studies. These difficulties include the range of surgical procedures studied with associated variations in threat they pose to the patient's life and the time before an indication of outcome is possible. The variety of knowledge and experience that subjects bring to surgery and the range of outcome measures used to assess recovery also contribute to the difficulty in arriving at any firm conclusions regarding types of psychological intervention. More well-controlled studies are needed to determine the efficacy of some of the techniques and whether other techniques are limited to certain types of surgery or patients.

A further difficulty is raised by the fact that many studies have compared the efficacy of an intervention technique to 'normal hospital procedures'. These procedures will not only vary from institution to institution, but will also be influenced by the changing traditions of medical practice. For example, it will be more difficult to indicate any effects of providing information in today's hospitals than it would have been twenty years ago. Surgical textbooks now place greater emphasis on providing patients with explanations and information, although the details of the information to be provided are frequently not specified (Frankel *et al.* 1982; Rains and Ritchie 1981). In some instances the guidance offered in these textbooks appears to be more indiscriminate than the current evidence would support. For example Rains and Ritchie (1981) writing in the current edition of Bailey and Love's *Short Practice of Surgery*, recommend providing explanations even to those patients who may be 'denying ostrich-fashion the realities of the operation'. The studies on the provision of information discussed above, suggest that with certain coping styles the provision of information may be counter-productive. This would suggest that a more careful assessment of the patient is required to obtain the maximum benefits from information.

None of the other forms of psychological intervention appear to be currently recognized in surgical textbooks or used in any routine fashion in hospitals. With further research the techniques that have the maximum ability to improve post-operative recovery may be integrated into normal hospital practice.

8　Satisfaction with health care

Ray Fitzpatrick

Introduction

With the benefit of historical hindsight it is clear that until the twentieth century health care depended almost entirely for its successes upon the placebo mechanism since few therapies were available that could be regarded as effective in modern terms. The very name of placebo, Latin for 'I will please', suggests that the satisfaction of the patient by the doctor or nurse was the crucial service that health care provided. Now, it may be said, the abundant scientific technology available to medicine makes such psychological devices as pleasing the patient archaic and almost unprofessional goals of care. Yet the last twenty years have seen intensified interest in the question of whether patients are satisfied with the treatment that they receive.

The significance of patient satisfaction

A number of analyses of the relations between medicine and society (Engel 1977; Freidson 1970; Kleinman 1980) converge in arguing that the very growth in scientific, technological approaches in medicine has had unforeseen and unfortunate consequences. Workers in the health care system, particularly doctors, are less sensitive to the concerns of their patients and to the personal significance for patients of the disorders that they present. According to this view the response of patients to this form of care has been increased dissatisfaction. The extent to which such an analysis is accurate, is something that can and should be examined by empirical investigation of patients' views.

CO-OPERATION WITH TREATMENT

One immediate consequence for health care of patient dissatisfaction has been clearly demonstrated. A sense of satisfaction with treatment received may be a crucial influence upon patients' co-operation with therapy. Disappointment or dissatisfaction upon leaving a clinic are likely to result in patients not following advice or taking prescriptions as indicated. Kincey, Bradshaw, and Ley (1975) found that, amongst patients attending a general practice in Liverpool, those who were dissatisfied with communication from their doctor were much more likely not to have followed the advice they received. A similar pattern was obtained when patients attending neurological out-patient clinics were asked their views about their consultation with the specialist and then followed up one year later (Fitzpatrick and Hopkins 1981a). Those who had been rated as dissatisfied with the information received from the doctor were subsequently much less likely to have taken medication as advised (see Chapter 6).

IDENTIFYING PROBLEMS IN HEALTH CARE

Increased effort has gone into identifying problems that patients experience with health care and into establishing how widespread or serious such problems are. A recent example in Great Britain is the investigation initiated by the Royal Commission on the National Health Service/Office of Population Censuses and Surveys (1978b). As one part of a general examination of the health services, the views of a sample of patients who had received hospital care were obtained on a number of aspects of their care. The results of such work identify serious problems associated with the working of a complex organization such as the National Health Service (NHS).[1] They concluded that two-thirds of the dissatisfaction expressed by respondents could have been eliminated by two elementary changes in hospital practice: making the time at which patients are woken up in the morning more reasonable and ensuring that patients are kept better informed about the progress of their illness.

THE EVALUATION OF HEALTH CARE

From the principles involved in obtaining patients' views in order to identify problems that they experience with health care, one can progress to more formal investigations where such views are systematically used as a measure in the evaluation of health care, and as a means of making better-informed decisions about changes in the way health care is provided. For obvious reasons the evaluation of health services has focused on morbidity and mortality. Nevertheless other possibilities exist. Sir Richard Doll (1973) identified three dimensions in terms of which the NHS could be evaluated: medical outcomes, economic efficiency, and social acceptability. Methods of evaluating medical outcomes have become increasingly exact, especially since the appearance of Cochrane's seminal work 'Effectiveness and Efficiency' (Cochrane 1972). Similarly, in recent years health economics has progressed as a discipline to examine economic efficiency (Culyer 1976). Doll argued that there were severe limitations in the sources of information for his third type of evaluation – social acceptability. The data from the complaints procedures of hospitals or family practitioner committees would offer only partial and limited evidence of patients' views. Doll therefore advocated the development of 'a medical equivalent of market research' (Doll 1983: 733). To the extent that methods could be developed for investigating patients' views with sufficient accuracy, then they could be incorporated as another element in decision-making about health services.

A random selection of studies from various countries attests to the variety of aspects of health care in which 'social acceptability' has been investigated. Varlaam, Dragoumis, and Jefferys (1972) examined patients' views in London of the care received from single-handed practitioners compared with partnerships of doctors. Breslau and Mortimer (1981) investigated parents' satisfaction in special clinics for disabled children and in particular were concerned with whether seeing one doctor continuously led to greater satisfaction than consulting several doctors. Romm, Hulka, and Mayo (1976) examined the outcomes of various forms of management of congestive heart failure and, in addition to assessing symptoms and levels of impairment of activity, also measured patient satisfaction. Adler *et al.* (1978) incorporated an assessment of views of patients and their families into a randomized controlled trial of early discharge from hospital for hernia and varicose veins. Several studies have been conducted in the United States to examine the differences between pre-paid insurance schemes for health care and fee for service (Ross, Wheaton, and Duff 1981; Tessler and Mechanic 1975). On a grander scale, Enterline *et al.* (1973) used measures of patient satisfaction as one of several means of evaluating the impact of the introduction of compulsory, universal health insurance in the province of Quebec, Canada. In each example the attempt is made to measure views accurately in order to contribute to the evaluation of a method or form of providing health care.

THE EXPERIENCE OF BEING A PATIENT

This field of research has also served a quite different purpose: it can be used to examine assumptions about the experience of being a patient. What are the major concerns of patients? How do patients approach and respond to medical consultations? It has been argued (Bloom and Wilson 1972) that both patient and doctor are governed by socially prescribed roles during consultations. One aspect of the patient's role is that, in response to questioning about his or her problems, the patient should reply with a description of the complaint rather than with a statement of expectations of the doctor in relation to the complaint. Stimson and Webb succinctly characterize respective roles thus: 'a doctor's instructions: "Now I want you to take these tablets three times a day" are not matched by a patient stating: "Now I want you to examine me and prescribe something appropriate" ' (Stimson and Webb 1975: 50).

One result of these rituals in the consultation is that many of the major concerns of patients remain unexpressed. Thus Korsch, Gozzi, and Francis (1968) interviewed mothers attending paediatric clinics, before their consultations. The consultations with the doctor were tape-recorded. Only 35 per cent of expectations and 24 per cent of main worries identified by the researchers were actually mentioned to the doctor. The formalities of deference and acceptance shown by the patient may disguise disagreements and disappointments. It is to research into patient satisfaction that one must turn for insights into the underlying experiences of the patient anticipating and reacting to medical consultations.

It is sometimes suggested that increased interest in patient satisfaction is one aspect of a wider social movement towards consumerism and that, furthermore, it is in many ways more beneficial for patients if they are thought of as consumers. More importance is likely to be attached to the patient's point of view, it is argued, if he or she is viewed as a consumer of health services. In fact this is not a completely convincing account of the origins of patient satisfaction research and it may not be particularly helpful to think of the patient as a consumer. The impetus towards investigating patients' views has come not so much from consumerist pressure as from the interests of third parties to the doctor–patient relationship such as the state which needs to know more about the value of services which it directly or indirectly funds. Increasingly, clinicians have also recognized the need to examine the impact of services from the patient's point of view (Barsky 1981). Stacey (1976) argues that it is misleading to think of the patient as a consumer: people do not normally retain concerns about health care beyond the time that they have to make use of them. Moreover, when someone seeks help from the health services, a more intimate relationship with the 'product' and the 'producer' is likely than is conveyed by the term 'consumer'. Thus the value of work in this field is more likely to be in its contribution to improving health care and more closely identifying patients 'needs' than in offering support for a new ideology regarding the patient's role.

Whatever the merits of consumerism in health care, it should be clear that patient satisfaction research contributes to a number of different issues: the task of identifying problems in health services from the patient's point of view; the need to evaluate comprehensively the impact of health services and a more general desire to understand how patients experience and respond to health care. These different tasks to some extent coincide but, at the same time, many of the difficulties in this new field, to which attention is drawn in this chapter, reflect the variety of demands that are made of the concept of patient satisfaction.

The concept of satisfaction and its measurement

It is quite remarkable that, despite wide agreement upon the importance of patient satisfaction as a concept, there is much less consensus as to its meaning. Locker and Dunt (1978) conclude a review of the subject by saying that 'it is rare to find the concept of patient satisfaction defined and there has been little clarification of what the term means either to researchers who employ it or respondents who respond to it' (Locker and Dunt 1978: 283).

One interpretation of the term is quite common. In much research the object of investigation has been an assumed attitude or set of attitudes held by the respondent in relation to such matters as the approach and manner of doctors or the quality of health care received (Linder-Pelz 1982). The assumption of such research is that people adopt relatively stable views in the form of attitudes that can be identified by the researcher. This sense of satisfaction shades into a slightly different use to which the concept is sometimes put – to identify respondents' views of the value of particular consultations or stays in hospital to specific health problems experienced by respondents. Although it is reasonable to imagine that evaluations of specific episodes form the basis of general attitudes to health care and that therefore the two aspects are part of a continuum, it is nevertheless useful to distinguish the two in trying to make sense of the field. Attitudes in general may be quite distinct from and independent of evaluations of the benefits of particular consultations. In this chapter consideration is given to both ways in which satisfaction has been understood and investigated.

It has been more often employed in its first sense – as an attitude. Although in everyday life we frequently and without difficulty infer attitudes from other people's remarks and behaviour, more rigorous identification and research into attitudes has proved more difficult. These difficulties are reflected in the field of patient satisfaction research.

One very obvious problem in investigating patient satisfaction is uncertainty as to whether respondents' answers to questions correspond to their real views. There would appear to be quite strong pressures on patients to express socially acceptable views when talking about health care. French reports from her study of patients undergoing surgery that she experienced 'a perceptible frosting of the atmosphere' when she asked patients for their views about their treatment (French 1981: 27). They wished to avoid implied personal criticism of the staff. It may be that patients make less use of socially desirable answers if the researcher is less identified with the health care service that is being discussed. Similarly it is reasonable to assume that patients express more frank views in the privacy of their own homes. However, one of the few studies that offers data on this question (Raphael 1969), found that patients asked to give their views after discharge from hospital at home expressed less dissatisfaction than a comparable group who took part in the study whilst still in hospital.

It is also possible to avoid misleading responses by more careful attention to methods of obtaining views. Several studies (Hulka *et al.* 1975c; Ware and Snyder 1975) have attempted to identify more precisely the dimensions into which patients' views about health care form. In Ware and Snyder's study the views of respondents with regard to a number of different aspects of health care were elicited. Respondents were asked to respond to items (some examples of which are given in *Table 11*) on what is known as a Likert format of choices, selecting

Table 11 *Ware and Snyder's Satisfaction Scale: examples of initial aspects investigated and of items used for each aspect*

aspect	number of items for aspect	example of item, attitude to which sought
information giving	4	doctors are careful to explain what the patient is expected to do
thoroughness	4	doctors examine their patients thoroughly before deciding what's wrong
cost of care	4	the cost of medical care is reasonable
courtesy and respect	4	sometimes doctors make the patient feel foolish
continuity of care	2	I see the same doctor just about every time I go

Source: Ware and Snyder (1975).

between 'strongly agree', 'agree', 'uncertain', 'disagree', 'strongly disagree'. Thus the respondent is given an equal opportunity to select
positive and negative views. Locker and Dunt (1978) suggest that less
critical comments are given in reply to open-ended questions (What do
you think about . . . ?) compared with specific questions (Did you get
the information that you wanted?). Increased confidence in methods may
be gained by testing questionnaires for reliability. Respondents can be
re-interviewed with the same questions or the correlations inspected
between questions thought to measure the same concept (Ware and
Snyder 1975). Despite greater care in methodology it has to be acknowledged that a wide variety of approaches are in use and this makes the
comparison of studies sometimes difficult.

The dimensions of patients' views about health care

One general question is of importance in this field: about which aspects
of their health care do people form views that the researcher may investigate? One argument might be that, as a layman is incapable of
appreciating any of the technical complexities of modern medicine, there
can be little of value that the patient is capable of judging. The responses
obtained in interviews would, in this view, be artefacts of the questions
posed.

   One way of approaching this problem is to obtain patients' views
about a particular health care facility on which one has an independent
source of data. In this way it is possible to see which, if any, aspects of
the facility are discerned and form the basis of patients' views. This
approach was adopted by DiMatteo *et al.* (1980). Seventy-one doctors
working in a New York community hospital were assessed by the
researchers for their sensitivity to human emotions. This was done by
means of two tasks that they were asked to perform. Firstly they had to
interpret the non-verbal emotions shown by subjects in a film designed
for the study. In the second task, they had themselves to demonstrate any
of four different emotions on a film that was subsequently rated by other
participants in the study. Patients consulting the doctors in the hospital
were then asked how satisfied they were with their doctor's technical
care and with such inter-personal skills as showing concern for the
patient. The doctors' inter-personal skills, as reflected in their scores, for
example, in tasks requiring the interpretation of emotions from non-
verbal cues, were found to be significantly associated with patients'
rating of their inter-personal qualities in clinical conditions but were not
associated with patients' ratings of doctors' technical skills. The study
is evidence that patients' views are formed in response to particular
experiences in their encounters with health care and are not therefore
random expressions of feeling.

Stiles *et al.* (1979) pursued a similar strategy to explore the objective events within consultations that might be linked to patients feeling satisfied with the inter-personal skills of their doctor. The consultations of nineteen doctors providing general medical care were tape-recorded and patients were interviewed to assess their satisfaction. Communication between doctors and patients was coded according to the supposed intention identified by the researchers, for example, disclosing information. The main conclusion reached when the two sets of data were combined was that satisfaction with the inter-personal or human qualities of a doctor was most associated with those forms of dialogue within the consultation that most enabled patients to describe their problems in their own words. The authors conclude that patients who had an opportunity to convey their own perspective, and felt the doctor had listened, were more likely to feel that the doctor had been interested and understanding. The more general significance of such work is to suggest that research can reveal views that form in response to particular experiences in health care and that such views are of potential value for the evaluation of health services.

A related concern in patient satisfaction research has been to identify the different dimensions of health care that appear to be distinguishable in the views of patients obtained in surveys and in terms of which people tend to form attitudes.

For this purpose Ware and Snyder (1975) interviewed people from a sample of Illinois households. Their views were obtained about the quality of their health care by means of a questionnaire. In the first stage attitudes to eighty different aspects of care were obtained by means of between two and four questions for each aspect. Some examples of the different aspects into which they enquired and the items by means of which they assessed attitudes have been given in *Table 11*. Thus respondents were asked their views about, for example, 'continuity of care' by means of two items, one of which was 'I see the same doctor just about every time I go.' For every item respondents had a Likert format of choices as described earlier. The replies on all eighty aspects of care were then examined by means of a factor analysis, the purpose of which was to show into how many common factors respondents' views clustered. They concluded that the sample evaluated their care in terms of four different dimensions:

1 The doctor's conduct
2 Availability of care
3 Continuity and convenience
4 Financial accessibility

In other words these were the separate criteria in terms of which people judged the quality of their health care.

Ware and Snyder (1975) conclude that although people may distinguish between different aspects of a doctor's conduct, such as his medical contribution to their problems versus his manner and friendliness, they nevertheless tend to develop a single global attitude regarding his conduct that merges technical and humane qualities. This interpretation clashes with the evidence cited above by DiMatteo *et al.* (1980) that patients form sharply distinctive views of the two aspects of their doctor. Support from surveys for this latter view comes from the study by Hulka *et al.* (1975). In their survey of attitudes, respondents did form distinctive views of doctors' professional technical qualities compared to more personal qualities. These issues are some distance from resolution. The work nevertheless is evidence that patients' views are discriminating and based on fairly complex judgements.

Satisfaction in relation to different aspects of health care

SATISFACTION WITH HEALTH CARE IN BRITAIN

A number of surveys of patients' attitudes to health care in Britain and in the United States suggest certain common themes. An important source for patients' views of primary care in England and Wales is the recent survey by Cartwright and Anderson (1981). They report that nine-tenths of their sample described themselves as satisfied or very satisfied with the care that they received from their family doctor. This very favourable overall view of patients in relation to health care is by no means unusual. High levels of general satisfaction are commonly found in such surveys and sharply challenge any simplistic notion of a profound and widespread disenchantment with modern medical care. The methodological problems have been acknowledged that might cast doubt on such results but it is all the more remarkable, given the diversity of methods used that consistently high levels of general satisfaction are recorded. It is with regard to specific dimensions of health care that greater variability in patients' views is found. Thus Cartwright and Anderson asked people whether their doctor was 'good' or 'not so good' on a number of different matters. The comfort of the doctor's waiting room gave rise to the highest proportion of critical responses – 30 per cent. The next most criticized aspect of the general practitioner was whether or not he explained things fully to the patient; 23 per cent felt their doctor was not so good in this respect. Far fewer were critical about whether their doctor examined them thoroughly or listened carefully to them. From a somewhat differently worded question 11 per cent were in some way critical of the way in which their doctor prescribed.

Just as the amenities of general practice are a common focus of criticism, so too in the Royal Commission's investigation (OPCS 1978b), amongst hospital in-patients 21 per cent and 19 per cent were dissatisfied respectively with food and washing facilities. The single most criticized aspect of hospital experience was being woken too early, with which 43 per cent were dissatisfied. This is not too surprising since nearly half the respondents had been woken at six o'clock or earlier!

The Royal Commission's study points to the same problems as did Cartwright and Anderson (1981) with 31 per cent of in-patients and 25 per cent of out-patients dissatisfied with the information they received about the progress of their illness. Indeed dissatisfaction with information is the single most common concern expressed by patients (Locker and Dunt 1978). Attention now needs to be devoted to the kinds of information that patients feel doctors ought to be giving. Kincey, Bradshaw, and Ley's (1975) study of general practice suggests that patients were more dissatisfied with the information they received about the causes of their illness than with information about the nature of their treatment. In the study of neurological clinics cited earlier (Fitzpatrick and Hopkins 1981a) dissatisfaction about information mostly focused on the lack of explanations about dietary, environmental, and psychological factors that might be involved in the causes of the headaches of which the patients complained. Far fewer expressed concern to know more about the 'underlying mechanisms' for the symptoms in the medical sense. Technical, physiological explanations were of less importance than discussion of factors in everyday life upon which the patient might act to avoid or reduce symptoms. Few expressed dissatisfaction with the explanations of treatment that they received.

SATISFACTION WITH HEALTH CARE IN THE UNITED STATES

There are many similarities in the perspectives of American patients as reflected in surveys. For example, in a study of people enrolled in either a pre-paid or fee for service health plan (Gray 1980), amongst both groups dissatisfaction was most commonly expressed about information given to the patient.[2] A study of subscribers to pre-paid health care only (Pope 1978) found that the proportion dissatisfied with information given was only surpassed by those dissatisfied with the time spent in getting appointments and with delays between obtaining an appointment and the appointment itself. In both studies the competence and technical performance of doctors gave rise to less dissatisfaction than other factors.

Forms of providing health care are more varied in the United States compared with England and Wales and in recent years have experienced several changes, especially away from traditional, single-handed, fee for service practices. Several studies (e.g. Tessler and Mechanic 1975) suggest that newer forms give rise to more dissatisfaction on whatever dimension measured despite the fact that a higher standard of care is generally provided. It has been suggested that large pre-paid clinics are more bureaucratic and less patient-oriented than the traditional fee for service practice. However an elegant study by Ross, Wheaton, and Duff (1981) showed that patients start with negative images of large pre-paid group practices and are more critical than are the patients of fee for service, smaller practices. When, however, patients who have had several years' experience of the respective types are compared, patients of pre-paid practices emerge as more satisfied. Ross and colleagues argue that over time the better psychosocial care of pre-paid practice is appreciated by patients and outweighs initial prejudices.

The technical and the personal dimensions of care

Hulka *et al.* (1975c) concluded from their interviews that whereas 27 per cent were to some extent dissatisfied or neutral in views about the costs and convenience of medical care, 14 per cent expressed such views about the personal qualities of their doctor, and only 6 per cent with regard to the doctor's skills and competence. This is one instance of the frequently reported contrast thought to exist in patients' attitudes to technical compared to other aspects of health care. One over-view of evidence concluded: 'The American public is generally more satisfied with the technical aspect of medical treatment than with the interpersonal component or with costs and accessibility' (Pope 1978: 293). Similar contrasts have been made about the focus of satisfaction and dissatisfaction in British reactions to health care:

'patients seldom criticize their doctor's clinical judgement or their technical competence. A not inconsiderable minority . . . will complain about the difficulty of consulting their doctor as soon as they would like. Even more will confess that their general practitioner is not so warm or friendly as they would like or that they have difficulty in telling him all that they feel he should know about them and their condition.'

(Jefferys 1977: 188)

Evidence to support this view has already been cited. However the idea that patients are more satisfied with the technical aspects of their care has to be treated with some caution. First, some surveys simply do not investigate those aspects of patients' views. The Royal Commission's survey argued:

'It was decided not to ask patients about their satisfaction with their actual treatment and with the standard of medical care they had received for two reasons: firstly there was no objective standard against which to set their answers and secondly it was felt that the patient's own views on his treatment would not be a sound basis on which to make recommendations for changes or improvements.'

(OPCS 1978b: 5)

Another difficulty is that respondents may be more uneasy about expressing frank views about the medical aspects of their care relative to such 'safer' subjects as the comfort of the waiting room. Finally it was pointed out by Freidson (1961) that patients may indeed normally assume a certain level of basic competence in health care professionals. Nevertheless what matters most to a patient is the *application* of that ability to the patient's presenting problem. This may be less taken for granted by patients at the time they actually seek help as it requires the doctor's interest and involvement in the patient as well as his technical abilities. It may be less easy to grapple with such complexities in the format of a survey.

Satisfaction and demographic factors

Patients' responses to health care may, of course, reveal much less about the quality or appropriateness of the treatment they receive and much more about the varying values and expectations that exist in different groups in society. Some investigations have therefore been careful to take account of the influence of social characteristics such as social class and demographic variables such as age and gender.

Perhaps the most consistent finding is that older people tend to be more satisfied with health care than the young. This is the case for example in Raphael's study (1969) of admissions to London hospitals and in Pope's study (1978) of American pre-paid group practice. One possible reason for older people expressing more satisfaction is that they are more aware of the changes in access to health care such as the NHS or Medicare and are less ready to criticize. Their expectations of health care may be more modest. Respondents over sixty-five years of age were found by Cartwright and Anderson (1981) to expect less information from their family doctor.

There may be real differences between the young and old in their encounters with medicine that account for differences in satisfaction. Older patients may have closer relationships with their doctor (Cartwright and Anderson 1981: 170). A small-scale study of one general practice found that patients less than twenty-five years of age were more likely to be dissatisfied (Bradley 1981). The author, as a general practitioner with knowledge of the content of consultations, concluded that it was the dynamics of the encounter between younger patients and the doctor, rather than higher levels of expectations held by the young, that led to their greater dissatisfaction. The author concluded:

'The feelings of these dissatisfied patients that they had not felt able to describe their trouble or discuss their problems fully, had not been told what was wrong and had not understood or agreed with what they were told were highly significant. Their consultations had clearly been unsuccessful: in particular they shared the common element of a patient frustrated in discussion, explanation and agreement rather than thwarted by the rejection of wild or unreasonable demands.'

(Bradley 1981: 423)

The relationship between satisfaction and social class or income level is less consistent across studies. In many studies (Breslau and Mortimer 1981; Korsch, Gozzi and Francis 1968; Larsen and Rootman 1976) socio-economic variables play a minimal role. Cartwright and Anderson's (1981) results show similar attitudes to most aspects of general practice held by middle-class and working-class respondents. However they do show that the general practitioners of middle-class patients are somewhat more likely than those of working-class patients to have smaller list sizes, more practice equipment such as an ECG machine, and more further medical qualifications. To the extent that such facilities represent some aspects of the quality of care from a general practitioner, then it might be argued that working-class respondents are expressing satisfaction with lower levels of care and, by inference, have somewhat lower expectations (Cartwright and Anderson 1981: 179).

Generally although the role of such characteristics in influencing attitudes to health care requires careful attention, there is little evidence that they alone play a consistent role. Moreover even in those studies (e.g. Pope 1978) in which social and demographic variables are significantly related to views, it is usually the case that they explain only a small amount of the variance in attitudes expressed.

Expectations

The term 'expectations' has already been invoked to explain differences in response to health care. There is intuitive sense in the statement that the degree of satisfaction expressed by a patient is very largely influenced by his or her initial expectations. The higher levels of dissatisfaction reported by younger or middle-class respondents can easily be interpreted in these terms. However the apparent simplicity of the concept of expectations in this context is misleading. Stimson and Webb observed in the course of their study of patients attending British general practices: ' "Expectation" seems to be a concept which, like so many others used in describing social aspects of medicine . . . is extremely difficult to examine analytically' (Stimson and Webb 1975: 27).

One problem is that, although it is very convenient to explain, for example, the differences in levels of satisfaction between one social group and another as being due to different expectations, there have been few attempts to clarify what is meant and to support the interpretation by the measurement of expectations separately from satisfaction. One has to assume that the concept here refers to some notion of 'standards' or 'aspirations' in relation to health care. There is very little clarity or consensus as to whether such attitudes exist as identifiable, stable properties of individuals or groups.

Most research has in any case concentrated on expectations in a quite different sense from 'standards'. The emphasis has been on the kinds of actions, approaches and treatments by the doctor that patients expect. These may be expectations held in relation to a specific illness episode and consultation or more generally. However the ambiguities of the concept have bedevilled research in the field. Expectations may refer either to hopes and desires for what ideally should happen or to guesses and predictions of what is likely to happen (Stimson and Webb 1975: 27). It is important to be clear about which is the focus of interest when patients are asked about their expectations. In practice the ideal and the probable are going to be intimately connected in a patient's views about treatment.

These problems are illustrated in a study by Fitton and Acheson who investigated the expectations of general practice held by English patients (Fitton and Acheson 1979). They considered whether patients preferred their doctor to be restricted in interest to their medical problems or to be more generally interested in them as persons. The majority preferred the doctor to be interested in them as a person as well as in their medical condition. Partly they felt that only with knowledge of the person could the doctor deal with many kinds of medical problems. One-third expected the doctor to confine his interest to the medical. However, this is a good example of the realities of expectations influencing notions of the ideal. Many felt that it was unreasonable to expect the doctor to take an interest in the person. One patient is quoted as saying: 'It is impossible to expect doctors to handle people as individual persons. The most you can ask for is medical competence' (Fitton and Acheson 1979: 78).

The same study also found that more patients preferred a 'business-like but friendly' approach from the doctor to a 'personal and friendly' or an impersonal and business-like style. Although the exact meaning of the choices made by respondents may not be clear, it would appear that the majority felt that their own doctor corresponded to the ideal. This could be either because patients select doctors who correspond to their role expectations or they adjust their expectations to reality. There are some similarities here with an American study of mothers' expectations of their paediatrician (Breslau *et al.* 1975). They were asked how comprehensive they expected the services and abilities of the paediatrician to be. Replies suggested that a narrow basis of technical competence was far more important than more general psychological skills. On the other hand the mothers preferred care by a single doctor and felt that this was likely to ensure that the doctor understood and had rapport with the individual patient. Thus the narrow, traditional, medical skills were expected to be complemented by seeing one doctor continuously. This combination, the authors conclude, is precisely the one that the profession has taught patients to expect. Thus expectations are heavily influenced by experience. Both Fitton and Acheson and Cartwright and Anderson show that the majority of respondents express a preference for the British referral system whereby a patient sees a general practitioner before seeing a specialist rather than having direct access to a hospital doctor. The reasons given by respondents appear to reflect as much the interests of the medical profession as of the patient. Thus one of Cartwright and Anderson's respondents says of the possibility of direct hospital access: 'From a selfish point of view it would be great. But from a practical commonsense point of view it could be a terrible waste of a professional man's time' (Cartwright and Anderson 1981). The quotation clearly shows the complexities behind the notion of expectations.

Images of the patient's experience of care

At the beginning it was suggested that patient satisfaction research has not only developed as a means of evaluating health services and of selecting more appropriate forms of care. It has also played an important role in offering concepts for understanding how patients seek help for their health problems and subsequently evaluate the help that they have received. At least some of the difficulties that are acknowledged to exist (Stimson and Webb 1975: 77–8) in the use of the concept of satisfaction have arisen because a number of different images, assumptions, or models have emerged about the experiences of patients, which although fundamentally contrasting in emphasis have been collapsed or confused under the single concept of satisfaction. Each set of assumptions draws attention to some important aspects of being a patient, but sometimes the assumptions have severe limitations. It is therefore worthwhile considering the images and assumptions separately.

THE NEED FOR THE FAMILIAR

This first approach emphasizes the importance of expectations, socially created and varying from one social group to another, that patients come to form of the role of the doctor and of the health care system. These general expectations are the primary determinant of the degree of satisfaction that a patient experiences from encounters with health care. The most graphic example of such influences appears where there are considerable cultural differences between patient and doctor. Kleinman, Eisenberg, and Good (1978) describe the case of a young Chinese man attending a Massachusetts hospital and presenting with various symptoms such as tiredness, back pains, and insomnia for which no specific causes could be found on investigation. He appeared depressed but did not define his problems in emotional terms. He refused psychotherapy on the basis that talk could be of no benefit but accepted psychiatric care provided that it included medication. His definition of his problem was 'wind' and 'not enough blood' which he attributed to over-indulgence in sexual relations. The authors argue that the patient's view of his symptoms and treatment can only be understood in terms of a Chinese theory of a balance of humours, which, when upset, results in 'not enough blood' and requires symbolically 'hot' foods as remedies. The patient accepted medication as potentially relevant to this balance between 'hot' and 'cold' but could see no value in the talk that formed one of the psychiatrist's main treatments for a diagnosis of depression. The authors conclude: 'Discrepancies between his culturally patterned treatment expectations and those of his doctors almost led him to drop out of professional care' (Kleinman, Eisenberg, and Good 1978: 253).

Henley (1979) in discussing the health care experiences of Asian communities in Britain describes numerous cultural differences between migrant and indigenous cultural expectations. Thus Henley points out that: 'Asian patients may be worried by the less personal style of health provision in Britain. Some, particularly East African Asians, may be upset for example, by the short and infrequent visits of doctors to the wards' (Henley 1979: 58). Henley argues that such expectations are based on the experience of more personal relationships with doctors than are the norm in their country of origin.

These are all examples of patients who, by virtue of migration, are confronted with the unfamiliar forms of western medicine (further examples are discussed in Chapter 4). To what extent within western culture are there differing role expectations of the doctor? Larsen and Rootman (1976) examined this question by asking people from a household sample in Alberta, Canada, to complete questionnaires about their expectations with regard to a number of aspects of the doctor's behaviour such as whether the doctor should avoid giving advice over the phone or should call patients in for regular check-ups. They were then asked whether their doctor conformed to each of these expectations. The authors then assessed overall satisfaction with the doctor and found that this was significantly related to whether patients reported their doctors as conforming to expectations. Such evidence supports Mechanic's view that people have 'an image of the physician's role and the way it should be performed'. In terms of this image 'the patient attempts to evaluate the professional qualifications and capabilities of the doctor' (Mechanic 1978: 407).

One potential limitation of this approach is that it adopts too static a view of the relationship between doctors and patients and implies that attempts to alter the relationship are particularly problematic. Marsh (1977) reports an effort in his general practice to reduce the amount of prescribing for minor self-limiting symptoms. In appropriate consultations, instead of a prescription or medication, patients were given reassurance about the nature of their symptoms, indications for reconsultation were explained and the limitations of medication were discussed. As a result, the rate of prescribing in the practice fell by 19 per cent. Although patients' views of this change were not systematically obtained Marsh felt that they responded favourably. If his impression is correct, then their role expectations of the doctor were not so fixed that a significant change in style of practice, if explained to patients, could not be accepted.

The example of prescribing holds another lesson. One of the most commonly reported expectations held by British patients in relation to their general practitioner is that the consultation should conclude with the prescription of a drug (Bradley 1981; Fitton and Acheson 1979; Rapoport 1979). However it is not clear whether such expectations are the patients' hopes or goals from the consultation or rather their predictions from past experience. Support for the latter view comes from a study by Rapoport (1979) in which it was shown that the total prescribing rate of the particular doctor consulted by the patient was the best predictor of whether patients in the general practice studied reported themselves as expecting a drug prescription at their consultation. Their expectations were thus in the main accurate predictions from past experience.

Generally this first approach makes clear that by virtue of belonging to a particular culture and through an accumulation of experiences of contacts with doctors, patients do come to hold expectations of doctors in the sense of stereotypic ways in which they are expected to act. This approach is less convincing at showing that such stereotypes always play the determining role in how a patient evaluates consultations with the doctor.

THE IMPORTANCE OF EMOTIONAL NEEDS

A very different approach argues that most problems patients bring to doctors involve an emotional or 'affective' component, for example arising from uncertainty and anxiety as to the seriousness of the problem. The patient is unable to judge how much the doctor's actions contribute to the solution of the problem because of lack of medical knowledge. On the other hand the way the doctor acts with regard to the patient, by for example showing interest and offering reassurance, can be observed by the layman. Hence, it is argued, the degree of emotional support felt by the patient and directed to his or her affective concerns will largely influence how satisfied he or she is with a consultation. Thus the doctor's 'affective' behaviour such as showing interest is a greater influence over the patient than his 'instrumental' behaviour – bringing to bear technical competence. Ben-Sira (1976) explored this approach in interviews with a sample of Israelis about their general practitioners. They were asked about their satisfaction in relation to treatment from their doctor and the doctor's technical skills and administrative aspects of his practice such as waiting times and the helpfulness of administrative staff. They were also asked for their views about the doctor's 'affective behaviour', such as showing interest in and giving sufficient time to the patient. Also an assessment was made as to how much respondents felt their doctor conceded to requests that were made to him. Results showed that satisfaction with treatment by the doctor was much more strongly related to perceptions of interest and devotion by the doctor (affective behaviour) than to the other factors measured.

Ben-Sira argues in a subsequent study (Ben-Sira 1980) that the link between the affective behaviour of the doctor and satisfaction on the part of the patient will be stronger in patients who are currently more concerned about their health, as they will be more emotionally involved in their presenting problems and more influenced by the emotional support received from the doctor. Also it is argued that the influence of affective behaviour upon patient satisfaction will be greater among the less well educated, who are less likely to be able to judge the doctor's technical actions. Both ideas are supported in the study where the strength of the original associations could be looked at within groups who differed in their level of concern about health and level of education.

This approach offers an interesting solution to the question of how patients respond to and evaluate their health care when they lack the expertise, according to this theory. However, the view that it is the degree of interest and concern from the doctor that influences the patient rests on evidence largely from interviews separate in time from actual episodes of seeking help for illness. Further examination is needed as to the extent to which patterns found in surveys indicate processes that are important at the time patients receive treatment.

THE GOALS OF HELP-SEEKING

The third approach looks more closely at how patients themselves describe the experience of anticipating and responding to health care. According to this approach, although patients may sometimes be able to express such experiences in terms of 'expectations' or 'satisfaction', such terms provide only limited insights into what matters most to patients when seeking help for health problems. It is more important to look at the major goals or concerns which patients have in relation to their health problems and their subsequent judgements as to whether treatment is helpful. The importance of this apparently minor shift in concepts should become clearer by examining the applicability of concepts to patients' own accounts.

How do patients themselves describe their expectations when they go to see a doctor? Stimson and Webb (1975) found that the majority of patients attending the general practices that they studied did express to researchers some kind of expectation prior to their consultations. A prescription was the expectation most frequently cited. However, as was discussed earlier, the meaning of expectations used by respondents was unclear: 'expectations can be used in the sense of how one actor hopes or would like the other to behave or act and again in terms of how he usually does act on the basis of past experience' (Stimson and Webb 1975: 28). The patients that they studied were more often expressing probable rather than ideal outcomes. These expectations were more concretely and clearly expressed where the patient already had some idea of the diagnosis, had already received treatment for the problem, or had more knowledge of the doctor.

Other studies suggest that patients may find it quite difficult to report expectations either when they are attending for a health problem about which they are quite unsure or when they are consulting a health service with which they are unfamiliar. Lipton and Svarstad (1974) examined the expectations of American parents who were about to present children to a multi-disciplinary diagnostic clinic. Three-quarters of the sample expressed a desire for some kind of tests or check-up for their children but generally could not specify any particular kind of investigation. The few who did cite a particular test qualified their remarks by deferring to the professional's judgement. Similar responses were given when asked whether they expected to see any particular kind of specialist. They often felt that they were guessing about their expectations or that it was not appropriate to have expectations. A typical remark was: 'Well, whatever they think is necessary to do. I'm not the doctor right?' (Lipton and Svarstad 1974: 164).

British studies have shown similar problems in identifying expectations in patients referred from their general practitioner to a hospital specialist. Skuse, investigating patients' views of referral to a hospital psychiatry clinic concludes: 'Three-quarters had no clear idea of what help might be offered them at the clinic, usually because they had no idea what psychiatrists did' (Skuse 1975: 470). In the absence of firm ideas, patients imagined possibilities: 'Mrs A. told me they put things on your head and give you shock treatment and examine your brain' (Skuse 1975: 470).

The same uncertainty was expressed by patients presenting headaches at neurology clinics (Fitzpatrick and Hopkins 1983). The majority of patients were unaware of the kind of specialist they were about to see. The lack of conviction behind expressed expectations was revealed in the way that respondents used the research interview itself to formulate ideas about the coming consultation. One patient, asked about the likelihood of tests replied: 'I didn't particularly give it too much thought but now you mention it, I wouldn't be surprised if they . . .'

The expectations that were expressed arose less out of stable views of the doctor's role of the kind discussed above in Larsen and Rootman's work and more out of their thoughts about their illness. In particular concepts of the possible psychological and dietary causes of headaches were the source of patients' speculations as to what to expect from the doctor.

There is some evidence of the terms in which patients tend to judge consultations afterwards. Stimson and Webb (1975) found it difficult to categorize patients' responses to general practice consultations in terms of satisfaction. They suggest that people's views fluctuate over time as they reappraise their consultations in the light of changes in their symptoms. It is misleading to summarize such complex, changing views in terms of satisfaction. The patients attending neurological clinics subsequently expressed a wide range of positive and negative comments about their doctor, especially with regard to the perceived thoroughness with which the history of the patient's problem had been investigated. However critical comments were frequently qualified, lest the patient appear ungrateful, thoughtless, or simply ignorant of the realities of medical work. As one patient explained: 'I know they are busy, I felt he didn't go deep enough into what was causing them, but, there again, I wasn't expecting him to when he's got other patients to see.'

Much more clearly recognizable in patients' comments were judgements of the success or value of their hospital visit in terms of their health problems. Three different reactions to the clinics were identified: 'a successful visit', 'a failure', or 'waste of time' and a more cautious 'wait and see' response. More negative responses to the clinics were most often associated with patients who had hoped to learn more about their illness or to increase their ability to avoid episodes of headaches. Positive or cautious responses were generally from patients seeking reassurance about the significance of their headaches or some form of symptomatic treatment.

It is now possible to consider the importance of expectations in determining such responses. If by expectations is meant the guesses and predictions tentatively expressed before their consultations, they played no role in determining patients' responses; patients, for example, cited expectations before the clinic which were not met in their consultations but did not become a matter of concern or comment afterwards. Expectations were frequently felt by patients to emerge in the course of consultations or afterwards. Three distinct problems were identified in patients attending the clinics: concern for reassurance, for symptomatic relief, and for preventive intervention. Expectations of how the clinics might relate to such concerns were equally unclear in all three kinds of problem. Patients with a concern for preventive intervention were most likely to be subsequently disappointed.

In summary it provided only limited insights to examine patients' experiences in terms of expectations and satisfaction. Patients rarely expressed firm expectations and were uncomfortable and uninterested in forming attitudes as such in relation to the clinics. Moreover if one remembers one central task of patient satisfaction research – to contribute to the evaluation of health services – attitudes expressed about the doctors and clinics were less revealing of the strengths and weaknesses of the clinics investigated than were patients' views of their health problems and of the extent to which clinic visits had been worthwhile. Clinics that were quite successful at reassuring patients concerned about serious disease did less well at giving people information of the causes of their symptoms, or at least of the limits of medical understanding of causes.

Conclusion

The need for the effectiveness of medical procedures to be more rigorously examined is steadily gaining acceptance (Bunker, Fowles, and Schaffarzick 1982). As attention has focused upon the outcomes of medicine and the methodology of their assessment, it has become clearer that a wider range of indicators of outcomes are essential to do justice to the aims of modern health care. Concentration on mortality statistics or changes in pathological processes too narrowly limits the focus. One broad range of indicators upon which medicine aspires to be judged are those concerned with the patient's quality of life. Many modern technological interventions, such as hip replacement operations, are partly judged in such terms. Yet a review by Najman and Levine (1981) shows that research evaluating the impact of medical interventions upon the quality of life is, for the most part, underdeveloped and that in particular, the patient's subjective perspective has yet to be seriously incorporated into such evaluative research. This chapter should have made it clear that methods of eliciting the patient's perspective are still evolving and that there are a variety of distinct approaches to the task of discovering the matters of greatest concern to patients. Nevertheless the investigation of patients' views about health care will become an increasingly central element in the development of health services.

Notes

1 For readers unfamiliar with the National Health Service, it is a system in which nearly all health care costs, with exceptions such as some of the costs of drugs and of dental and optical services, are met out of national taxation rather than privately paid fees. The distinction between hospital-based specialists and the community-based general practitioner is much sharper than in the United States. Access to hospital services can normally only be obtained through the general practitioner on whose 'list' the individual is registered.
2 Traditionally the doctor in the United States worked in a single-handed ('solo') practice and earned an income from fees paid by the patient at each consultation. Although the majority of doctors still work independently, there is a growing trend towards group practices in which several doctors share facilities. Similarly only one-third of personal health care is paid for by patients in the traditional 'out of pocket' way and many practices are involved in schemes in which the individual's insurance covers most costs. Hence the term 'pre-paid' practice.

Part 3
Chronic and terminal illness

9 The psychological consequences of cerebrovascular accident and head injury

Stanton Newman

Introduction

The need for an explanation of the experience of illness that integrates biological, psychological, and social factors is clear (Engel 1977). Nowhere is the urgency for such an integration more apparent than in the chronic disabilities arising from catastrophic brain damage. The argument in this chapter is that such disabilities have serious consequences for the individual at a number of levels. There are of course immediate tissue damage and resultant physical restrictions. There are direct cognitive and emotional problems arising from the cerebral lesion. The illness may involve further psychological problems. Difficulties occur in employment and in social contacts. More importantly, the illness has serious emotional and social effects on the individual's family.

The aim of a psychosocial perspective is, in particular, to examine psychological and social consequences. However, it will be apparent from this chapter that an adequate explanation of the experience of disabilities arising in problems such as head injuries and strokes needs to incorporate a careful consideration of the physical aspects of damage.

The significance of chronic illnesses and disabilities for health care systems can be established from surveys of prevalence. The General Household Survey in the United Kingdom found that approximately 17 per cent of people considered themselves to be affected by a chronic illness. Using a different definition, the US Commission on Chronic Illness found approximately 12 per cent of Americans experienced some degree of limitation on their activities because of chronic illness (Strauss and Glaser 1975). The rates of chronic illness in the United Kingdom differ by occupation and sex (see *Table 12*).

Conditions commonly found in surveys of chronic illness include heart conditions, arthritis and rheumatism, impairments of the back, spine, and lower extremities, visual impairments, mental and nervous conditions.

The social and psychological consequences vary for different illnesses. For many chronic illnesses reduced mobility results in multiple handicaps: from difficulties in performing domestic tasks around the house to loss of employment and social contact (Blaxter 1976). The effort to maintain some level of normal activity within functional limitations may be frustrating and tiring (Bury 1982). Less obvious, but no less central to the experience of illness, are the uncertainties and worries about prognosis of variable and fluctuating disorders such as multiple sclerosis (Stewart and Sullivan 1983) and rheumatoid arthritis (Weiner 1975). Other problems, such as ulcerative colitis, may necessitate development of special strategies by the sufferer to avoid public exposure of embarrassing problems (Reif 1973; Chapter 10, this volume).

Head injuries and cerebrovascular accidents (CVAs) or strokes, the focus of this chapter, present a wide range of physical, psychological and social consequences. A major theme in examining these is the need for careful attention to different levels and sources of explanation in unravelling the multiple difficulties that may ensue.

Both problems tend to have an impact on the physical, cognitive,

Table 12   *Chronic illness by socio-economic group and sex*
(Rates per 1,000)

	male	female
professional	111	111
employers and managers	131	136
intermediate and junior non-manual	157	169
skilled manual	175	170
semi-skilled manual and personal service	196	234
unskilled manual	233	282
all persons	168	185

Source: Social Trends, 12: derived from the General Household Survey, 1979 and 1980; HMSO, 1982, p. 123.

emotional and social functioning in those who survive the initial trauma and thus require an adjustment to be made to some form(s) of disability. As will be demonstrated in this chapter, the adjustment is not only required by the patient, but also by their family, friends, and, in some instances, their work colleagues. The adjustment is all the more complex, because it extends beyond coping with certain physical limitations of the patient and frequently involves accommodating to the patient's changes in cognitive functioning and alteration in mood. Frequently the cognitive and affective changes may be subtle and only become evident to an outsider with a careful assessment or long-term observation of the patient.

The following discussion will attempt to distinguish the impact of CVAs and head injuries on the physical, cognitive, emotional, and social functioning of the patient. These divisions are somewhat artificial as the effects on one function are not independent of others. The emphasis will be placed on affective and social changes and detailed discussion of cognitive effects will be limited to those which appear to have some specific bearing on the affective or social functioning of the individual.

CVAs and head injuries differ from many other diseases of the nervous system such as multiple sclerosis or Alzheimer's disease in two important ways. The onset of CVAs and head injuries is occasioned by a traumatic event. Multiple sclerosis and Alzheimer's disease are both slow developing and insidious. The course of CVA and head injury survivors is one in which they show varying degrees of recovery of functioning from the time of incident. This recovery then plateaus and frequently remains relatively stable for the duration of the patient's life. In cases of multiple sclerosis and Alzheimer's disease, the disease tends to progress gradually over time with the patient becoming increasingly disabled. These differences in the rate and direction of progression, as well as the form of onset, need to be considered in any attempt to draw conclusions from the studies of CVA and head-injured patients to other forms of neurological illness.

The long-term management of head injury and CVAs commonly rests with the family and occurs with little or no assistance from the medical or paramedical services. Medical input is largely confined to the acute stages when the patient is admitted to hospital or arrives in the accident and emergency clinic. The primary task is to cope with the immediate physical threat. In the case of CVAs this would customarily extend to attempting a diagnosis of the cause and trying to exert some control over the patient's blood pressure as well as considering other forms of intervention, such as anti-coagulant therapy (Marshall 1976). The patient may also receive speech therapy, physiotherapy and an assessment of their cognitive functions by a psychologist. These may continue far beyond the period of hospitalization but would tend to cease when the patient appears to have reached a plateau in their abilities. With the exception of out-patient visits to the hospital or appointments with the general practitioner most patients would receive no further assistance from the medical services unless they were sufficiently disabled to warrant hospitalization or other institutional care. With head injuries the pattern of medical intervention is similarly concentrated in the acute stages but the forms of investigation of neurological damage will frequently be more extensive than that which occurs with CVAs. The long-term adjustment of both these groups of patients, after the acute phase and when the major portion of recovery is complete, occurs in the absence of any medical or paramedical support. There are a few exceptions to this pattern where specific head injury units or stroke units have been established and care extends for a longer period and may include other family members.

Forms, incidence and mortality rates

CEREBROVASCULAR ACCIDENTS

Cerebrovascular accidents involve an acute disturbance of the vascular system in or near the brain. The two major forms that may be distinguished are cerebral infarction and cerebral haemorrhage. Cerebral infarctions occur approximately three times more frequently than cerebral haemorrhages. Cerebral haemorrhages differ from infarctions in that they occur extremely rapidly, with maximal neural damage occurring in a few minutes and they are normally accompanied by a loss of consciousness. Cerebral infarctions on the other hand are not as abrupt in onset and consciousness is frequently not lost.

The incidence of cerebrovascular accidents has been estimated to be in the region of 2 per 1,000. There is an increasing incidence with age. It is important, however, that almost one-quarter of all CVA victims are under the age of sixty-five (Lishman 1978). When only survivors are considered the impact of age is somewhat reduced as mortality occurs with greater frequency in older patients (Sacco *et al.* 1982).

CVAs rank third as a cause of death in the western world, behind heart disease and cancer. Mortality rates have been found to vary from country to country (Acheson, Acheson, and Tellwright 1968; Stallones 1975). This has been variously ascribed to environmental factors, differences in medical facilities, and also to differences in diagnostic procedures (Kurtze 1969; Marshall 1976). In the United Kingdom, mortality rates for the years 1954–58 were placed at 1,333 per million for males and 1,838 per million for females (Hutchinson and Acheson 1975). The number of patients who succumb in the early stages has been found to range from 22 per cent in a study of all CVAs in the town of

Framingham in the United States (Sacco *et al.* 1982), through 20–26 per cent in a general hospital study in the United Kingdom (Carter 1964), up to 44 per cent in an Israeli study (Geltner 1972).

The net effect of this pattern of incidence and mortality is that CVA survivors constitute a large proportion of the severely disabled in western societies. They are generally over the age of sixty but a proportion will still be of an age when they would expect to be in full-time employment. The family who may be able to offer support will tend in the main to be the patient's elderly spouse and children.

HEAD INJURIES

Head injuries may be subdivided into a number of different categories. A general division is that between closed and penetrating head injuries. In the former, penetration of the dura mater does not occur, and the patient may have extended periods of unconsciousness. Closed head injuries occur primarily due to motor vehicle accidents, assaults, and other accidents. Penetrating head injuries result from an object penetrating the skull and occur most frequently during times of military conflict. In contrast to CVAs, head injuries tend to produce more diffuse damage to the brain.

An overall level of incidence of head injuries is difficult to establish, because, by their very nature, many head injuries may not be reported. It has been estimated that in the region of 2.5 per 1,000 of the population receive treatment for a head injury per annum. The incidence of head injury, especially severe head injury, has been found to be on the increase (Lishman 1978). This has largely been ascribed to an increase in motor vehicle accidents.

The likelihood of death is related to the severity of head injury. The term severe head injury is used to refer to those patients who experience a post-traumatic amnesia of twenty-four hours or a coma of more than six hours' duration. Mortality rates in these cases have been estimated to be 50 per cent over five years (Trimble 1981).

In contrast to CVA patients, those who receive head injuries tend to be relatively young, on average in their twenties. Consequently, the social support available to head-injured victims will differ considerably from CVA patients. Parents tend to play a primary role in their long-term care. Where there is a spouse, they also contribute to care.

There are features, other than age, of the head-injured population which distinguish them from the general population and also therefore from CVA patients. Prior to the head injury they tend to have experienced a higher than average incidence of accidents, they have exhibited more anti-social behaviour and derive from families with more than average disturbance (Jamieson and Kelly 1973). They also have, at the time of injury, a lower than average educational level (Tobis, Puri, and Sheridan 1982). These differences to the general population are important to bear in mind when the social adjustment of these patients is considered.

Consequences of CVAs and head injuries

The need for a broad approach to the problem of both CVAs and head injuries is apparent when one examines the broad range of functions that may be affected. A general picture of the frequency of physical deficits following CVAs may be seen in the results of the longitudinal study of the residents of the town of Framingham in the United States. The study initially considered 5,209 individuals, aged 30–62, between 1948 and 1952. Gresham *et al.* (1979) examined 148 of the 155 surviving CVAs and listed the percentage who had certain major neurological deficits. These findings are displayed in *Table 13*. CVAs also produce a variety of cognitive changes including memory disturbance, attentional disorders and a variety of perceptual disorders.

One of the most comprehensive studies of head injuries in recent years was conducted by Roberts (1979) on 291 survivors of head injury. The sample included a majority of closed head injuries, the remainder had received penetrating wounds. In 26 per cent of cases, surgical treatment was required. All of the patients had a post-traumatic amnesia of twenty-four hours or more and can thus be considered a sample of severe head injury. The physical consequences included various degrees of paresis, ataxia, spasticity, inco-ordination, loss of physical power, loss of balance, epilepsy, and dysarthria. In 12 per cent of cases the physical disability was sufficiently severe to prevent, or severely limit, normal domestic, social, or occupational life.

Post-traumatic epilepsy is a frequent consequence of head injury. The probability with which it is likely to occur is dependent upon the nature and severity of the injury, as assessed by post-traumatic amnesia and the

Table 13   *Framingham study: percentage of patients with selected neurological deficits following CVA*

neurological deficits	percentage of patients (%)
left/right/bilateral hemiplegia	48
hemisensory defect	24
dysphasia	18
dysarthria	15
hemianopia	13

Source: adapted from Gresham *et al.* (1979) [(*n* = 148)].

duration of coma. Head injury frequently results in some degree of amnesia, which has been found to persist for many months following injury (Brooks 1976; Hpay 1971). Dysphasia was found to occur in 7 per cent of a sample of 345 patients with penetrating head injury (Lishman 1968). In closed head injury, the classic forms of fluent and non-fluent dysphasia do not occur with any regularity although nearly half of a series of sixty patients were found to make anomic errors and to have word-finding difficulties (Levin *et al.* 1976).

The particular psychological changes that occur in head injury are those of personality. On both formal assessment and reports by relatives, a large proportion of the head injured experience a change in their character. Owing to the controversy surrounding the concept and measurement of personality, it is not possible to give an accurate figure on the number of patients who experience changes in personality without a consideration of the forms of measurement. Brooks and McKinlay (1983) asked close relatives to rate the severely head-injured adult, at various points in time, on a series of bipolar adjectives, descriptive of personality (e.g. excitable – calm; irritable – easy going). At twelve months following the head injury, 60 per cent of relatives judged the brain-injured adult to have changed in personality.

An area of the brain which is frequently damaged in head injuries is the frontal lobe area. This has long been associated with dramatic changes in personality and termed the frontal lobe syndrome. More recently, two types of consequences of frontal lobe damage have been distinguished (Blumer and Benson 1975). The first group tend towards indifference and apathy and have been termed 'pseudo-depressed'. The second group become coarse, irritable, facetious, and may become anti-social. These have been termed 'pseudo-psychopathic'. These types of changes associated with frontal lobe damage have been found to occur frequently in unselected groups of head injuries. Roberts (1979) found in a large sample of head injuries that 40 per cent demonstrated some of the changes associated with frontal lobe damage on a follow-up examination 3–25 years after injury.

Other forms of personality changes found in the head injured and, in some cases, CVA patients include irritability, emotional lability, stubbornness, restlessness, pathological laughter, and weeping, outbursts of rage and aggression, self-centredness and childish behaviour (Blyth 1981; Coughlan and Humphrey 1982; Roberts 1979; Thomsen 1974; Weddell, Oddy, and Jenkins 1980).

Emotional reactions to chronic illness or disability – depression

The advent of chronic illness has been described as a period of crisis. The most frequently occurring emotion following chronic illness is depression. Studies over a wide range of illnesses have indicated that a large proportion of individuals become mildly and in some instances severely depressed (Hughes 1982; Maher 1982; Rodda, Miller, and Bruten 1971; Westbrook and Viney 1983). Individuals have also been found to express anger at having been afflicted with the illness. In some cases they feel that they have contracted the illness because of past misdemeanours (see e.g. Abrams and Finesinger 1953).

In a recent study, interviews with 126 patients admitted to hospital for a range of illnesses, all of which would become chronic, were compared to a control group (Westbrook and Viney 1983). The patients were found to express more depression, anxiety, and anger in contrast to the non-patients. Depression and anxiety were particularly high in those patients who perceived their illness as interfering with their ability to care for themselves and to conduct inter-personal relationships. This finding emphasizes the central role that the patient's evaluation of the consequence of their illness plays in the determination of the emotional response. The emotional reactions seen in response to chronic illness and disability, in particular depression, may be due to a range of factors including the perceived loss of function(s), alterations in self-concept, frustration of ambitions, modification of social roles, stigma associated with the illness/disability, and, in some instances, the likelihood of an early demise. In case of brain damage, the reasons for depression are more complex than in other cases of chronic illness, as the following discussion will reveal.

Following cerebrovascular accidents, depression has been found to occur in many patients. The research studies have used a variety of techniques of assessment of depression and subjects who have differed on a number of variables. This may account for the range of patients who have been considered depressed in any study (see *Table 14*).

Depression has been found to follow head injury but with less frequency than that observed in cerebrovascular accidents. In Lishman's (1968) study of 345 patients with penetrating head injuries, 17 per cent developed depression. In a large study of head injuries Achte, Hillbom, and Aalberg (1969) found 1.3 per cent of patients to have developed a psychotic depression.

Table 14   *Frequency of depression following CVA*

	% depressed
Feibel and Springer (1982)	26
Robinson and Price (1982)	29
Coughlan and Humphrey (1982)	34
Folstein, Maiberger, and McHugh (1977)	45
Robinson and Szetela (1981) (left hemisphere only)	61

A more direct comparison between cerebrovascular accidents and head injuries was made by Robinson and Szetela (1981) who compared a group of patients who had a diagnosis of cerebral infarction (n = 18) with a group of patients who had received brain injuries. While the two groups had a similar incidence of neurological impairments and cognitive functions, significantly more CVA patients were found to be depressed (61 per cent) than head injured (18 per cent).

LOCATION OF LESION

Problems for any health professional and family members in coping with the many aspects of disability arising from CVAs and head injuries partly derive from an uncertainty as to whether the location of the lesion is directly implicated in the depression or whether it arises out of the patients' reactions to aspects of their disability. While the study mentioned above suggests, superficially, a greater incidence of depression in cerebrovascular accidents, the reason for this may be due to the location of the lesion, as suggested by the authors (Robinson and Szetela 1981). While the size of lesion was similar for both groups, the location of lesion was different. The CVA lesions tend to be more anterior in the brain, in the fronto-parietal area, while in the head injured, the lesions were towards the parieto-occipital areas. The authors examined whether the location of lesion was the important factor by matching of a CVA and head-injured patient for size and location of lesion. Although the analysis contained only seven pairs, no differences were found on measures of depression between CVA and head-injured patients. The importance of the location of lesion and depression was emphasized by further analysis which indicated higher depression scores as the lesions approached the frontal pole.

A more widely held view of the influence of lesion location on the incidence of depression concerns the lateral dimension. Lesions in the left hemisphere are considered more likely to result in a depressive reaction than lesions in the right hemisphere (Vallenstein and Heilman 1979). In a study of 103 CVA patients, Robinson and Price (1982) found depression to be both more frequent and more severe following left hemisphere damage as opposed to right hemisphere damage. In contrast, a study on ninety-one community-based CVA patients found roughly similar proportions of left and right hemisphere damaged patients to be depressed (Feibel and Springer 1982).

The apparent contradiction between these two studies may be resolved when both the methods of depression and the clinical descriptions of depression are compared. The first study administered a questionnaire to the patients that was found to correlate with a number of widely used depression inventories. The second relied on nurses' ratings of mood, behaviour, and somatic complaints. Robinson and Price (1982) describe their patients' symptoms as including depression, anxiety, hopelessness, irritability, social withdrawal, sleep disturbance, appetite disturbance with weight loss, decrease in libido, agitation, loss of interest, and loss of energy. In contrast, Feibel and Springer's (1982) reliance on nurses' views may have led them to stray from the accepted views of depression. The nurses described the depressed patients as 'having loss of purpose, crying often, has the blues and has trouble accepting illness'. These rather global terms may not be sufficiently specific to specify depression. In addition, the one feature described, 'trouble accepting illness', tends to be associated with right hemisphere lesions (Indifference Reaction). Thus it appears that left hemisphere lesions may more frequently lead to what is commonly understood by depression in clinical practice (see also Gainotti 1972; Gasparrini *et al.* 1979).

PHYSICAL AND COGNITIVE CHANGES AND DEPRESSION

Although the evidence above suggests that the location of the brain lesion may be an important influence on whether patients develop depression, this does not necessarily imply that the lesion has damaged an area of the brain responsible for emotions. It may be that the depression seen in these patients is a reaction to the physical loss and/or cognitive loss and the restrictions these impose upon the individual. As will become apparent in the discussion below on the studies that have attempted to separate the role of these factors, it is not strictly possible to determine the relative role of the location of the lesion, the physical loss, and the cognitive disturbance, in the depression seen in many neuro-logically damaged individuals.

One of the frequently occurring physical disabilities following CVA is a restriction in motor ability due to paresis (see *Table 13* above). It is conceivable that the depression seen in CVA and head injury patients may be, in part, a reaction to the physical restrictions resulting from paresis. Restrictions in motor activities are seen in other chronic illnesses, such as rheumatoid arthritis. In an attempt to examine the extent to which the brain lesion *per se* produces a depressive response in CVAs as opposed to a reactive depression to physical disability, Folstein, Maiberger, and McHugh (1977) compared the frequency of depression in CVA and orthopaedic patients. The two groups of patients were equated for demographic variables and for their ability to perform physical activities. The frequency of depression in orthopaedic patients was found to be 10 per cent, in contrast to 45 per cent in CVA patients. The authors conclude that the depression in CVA patients is more than a reaction to physical disabilities.

There was, however, an important difference between the two groups. The neurological patients were assessed shortly after their CVAs, while the orthopaedic patients were seen almost one year after the onset of their illness. This difference may well have reduced the frequency of depression in the orthopaedic patients, who would have had some time to consider the development of their disease and its possible ramifications. In contrast, the CVA patients would have had no possible time to prepare for their disability.

There are other difficulties in assuming that studies such as these may enable an analysis to be made of the separate contributions of location of lesion and physical and cognitive changes in the frequency of depression in CVA patients. In order to make a comparison with orthopaedic patients, only those brain-injured patients with motor involvement may be selected for study. This would make the group selected unrepresentative of the population of CVA patients and, more important, it would reduce the sample to those with lesions in a restricted area of the brain. As a result, these patients would also tend to have a particular range of cognitive disturbances. Thus, any differences in the frequency of depression between orthopaedic and CVA patients may be due to either the lesion and its specific location, or the CVA patients' reaction to the cognitive loss they have incurred, or it may be a combination of these.

An alternative method of teasing out the relative contributions of physical and psychological changes from the direct effects of the lesion is to examine the differences between those brain-damaged patients who become depressed and contrast them with those who do not. Feibel and Springer (1982) examined ninety-one CVA patients for depression, cognitive abilities and self-care, work, social, and leisure activities. Although the depression assessment they applied was limited to nurses' observations and may not conform to other clinical measures of depression, the study did yield interesting results. The depressed patients had experienced a significantly greater decrease in their social activities since their CVAs than the non-depressed group. On all the other measures, such as cognitive status, age, and marital status, the two groups were not found to be different. As the authors acknowledge, this association does not imply that the reduction in social activities caused the depression. It may well be that the depression led to a reduction in social activities, or, indeed, that they merely occurred together. The phenomenon of social isolation has been found to occur in many chronic illnesses and will be discussed in more detail below.

That damage to the left hemisphere results in depression more frequently than damage to the right hemisphere may be due to the different cognitive functions subserved by the two hemispheres of the brain. The left hemisphere, in most people's brains, tends to be intimately involved in language functions. The right hemisphere tends to subserve visuo-spatial functions (see e.g. Dimond and Beaumont 1974). Consequently, lesions in the left hemisphere frequently lead to dysphasia. A reduction in the ability to communicate has enormous repercussions on an individual's life and serves to restrict and limit their social interactions considerably. It would not be surprising if the greater frequency of depression following left hemisphere damage were largely attributable to a reaction to the loss of ability to communicate through language. For many patients, the frustration of not being able to communicate might lead to feelings of helplessness and depression (Benson 1973).

Benson (1973) claims that the form of dysphasia will influence the likelihood of depression. He suggests that non-fluent dysphasia, with slow effortful speech and reasonable comprehension, are more likely to lead to depression than fluent dysphasias which are primarily disorders of comprehension. Some support for this view was found in a study of dysphasics with a variety of aetiologies by Robinson and Benson (1981). Fluent dysphasics, non-fluent dysphasics and a group of global dysphasics who had both production and comprehension deficits, were examined for depression. The three groups did not differ significantly on demographic variables and the time since the onset of their illness. The non-fluent patients showed a greater frequency and severity of depression than those in the other groups, although depression was apparent in both fluent and global dysphasics. One explanation of this finding is that the non-fluent patients become more depressed because they are aware of their language deficit. In contrast, many fluent patients are not aware of the extent of their language deficits. While his explanation appears cogent, there are competing explanations. One of these concerns the locations of the lesions typically found in fluent and non-fluent dysphasia. In non-fluent dysphasia the lesions are towards the anterior of the brain, in and around Broca's area, while in fluent dysphasia they are towards the posterior of the brain. Other studies have suggested the proximity of the lesion to the frontal lobes increases the likelihood of depression (Robinson and Szetela 1981, see above). These two competing explanations of depression, one being a direct consequence of the lesion, the other being a reaction to the form of disruption to cognitive functions, cannot be distinguished in this, or for that matter any, study of this type.

The emotional response of the family and the illness

One of the most common approaches to understanding the response of family members to chronic illness has been to characterize the development of emotions in terms of stages. These stage models do not offer an explanation but are limited to describing the typical course of the emotional response of the family. In general, they tend to begin with the crisis of the diagnosis and culminate with the adjustment to and acceptance of the illness (see e.g. Burr, Good, and Del Vecchio-Good 1978). Lezak (1982) has proposed a stage model to describe the changing emotions of the family of head-injured patients and Newman (1981, 1984) has suggested a model for the family of CVA patients. In both of these models, the families' emotional responses are related to the expectations they have regarding the patient's recovery following the catastrophic life-threatening event. There are, however, important differences between head injuries and CVAs and many other chronic illnesses.

Most chronic illnesses show a downward trajectory where the individual deteriorates physically over time. This may be a rapid process or may be characterized by plateaux where no physical changes occur for long periods of time. In contrast, CVA and head injury patients begin with a clear onset where they are at their most vulnerable. This tends to be followed, in the survivors, by a steady improvement. In other words, in CVA and head injury, the trajectory is upwards. The expectations of family members are, not surprisingly, influenced by the speed of the illness trajectory. In CVAs and head injuries, the most rapid improvements tend to occur in the first three months when patients may move from a comatose state to one where they may be mobile and able to converse with others. This rapid rate of recovery in the early stages frequently establishes expectations in the family that the patient will be left with no residual deficits. When the recovery slows down and where residual deficits remain, the family have difficulty in adjusting their expectations. Thus for the families of brain-damaged individuals, the most difficult period occurs when the realization takes place that the patient has reached a plateau and may not fully recover (see Lezak 1982; Newman 1984).

In the longer term, the stresses and adjustments caused by a CVA or head injury in the family may result in some emotional disturbance, in particular depression, in other family members. For example, Coughlan and Humphrey (1982) examined the emotional state of spouses of CVA patients 3–8 years after the CVA; 25 per cent of the spouses, who prior to the CVA had not received any psychiatric treatment, had received some treatment for depression or tension in the follow-up period. Kinsella and Duffy (1979) performed a similar study on the spouses of seventy-nine CVA patients, three to thirty-six months after CVA. An inventory for depression given to each spouse indicated that 42 per cent may have been suffering from depression. In the follow-up period 78 per cent had received tranquillizers or sleeping pills.

A similar picture is apparent in the relatives of head-injured individuals. Panting and Merry (1972) examined the relatives of thirty brain-damaged individuals of between two and seven years' standing and found that 61 per cent had received tranquillizers or sleeping pills. Oddy, Humphrey, and Uttley (1978a) examined the frequency of depression in the parent or spouse of fifty-four young brain-damaged individuals. Twelve months following the incident, 24 per cent of the spouses or parents were found to be depressed.

One of the few studies that has compared the family response to both brain-damaged and non-brain-damaged individuals compared the spouses of soldiers who had suffered penetrating brain injury to those of paraplegics (Rosenbaum and Najenson 1978). Symptoms of low mood were found to be highest in the spouses of the brain injured. The spouses of the paraplegics in turn experienced significantly more symptoms of low mood than a control group.

The possible reasons for depression in the families of the brain injured, as with the patients themselves, include a range of factors. These include the increased physical burden, loss of a close relationship, possible economic difficulties, coping with psychological changes, and social and sexual difficulties. Some of these factors will be discussed in more detail below.

Effects of chronic illness or disability on family relationships

The occurrence of chronic illness or disability in a family places great strains on the previously established intra-familial relationships, which frequently have to adjust to the new circumstances. These adjustments occur with varying degrees of difficulty according to the degree and type of disability, the nature of the relationship and the activities previously performed by the patient, amongst many other factors.

Most studies have shown that the disruptive occurrence of a chronic illness in a family has a detrimental effect on marital relations (Blaxter 1976; Kinsella and Duffy 1979; Sainsbury 1970; Tobis, Puri, and Sheridan 1982) although some studies, particularly of illness in children, have found families to be drawn together by illness (Haggerty 1968).

Blaxter's (1976) study of disablement found different effects on marital relationships according to sex or, more particularly, who occupied the work role. When the illness affected a male, a more radical change occurred in the relationship than when the illness affected a female. The greater discord in the case of males appeared to result from a failure, primarily on the husband's part, to adjust to being confined at home most of the time.

With CVAs and head injuries, the spouse is required to adjust to both physical and mental changes of the partner. Thus not only is the pattern of the relationship altered but its very quality may be changed. Studies of both head-injured and CVA patients have shown a deterioration in the marital relationship (Lawrence and Christie 1979; Tobis, Puri and

Sheridan 1982). One study compared the relationships in the home in severe and moderately physically disabled CVA patients. Three years after the CVA, none of these patients had communication difficulties. In one-third of the instances of minimal physical disability and two-thirds of the severely disabled, the home relationships had deteriorated (Lawrence and Christie 1979). When communication is rendered more difficult by dysphasia, marital relationships suffer to a greater extent. Kinsella and Duffy (1979) examined the amount of friction between CVA patients and their spouses. Those relationships which included a spouse with dysphasia had significantly greater friction than where dysphasia was absent. These studies suggest that the degree and the nature of disability may have a determining effect on the marital relationship.

Before turning to those elements with which the relatives have most adjustment difficulties, it is necessary to consider the one technique of coping available to the spouse namely that of separation or divorce. In terms of models of the family unit as central to adjustment to chronic illness or disability, separation or divorce are not real solutions. For the individual, however, separation must be seen as one method of coping with the change in their partner. The frequency of divorce has been used as an index of marital disharmony following disability. Sainsbury (1970) found a higher frequency of divorce following disability and considered the marriage to be particularly at risk in the first year following the onset of disability. When looking at CVAs and head injuries, it is important to bear in mind that they tend to occur at different ends of the life cycle. Strokes occur relatively late in life, beyond the time when many individuals would contemplate dissolving a relationship, especially one of a long duration. In the case of head injuries, the partner may well be of an age and a generation where divorce is more easily contemplated. Studies do suggest a higher incidence of divorce for this group than that found in the general population (see e.g. Panting and Merry 1972).

Divorce rates can, however, only be a crude indicator of marital dysfunction, as the decision on whether to dissolve a marriage is influenced by a number of factors other than the quality of the relationship. These would include economic considerations, the presence of children and the lack of employment opportunities. In the case of wives looking after disabled husbands, the lack of any alternatives to remaining with the husband has been found to be an important factor in restricting the number of separations and divorces (Oliver 1983).

Sexual activity is one area of particular concern for both partners in the marital relationship. Studies of the chronically ill or disabled have shown this to be particularly susceptible to change. In situations where no movement disorders or reductions in physical sensation occur and even where a good physical recovery occurs, a large proportion of patients reduce sexual activity.

A sizeable proportion of couples cease sexual activity following CVAs. Kinsella and Duffy (1979) found 83 per cent of their sample of seventy-nine married CVA patients to have ceased sexual intercourse. In all these cases, the individuals were sexually active until the time of the CVA. While there may be particular physical problems with some CVA victims in achieving an erection, measures of the overall degree of motor impairment were not found to be related to the likelihood of ceasing sexual activity (see *Table 15*).

While overall motor functioning cannot account for the cessation of sexual activity, those CVA victims whose sense of touch was disturbed did tend to decrease or reduce sexual intercourse. Studies of sexual activity following head injury have not always indicated a reduction (Oddy, Humphrey, and Uttley 1978b). Rosenbaum and Najenson's (1976) study of paraplegic and brain-injured soldiers' wives found dramatic reductions in sexual activity in both groups. While the authors felt that the reduction in the paraplegics was due to spinal cord injury, they could only speculate that the reduction for the brain injured was due to the direct effects of the injury, anti-convulsant drugs or the relationship between husband and wife. The last factor appears to be important and will be discussed below.

Parent–child relationships may also become affected following a chronic illness or disability in one of the parents. This is likely to have wide-ranging effects when the parent is unable or unwilling to fulfil a parenting role. Blaxter's (1976) study found that a number of wives complained about their disabled husband's failure to take any interest in the children. These wives referred in particular to the husband's irritability. In brain injury, where cognitive and emotional changes have occurred as well as physical changes, it would be expected that particular problems of the parent–child relationship may result. Lezak (1978) reports brain-injured parents ignoring their children or bullying or belittling them. There is an attempt to re-establish their self-esteem as their child's skills begin to surpass their own. This type of behaviour has broader ramifications, as it either leads to an increased burden of child

Table 15   *Degree of motor impairment and cessation of sexual activities following CVA*

motor impairment	cessation of sexual activity
severe	38%
marked	36%
moderate	18%
slight	50%

Source: adapted from Fugl-Meyer and Jaasko (1980)

rearing for the physically well spouse or disagreements as to child rearing between the parents. Over and above the alteration in the quality of the relationship, in the case of CVAs and head injuries, the relationship may well have suffered some discontinuity during the period of hospitalization. This may be particularly disruptive for younger children (Coughlan and Humphrey 1982).

Having a brain-damaged partner has also been found to be a disturbing influence on the relationship between the physically well spouse and the children. Many spouses of CVA patients report a deterioration of their relationship with their children (Kinsella and Duffy 1979). Problems in this relationship were found to be influenced by the degree of severity in the CVA victim. Where dysphasia and hemiplegia were both present, the relationship was more disturbed than when only one of these was present.

Head injuries occur in a younger population in comparison to CVAs and, in a proportion of cases, the brain-injured individual will be living, on return home, with their parents. The evidence suggests that in these cases the relationship does not suffer as markedly as the marital relationship (Blyth 1981; Humphrey and Oddy 1978). A number of factors may account for the durability of this relationship. An important element concerns the nature of the previously established relationship. The parent–child relationship that has been established prior to the head injury involves dependency to a greater or lesser extent. With the advent of the head injury, both parties may find it comparatively easy to fall back into these roles. In contrast, the male adult CVA patient who has always led an independent life is likely to find it difficult to accept a dependent role, as indeed may his partner. Two additional reasons may also account for the durability of the parent–child relationship: the burden of care is spread between two adults, enabling some distribution of and relief from the caretaker function and, finally, recovery from brain damage in younger children is more extensive than in adults. This factor may encourage parents to withstand the pressures of the caretaking role, as they may gain a degree of satisfaction at seeing recovery take place.

Stress of physical and mental changes

An increase in the physical burden of the physically well partner is a feature common to many chronic illnesses or disabilities. The need to ensure that a partner maintains a particular diet or that a diabetic monitors his blood sugar levels, or assisting an arthritic partner with their daily activities, all require time and energy. In many cases of brain damage the patient becomes dependent on their family for self-care and the daily activities of cooking and housekeeping (Belcher *et al.* 1982; Hamrin 1982). One study of CVA patients compared the proportion of CVA patients dependent on others for activities required for independent living with a group of matched controls (Gresham *et al.* 1979). As opposed to 32 per cent of the CVA patients, 9 per cent of the control group were found to be dependent.

One may have expected the increased physical burden to be a particular cause of concern of the families of the brain damaged. Studies of both head injuries and CVAs emphasize that the relatives are more concerned with mental changes and current behaviours than with the additional physical burden (Bond 1975; Brocklehurst *et al.* 1981; Fahy, Irving and Millac 1967; McKinlay *et al.* 1981; Oddy, Humphrey, and Uttley 1978a). Thomsen (1974) found that most of the relatives of severely head-injured patients complained of difficulties in coping with the patient's personality problems and only a few were concerned about motor problems.

When relatives are asked to describe the changes they have observed in a head-injured family member, they tend to concentrate on the mental changes. In a study of fifty families with a severely head-injured member, relatives were found to mention mental changes (such as poor memory, slowness) and emotional changes (such as mood swings, irritability, impatience) significantly more frequently than other categories. Those relatives who reported the greatest amount of changes in these areas were the ones who appeared to be under the greatest amount of stress. Brooks and McKinlay (1983) asked relatives to assess the change in personality of a group of brain-injured adults. Those who noted the greatest amount of personality change also rated themselves highest on the amount of psychological stress they were currently encountering. There was also a suggestion in this study of a decrease in the ability of the relative to cope with personality changes as time progressed.

The fact that relatives find the mental and emotional alterations of the patient particularly stressful has only recently been recognized (Lezak 1978). What is of particular concern for the relatives is that in most instances there is no individual, medical or paramedical, who is available to assist or counsel them with these difficulties. As these problems have become recognized more and more, attempts have been made to establish centres for the families of brain-injured patients and to redirect some of the efforts of rehabilitation towards the family (Brooks and McKinlay 1983; Lezak 1978; Newman 1984).

Social contacts and leisure

It is not surprising that loss of social contacts and isolation is a consequence of chronic illness or disability where severe physical limitations are present. Reductions in mobility, difficulties with communication, and problems with hearing or vision would all tend to place restrictions on an individual's ability to retain old friendships as well as establish new ones. Even in cases where the illness reduces the energy and time available to an individual, friendships may suffer. These types of difficulties have a direct effect on friendships and social contacts and are involuntary to the extent that the chronically ill or disabled individual has no alternative but to accept these restrictions. They are to be distinguished from a voluntary social withdrawal that some individuals engage in as a result of their attitudes towards disability and of the disabled individual's own withdrawal from others (see Chapter 10).

Studies have found that a proportion of both males and females of all ages become completely socially isolated after becoming disabled (Blaxter 1976; Miller 1978). Blaxter (1976) found that those individuals who had become socially isolated did not have a firm base in the community in which they were living and, in particular, did not have any family members living in the close vicinity. Extreme social withdrawal appeared to affect the severely disabled and those with communication difficulties more than others. However, even in studies where there is minimal physical disability, a proportion of individuals do suffer from social isolation (see e.g. Heller, Frank, and Kornfield 1974).

With CVA patients a reduction in social contacts and leisure activities has been found to occur, even in cases of minimal disability. In a series of studies that matched CVA patients for age and sex to controls, a significantly greater reduction in leisure and social activities occurred with CVA patients (Gresham *et al.* 1975, 1979; Labi 1980). The extent of this reduction was found to be related to the degree of neurological impairment. However, what was notable was that even in those who had made a good neurological recovery, a significant decrease in social and leisure activities had taken place. Dysphasia has been found to be a particularly restricting disability with CVA patients as far as social contacts are concerned but even when no dysphasia is present social activities have been found to be reduced.

With head injuries, a younger group in contrast to CVA patients, the picture is very similar. A large proportion suffer a reduction in leisure activities (Bond 1975; Oddy and Humphrey 1980) and social contacts (Hpay 1971; Lezak *et al.* 1980; Lundholm, Jepsen, and Thornval 1975). This reduction does not appear to be reversed with time (Lezak *et al.* 1980). The extent of the reduction in both social and leisure activities is related to the degree of physical disability but, as with CVAs, even in cases of minimal physical disability social and leisure activities are reduced (Bond 1975; Lundholm, Jepsen, and Thornval 1975; Oddy and Humphrey 1980).

The finding of reduced social and leisure activities in the absence of severe physical restrictions has led to the suggestion of a lack of motivation on the part of the brain damaged. There is evidence to suggest that damage to the frontal lobes of the brain may result in a form of apathy (see above). However, this may only partly account for reduced social and leisure activities. Social isolation appears to affect other chronically ill or disabled individuals and there is every reason to assume that the brain damaged are influenced by the same factors as well as ones peculiar to their state. The common factors would include the attitudes of others, lack of confidence in one's abilities and concern about appearance.

Not only does the frequency of social contacts decline with head injury but also the quality of the relationships appears to change. The number of reported acquaintances does not change but the head injured appear to lose some of their close friends over time (Weddell, Oddy, and Jenkins 1980). The features of the head-injured individual which have been suggested bring about the loss of social contact and friendships are the personality changes of the individual (Hpay 1971; Weddell, Oddy, and Jenkins 1980) and cognitive changes, in particular memory changes (Oddy and Humphrey 1980).

These effects on social contact and leisure are not limited to the chronically ill or disabled individual. One study compared the social effects on the wives of soldiers who suffered penetrating brain injury or paraplegia. The wives of the brain-injured soldiers suffered a greater reduction in social activities than the wives of paraplegics. These wives felt their husbands' condition was a social handicap and also considered that their friends were deserting them (Rosenbaum and Najenson 1976). The spouses of CVA patients appear to have similar experiences to the head injured. The reduction in leisure activities, contacts with friends and other social contacts is experienced most acutely by those whose spouse has dysphasia (Kinsella and Duffy 1979). The effect of this objective reduction in social contacts is that both the spouses and the brain-damaged individual complain of boredom, loneliness and social isolation (Kinsella and Duffy 1979; Thomsen 1974; Weddell, Oddy, and Jenkins 1980).

Table 16   *Proportion of registered disabled unemployed for more than one year in comparison to the general population in the United Kingdom (1980)*

population	disabled %	general %
young people	11.0	4.4
women	47.3	17.8
men	51.5	25.4
total	50.1	19.2

Source: House of Commons Hansard 23/7/81, col 230.

These findings on the social effects of CVAs and head injuries emphasize that, despite relatively good physical recovery, a large proportion of brain-damaged individuals become isolated and lose social contact. The effects also extend beyond the disabled individual to the spouse. Any attempt to limit consideration of the brain damaged to physical and cognitive deficits will ignore the social disabilities they suffer. In addition, an approach which fails to take cognisance of how the family is affected will not have appreciated the ramifications of such a disability on those that live with the brain damaged.

Employment

The restriction in social contacts outlined above is compounded by the fact that a large proportion of the chronically ill or disabled have difficulties in the area of employment. When the figures for unemployment are considered, a disproportionately large number of the disabled tend to be represented. *Table 16* indicates the proportion of the disabled in the United Kingdom who registered as unemployed under the Disabled Persons Employment Act and who had been unemployed for more than one year, in comparison to the general population. The figures are for the year of 1980. The figures for the registered disabled are known to underestimate the real numbers of disabled in the population (Lonsdale 1984).

These figures and other surveys have indicated the tendency for unemployment to affect elderly men in particular (Blaxter 1976). This factor is also in evidence when the unemployment rates following head injuries and CVAs are considered. The level of unemployment for head injuries tends to be lower than that for CVA groups who tend to be both elderly and male (see *Tables 17* and *18*).

Other factors will tend to lead to higher unemployment following CVAs in comparison to head injuries. One of these is that for older workers the opportunity for early retirement is frequently a more satisfactory alternative than continued job seeking. In addition those that receive brain damage earlier in life tend to exhibit a greater level of recovery and thus may physically be more capable of work than older individuals.

Return to work has frequently been used as an index of recovery from illness or injury. Other factors impinge upon employment levels rendering this at best only a crude indicator of recovery from illness. Return to employment is influenced by the age of the individual, their economic resources, the type of work they perform and whether it may be easily modified, their occupational status as well as current legislation regarding employment of the disabled, and the general economic climate (Bond and Brooks 1976; Lonsdale 1981; Lonsdale and Walker 1983). Despite these concerns, with the head injured at least, a general relationship

Table 17   *Work status following head injury*

authors	severity	follow-up (years)	% out of work
1 Steadman and Graham (1970)	most pta 24 hrs	5	1
2 Rowbotham, McIver, and Dickson (1954)	—	3–4	4
3 Grosswasser *et al.* (1977)	u/c 1 day	2	5
4 London (1967)	hospital 7 days	1	9
5 Miller and Stern (1965)	pta 24 hrs	3–11	12
6 Adey (1967)	u/c 24 hrs	5–15	12
7 Hpay (1971)	u/c 24 hrs	3–5	17
8 Humphrey and Oddy (1978)	pta 24 hrs	1–2	18
9 Brennan (1981)	u/c 6 hrs	0.75	20
10 Najenson *et al.* (1974)	u/c 24 hrs	+1	25
11 Lewin (1968)	u/c 1 month	—	28
12 Gerstenbrand (1969)	moderate–severe	1–5	32
13 Bruckner and Randle (1972)	pta 24 hrs	3–14	36
14 Panting and Merry (1970)	most u/c 24 hrs	1–5	43
15 Weddell, Oddy, and Jenkins (1980)	pta 7 days	2	45
16 Heiskanen and Sipponen (1970)	u/c 24 hrs	3–5	47
17 Richardson (1971)	unselected	5–6	50
18 Blyth (1981)	pta 24 hrs	0.5–2.0	50
19 Lezak *et al.* (1980)	Unselected	3	53
20 Thomsen (1974)	u/d 24 hrs	1–6	72

pta = post traumatic amnesia
u/c = unconscious

appears to exist between measures of severity and the likelihood of unemployment, as may be seen at the extreme ends of *Table 17*. Both physical and psychological factors have been implicated as determinants of a failure to return to work (Bond 1975; Bruckner and Randle 1972; Oddy and Humphrey 1980). The particular forms of disability found to restrict the likelihood of employment with the head injured include memory problems, dysphasia, hemiplegia, epilepsy, sensory loss, emotional lability, and general disturbance of cognitive functions.

Table 18   *Work status following CVA*

author	follow-up (years)	% out of work (of those previously in work)
Lawrence and Christie (1979)	3	68
Coughlan and Humphrey (1982)		
males	4–8	70
females	4–8	76

The effects of brain damage do not only effect the employment prospects of the individual sufferer. If the disabled individual is at home, as is frequently the case, a member of the family may have to sacrifice their employment to assist in caring for the disabled individual. For example, a study of CVA patients indicated that 14 per cent of carers who had previously been in employment had to give up their jobs in the year following the CVA to act as full-time carers (Brocklehurst *et al.* 1981). Not only are the chronically sick or disabled particularly susceptible to unemployment, but even when in employment they suffer from disadvantage. They tend to have lower earnings than the general population (Townsend 1979). The net effect of the levels of unemployment, disadvantage in employment, as well as the relatively low levels of social security benefits available to the disabled, results in them forming a disproportionately large percentage of those living in poverty (Townsend 1979).

The effects of unemployment are not restricted to economic factors. Not having a place of work reduces the likelihood of meeting people and thus being able to establish social contacts and friendships. Therefore unemployment compounds the social effects discussed in the previous section. In addition unemployment carries a stigma in its own right. Thus the disabled may be doubly penalized by the stigma of disability and unemployment (see Chapter 10).

The effects of chronic illness or disability outlined in this and the previous section would be likely to produce feelings of isolation and depression even in the absence of any disability. Although it is unlikely they are the sole cause of the incidence of depression in CVAs and head injuries they can only serve to increase the numbers of depressed and to exacerbate the difficulties this group experiences.

Conclusion

Chronic or disabling illness illustrate an area of illness where the value of a bio-psychosocial approach is most obvious. As this chapter has illustrated the range of effects of chronic illness or disability, in particular CVAs and head injuries, is considerable. These invade the individual's cognitive, emotional, and social functioning as well as those of the immediate family. The extent to which the individual and the family are able to cope with chronic or disabling illness is dependent upon their physical, psychological, and financial resources. Although the form the response takes will vary considerably from individual to individual they may be modified and assisted by a co-ordinated effort at a number of different levels. The concerns of the medical and paramedical staff should extend into the family, where they may be able to attempt to assist the individual and the family in coping with the physical and psychological pressures resulting from chronic or disabling illness. In particular, with head injuries and CVAs, the need to establish groups for the patients and relatives to discuss their difficulties and consider various strategies to cope with particular problems has been a useful recent innovation. In addition the formation of voluntary groups of patients and others has not only added to the assistance available, but also served to enable the disabled to form powerful lobby groups. It is at the level of social and economic policy where, despite some significant changes in recent years, a large amount of legislation is required if the economic and social deprivation of the chronically ill or disabled is to be overcome. Some examples include legislation to improve the access to buildings and to public transport to reduce the social isolation experienced by many individuals. At the economic level, enlightened legislation that improves employment prospects and restricts discrimination in employment is still required in many countries.

10 Perceiving and coping with stigmatizing illness

Graham Scambler

Introduction

The word 'stigma' is now ordinarily used in a rather broad sense to refer to the disgrace associated with certain conditions, attributes, traits, or forms of behaviour. Precisely which of the latter are publicly regarded as signs or marks of disgrace and to what degree, has of course varied historically and continues to vary between cultures. By way of illustration, consider the divergent experiences of two eminent European philosophers who also happened to be homosexual, Socrates and Wittgenstein. In Greece in the fifth century B.C. homosexuality was an acceptable and expected form of love between normal males, deemed to be most appropriate between youths and older men in a position to set them a good example. We are told that Socrates, 'whose insatiable love of boys is frankly emphasized by his disciples Plato and Xenophon, who were yet at pains to clear him of any charge of corrupting the young, spent much of his time hanging round schools and gymnasia' (Wilkinson 1979: 120). Contrastingly, Wittgenstein, in the very different moral climate of Austria in the first quarter of the twentieth century, was close to despair, even suicide, when he found himself drawn again and again to the dark alleys of towns 'where rough young men were ready to cater to him sexually'. He wrote to a friend in 1921: 'My life has really become meaningless and so it consists only of futile episodes. The people around me do not notice this and would not understand what I am writing here' (Bartley 1977: 27). While Socrates' homosexuality was open and acceptable, Wittgenstein's was clandestine and brought with it the omnipresent threat of exposure and disgrace.

An appreciation of this kind of historical and cultural variability in the criteria of attribution of stigma is important. It compels acknowledgement, for example, that the complex of values pertaining to stigma in contemporary Britain could well have been other than it is and will almost certainly change in the future. (Arguably, it suggests also that *all* such value-complexes are best interpreted as 'social conventions'; it does not follow of course that they are entirely arbitrary.) The present chapter concentrates on stigma in modern western societies like Britain and the United States and has three main sections. In the first, a provisional, somewhat tentative response is offered to the general question, 'How might we characterize those infringements or "offences" against cultural norms which threaten or result in disgrace and ignominy?' The second focuses on how individuals in predicaments like Wittgenstein's perceive their stigma and endeavour to cope or come to terms with it. Particular attention is paid to the stigma associated with epilepsy. In the final section, some of the implications of social scientific research on stigma for health policy and practice are discussed.

Stigma and the social order

STIGMATIZING ILLNESS

Clearly not all those infringements against norms associated with disgrace are wilful, or even avoidable. After studying the lot of the blind in the United States, for example, Scott (1969, 1970) concluded that many were regarded as deviant simply because they could not see. Mankoff (1971) has referred in this context to 'ascribed' as opposed to 'achieved' deviance or rule breaking. An ascribed rule breaker acquires his or her deviant status independently of any purposeful activity: thus, for example, an ugly person might be considered an ascribed rule breaker. By contrast, an achieved rule breaker can be said to have 'earned' his or her deviant status: the young delinquent or the alcoholic have both achieved rule breaking status, at least to some extent, on the strength of their own actions. It has often been assumed that less stigma attaches to ascribed than to achieved rule breaking (e.g. Haber and Smith 1971). However, Albrecht, Walker, and Levy (1982) found that 'the perceived disruption to social interaction a stigma causes, rather than attribution of responsibility, appears to be a better explanation for differential social distance from individuals with various types of stigmas' (Albrecht, Walker, and Levy 1982: 1325). For example, individuals with heart disease (and 'ex-convicts') were considered more responsible for their condition than the mentally ill and yet respondents expressed greater social distance from the mentally ill. A recent study by Furnham and Pendred (1983) suggests that people generally tend to have more positive attitudes towards the physically disabled than they do towards the mentally disabled.

Many accounts of the stigma attaching to particular mental or physical illnesses are personal or impressionistic (e.g. Hunt 1966). However, a number of more formal studies have also accumulated and these now cover a wide range of conditions from severe physical deformities to mild obesity, pimples, and 'bad breath' (Safilios-Rothschild 1970). This range of conditions is matched by the range of researchers' interests, of which the following are selective illustrations: Goffman (1968) has provided a classic and pioneering statement about the concept of stigma and its implications for possessors and others, drawing on many published and unpublished American studies of illness. Edgerton (1967), Higgins (1980) and Scambler (1983) have given general accounts of the impact of the stigmas associated with mental subnormality, deafness and epilepsy respectively on the perspectives and life activities of sufferers. Reif (1973) has shown how people with ulcerative colitis develop strategies to manage both embarrassing social situations due to their diarrhoea and its odours and constraints on their time imposed by illness-related concerns. Jobling (1977) and Knudson-Cooper (1981) have focused on problems of psychosocial adjustment to, respectively, psoriasis (a skin abnormality) and severe burn injuries sustained in childhood. Hopper (1981) has analysed how diabetes, itself stigmatizing, can bring about changes in sufferer's circumstances that are stigmatizing in their own right (e.g. special diet, loss of sexual activity, peripheral neuropathy, and retinopathy, leading to amputations and blindness, broken friendships, and unemployment). Following Goffman, Hilbourne (1973) recounts how stigmas can 'spread' to despoil the identities of friends and relations. Scott (1969, 1970) has looked at the role of health agencies and bureaucracies in constructing and imposing particular notions of blindness and Volinn (1983) has done the same for alcoholism and leprosy. Finally, Ablon (1981) has examined the emergence of pressure groups in the United States to combat popular stereotypes and stigmatization in relation to dwarfism.

STIGMA AS A THREAT TO THE SOCIAL ORDER

Scott (1972) has proposed a framework within which he believes a number of theoretical questions concerning both ascribed and achieved deviance might one day be answered. A brief summary of this frame-work, which owes much to the work of Berger and Luckmann (1966), will provide a rationale for regarding illnesses that are stigmatizing as in some sense constituting a threat to the social order. An attempt will then be made to specify just how this might be so.

Scott begins by suggesting that man differs from other animals in that his relationship to the environment is not determined genetically. He has the capacity to

'apply his basic biological "equipment" to a very wide, continually changing range of activities and experiences. Berger and Luckmann term this quality "world-openness". Because of it, man is a highly adaptable animal but at the same time he lacks any innate mechanism that can provide him with stability in relationships with other men . . . One reason, therefore, why the human animal requires a symbolic framework for ordering social reality is because he is basically an unstable being. What social order does, in effect, is provide him with a stable environment by effectively pre-empting his capacity for world-openness and transforming it into a kind of "world-closedness".'

(Scott 1972: 18)

Social order is accomplished through man's tendency to habitualize his actions. Berger and Luckmann write: 'Any action that is repeated frequently becomes cast into a pattern which can be reproduced by its performance as that pattern' (Berger and Luckmann 1966: 50). Habitual-ized patterns become social institutions – commonly accepted or established ways of doing things – when transmitted by their initiators to the next generation. 'The child who acquires these patterns as established ways of doing things comes to view them as real. They confront him as things that are external and constraining and they resist his efforts to modify them' (Scott 1972: 19). These patterns or social institutions, which constitute a kind of 'institutional order', are further buttressed by elaborate modes of justification, or 'legitimations', con-structed over time by their initiators, as well as by mechanisms of social control to employ against the inadequately socialized.

'The most abstract level of legitimation', writes Scott, 'entails the effort to integrate the entire institutional order into a symbolic totality' (Scott 1972: 19). Berger and Luckmann refer in this context to 'the symbolic universe': 'In a symbolic universe, all the sectors of the established order are integrated in an all-embracing frame of reference, which now constitutes a universe in the literal sense of the word because all human experience can now be conceived as taking place within it' (Berger and Luckmann 1966: 89). This symbolic universe 'hardens' and 'thickens' and gradually takes on the mantle of objective reality. It should be remem-bered, however, that the symbolic universe involves the genesis of a sense of order out of things that are by their nature untidy. Social order, in short, exists in the midst of uncertainty and may at any time be undermined and have to yield to chaos. Berger and Luckmann again: 'All social reality is precarious. All societies are constructed in the face of chaos. The constant possibility of anomic terror is actualized whenever the legitimations that obscure this precariousness are threatened or collapse' (Berger and Luckmann 1966: 96).

Scott interprets 'deviance' as a property of social order. 'This property', he writes, 'is conferred upon an individual whenever others detect in his behaviour, appearance, or simply his existence, a significant transgression of the boundaries of the symbolic universe by which the inherent disorder of human existence is made to appear orderly and meaningful' (Scott 1972: 22). Such an individual is perceived and treated as something of an 'anomaly'. The contemporary homosexual is an anomaly in this sense: according to Plummer, for example, he represents a threat to taken-for-granted assumptions about the institution of marriage and the family unit, the simple gender dichotomy of 'male' and 'female' and the link between sex and procreation (Plummer 1975: 119–20).

Every social order, Scott argues, develops what Berger and Luckmann call 'universe-maintaining mechanisms' as protection against the chaos implied by anomaly. He goes on to identify and describe several universe-maintaining mechanisms which he regards as common to most modern western societies. Two of these warrant a mention here. The first is 'normalization', which refers to attempts to force anomalous individuals to change so as to become more like normal people. The educators of the deaf, for example, have traditionally emphasized 'oralism' and suppressed 'signing' among deaf children (Becker 1981; Higgins 1980). The second is a class of techniques of social control for use against deviants who cannot be changed. 'The symbolic universe may be threatened by a madman but its ultimate superiority may nevertheless be reaffirmed if the social order can render him harmless. There are several ways in which the madman can be 'defused', the most common being confinement. By putting the madman or criminal away, a social order removes the symbolically noxious element from its midst and at the same time demonstrates its capacity to master those whom it cannot domesticate' (Scott 1972: 27).

Finally, Scott shares the view, expressed most forcibly by Erikson, that deviance is not invariably an alien element in society, that it can also be, 'in controlled quantities, an important condition for preserving stability' (Erikson 1964: 15). It can preserve stability or social order by providing occasions for clarifying or reasserting the boundaries of the symbolic universe. It may even be the case that these boundaries can only remain salient for people if they are regularly tested by those on the fringes of society and defended by those who represent society's 'inner morality'.

It must be stressed that Scott's own account is tentative and replete with statements of qualification and is, hence, less dogmatic and all-embracing than this summary may have suggested. He is well aware, for example, that there can be more than one symbolic universe in a society and that there are often a number of sub-universes of meaning, which may occasionally represent genuine counter-cultures. His limited ambition is to propose a framework for analyzing deviance as a property of social order; in his own words, this framework 'only recommends to us the kinds of questions we ought to ask and answer in order to produce a theory to explain this social property' (Scott 1972: 29). Scott's disarming admission that his contribution does not amount to anything like a 'theory of deviance' does not of course render it immune from criticism. It might be objected, for example, that it incorporates unduly pessimistic assumptions about human nature or that it is seriously misleading in that no explicit reference is made to the importance of power in the emergence, development, and maintenance of social order. There is some justice in these hypothetical criticisms but this is not the place to discuss the complex issues they raise.

As the focus in this chapter is on ascribed rather than achieved deviance, consideration will be limited here to ways in which people with certain conditions of the body or the mind may be said to threaten the social order. It will be suggested, in fact, that they pose a threat in at least two major ways. They do so, first, by their failure to conform to a particular class of cultural norms – namely, those pertaining to how people should *be* rather than how they should *act*. Goffman refers in this context to norms of identity or being; he writes:

'Failure or success at maintaining such norms has a very direct effect on the psychological integrity of the individual. At the same time, mere desire to abide by the norm – mere good will – is not enough, for in many cases the individual has no immediate control over his level of sustaining the norm. It is a question of the individual's condition, not his will; it is a question of conformance, not compliance.'

(Goffman 1968: 152–53)

It is not that an individual who infringes against such norms stands condemned for a misdemeanour of some sort – he or she is not *morally* culpable – but rather that that individual is judged an essentially 'imperfect being': the nature of his or her 'offence' is perhaps best characterized as *ontological* (from 'ontology', the study of being). Although it would of course be quite wrong to deny that some stigmatizing conditions – like the sexually transmitted diseases – carry strong connotations of moral failure, it is suggested that it is *generally* the case that such connotations are secondary to those of ontological deficiency.

The second way in which such people jeopardize the social order is by violating cultural norms governing routine social intercourse, by causing what Albrecht, Walker, and Levy (1982) refer to as 'ambiguity in social interaction'. In their study of the attitudes of normal people this was the most frequent reason given for distancing from the stigmatized; respondents said things like, 'We are usually afraid of those things which we don't understand and things that are new or foreign to us,' 'The person doesn't know how to cope and feels uncomfortable with the disabled,' 'They don't know what, if anything, they should do to help,' and so on (Albrecht, Walker, and Levy 1982: 1324). Concluding her review of studies of the physically disabled, Safilios-Rothschild comments: 'Interactions between physically disabled and physically normal people are anxiety-laden, tend to cause emotional discomfort and usually take on the form of "stereotyped, inhibited and over-controlled experiences" (Safilios-Rothschild 1970: 122). In his autobiography *Journey Into Silence*, Labour MP Jack Ashley recalls several unhappy sequelae to his return to the House of Commons after becoming totally deaf. Among these is the following:

> 'On one occasion in the tea-room, I took my cup of tea to a table to join four friends. When one of them asked me a question which I could not understand, the others repeated it for me but I was still unable to lip-read it. They paused while one of them wrote it down and I was aware that the easy-going conversation they had been enjoying before my arrival was now disrupted. When I answered the written question it was understandable that none of them should risk a repeat performance by asking another. Within a few moments two of them had left and after a brief pause the others explained that they had to go because of pressing engagements. They were genuinely sorry and I understood but it was small solace as I sat alone drinking my tea.'
>
> (Ashley 1973: 149)

These suggestions, admittedly somewhat speculative and provisional, provide a backcloth for a consideration of the impact of stigmatizing conditions on the lives of their victims. What is it like to fall foul of culturally entrenched criteria of ontological normality and to be abused, pitied, or simply avoided as a result? How does it feel to embarrass others and unwittingly to disrupt normal social interaction? How does living with a stigmatizing condition alter one's ideas of self and self-worth? It is to questions like these that this chapter now turns.

Perceiving and coping with stigmatizing conditions

VISIBILITY

If people with stigmatizing conditions share a capacity to threaten the social order in specifiable ways, they have little else in common: in almost all other respects they are likely to be as heterogeneous as the population as a whole. Nor is there much that is uniform about their conditions. There is enormous variation, for example, in what Goffman (1968) calls the 'visibility' (or 'evidentness') of stigmatizing conditions. Goffman also distinguishes usefully between a stigma's visibility and its 'known-about-ness', its 'obtrusiveness' and its 'perceived focus'.

The need for a distinction between a stigma's visibility and whether or not it is known about is readily apparent: an individual's diabetes may be invisible yet widely known about. Of the distinction between a stigma's visibility and its obtrusiveness, Goffman writes: 'When a stigma is immediately perceivable, the issue still remains as to how much it interferes with the flow of interaction' (Goffman 1968: 66). He cites the example of a man in a wheelchair attending a business meeting; his stigma is obvious and yet, around a conference table, unlikely to be obtrusive. Compare his situation with that of another participant with a speech impediment; the latter's stigma is relatively minor but 'the very mechanics of spoken encounters constantly redirect attention to the defect, constantly making demands for clear and rapid messages that must constantly be defaulted' (Goffman 1968: 66).

The visibility of a stigma also needs to be distinguished from its perceived focus. Goffman points out that normal people tend to 'develop conceptions, whether objectively grounded or not, as to the sphere of life-activity for which an individual's particular stigma primarily disqualifies him' (Goffman 1968: 66). A facial deformity, for example, might be regarded as imposing an unpleasant burden on face-to-face communication but be considered irrelevant to an individual's employment status or competence. By contrast, a condition like diabetes may be felt to have little or no effect on social interaction but be acknowledged as a proper justification for negative discrimination in employment.

THE DISCREDITED

Clearly, whether or not someone's stigmatizing condition is known about is of fundamental importance. Goffman's describes the individual whose stigma is known about as '*discredited*' and the individual whose stigma is not known about as '*discreditable*' (Goffman 1968: 14). He suggests that one of the main problems confronting the discredited person is the 'management of impressions', the impressions others have of him or her. Davis, for example, has claimed that people with visible physical handicaps typically pass through three stages when building sociable relationships with normal people: the first is one of 'fictional acceptance' – they find they are ascribed a stereotypical identity and accepted on that basis; the second stage is one of 'breaking through' this fictional acceptance – they have to induce others to regard and interact with them as normal persons; and the third stage is one of 'consolidation' – they work to sustain the definition of themselves as normal. Davis refers to the unfolding of these three stages as a process of 'deviance disavowal' (1964: 126).

Appealing though Davis's account of deviance disavowal is, it should not lead to an over-simplified view of impression management. Scott (1969) has shown in relation to the discredited blind, for example, that the reality is often more complex. He is at one with Davis in arguing that blind people are initially accepted on a fictional basis, both because they are popularly stereotyped as helpless, dependent, and so on and because blindness is a stigmatizing condition implying inferiority. He differs from Davis, however, in his insistence that few blind people have the strength of will and psychological stamina to consistently engage in deviance disavowal: 'Even those who follow this road successfully are left with a certain bitterness and frustration that is the inevitable residue of any attempt to break the stubborn moulds into which the blind man's every action is pressed' (Scott 1969: 24). Some blind people, whom Scott terms 'true believers', actually come to concur with the verdict reached by the sighted: 'They adopt as part of their self-concept the qualities of character, the feelings and the behaviour patterns that others insist they must have' (Scott 1969: 22). Many others develop and deploy strategies not predicated on an explicit disavowal of their deviance (e.g. they may 'pretend' to comply purely to ease interaction). The psychologist, Allport (1958), has listed no fewer than fifteen 'ego defences' that individuals may develop as a reaction to prejudice and discrimination. In a study which parallels Scott's in many respects, Higgins (1980) has shown how the discredited deaf sometimes adopt the expedient of 'avowing' their deviance, and even extending it by acting mute, in order to simplify their dealings with the hearing: written messages can minimize mis-understandings and save time and trauma.

Scott also differs from Davis in stressing the influence of other kinds of factors on impression management. Two are given special emphasis: the fact that, because of the critical importance of eye contact in human communication, personal interaction is deeply disturbed when one of those involved cannot see, and the fact that interactions between the blind and sighted tend to become relationships of social dependency. Scott maintains that these two factors, both of which relate to the mechanics of inter-personal contact, affect the outcomes of socialization in three ways:

'They force upon blind people further evidence of their difference; they deny them the kind of honest, uncluttered feedback about self that is commonplace to the sighted; and they place them in a subordinate position, making it difficult for them to form intimate

relationships with those they regard as their intellectual and psychological equals.'

(Scott 1969: 38)

THE DISCREDITABLE

If one of the primary problems facing the discredited person is the
management of impressions, the most pressing problem for the discreditable person is often the 'management of information' about
himself or herself. In Goffman's words, the main quandary is: 'To display
or not to display; to tell or not to tell; to lie or not to lie; and in each case, to
whom, how, when and where' (Goffman 1968: 57). The person with
epilepsy is typically in this position and a fairly full account of the impact
of epilepsy as a stigmatizing condition will lead, first, to an appreciation
of some of the stresses associated with information management and,
second, to an examination of a number of other aspects of perceiving and
coping with stigma.

FOCUS ON EPILEPSY

There is a widespread but largely untested assumption amongst those
occupied with the health and welfare of people with epilepsy that crude,
erroneous stereotypes of epilepsy and epileptics are commonplace and
that much of the unhappiness experienced by epileptics derives from
the fact that they are routinely subject to negative discrimination by
employers and others. The authors of the 'Reid Report' write: 'Through
ignorance and prejudice about the nature of the disease, there is a
reluctance to give them a home, a job, or to accept them as relations by
marriage or as fit to become natural or adoptive parents' (CHSC 1969: 16).
This will be referred to as the 'orthodox viewpoint'. It is against this
background that the study reported here – based on interviews with
ninety-four adult epileptics living in and around London – should be
considered (Scambler 1983). It represents something of a challenge for
advocates of the orthodox viewpoint. For convenience the discussion is
split into five parts.

1   *The application of the label*

In only a fifth of cases had the possibility of a diagnosis of epilepsy been
anticipated and, almost without exception, people were extremely upset
when the diagnostic label was applied. The following exchange was
typical:

> *GS:* 'How did you feel when he said it was epilepsy?'
> *Mrs X:* 'I cried for two days. I think it was the word that frightened me
> more than anything.'

GS: 'Why was that?'

Mrs X: 'Oh, I just don't know. It was the way I felt I suppose. It's not a very nice word, is it? I can't describe it really. I just can't describe how I felt.'

GS: 'It was something about this word "epilepsy" that sparked that reaction off in you?'

Mrs X: 'Mm. Because, to me, when you tell people, they sort of shun you, that's the way I look at it. They, you know, they don't want to know; in fact, my mother doesn't for one. If you go for a job and its on a form – and you've got to put down 'yes', more often than not – you don't get the job, you know.'

GS: 'Have you actually found this, or is this something that you understood would happen?'

Mrs X: 'I understood would happen, because those who I work with don't know I have them anyway.'

GS: 'What made you think this sort of thing does happen to people with epilepsy?'

Mrs X: 'I don't really know, to be truthful. I just don't really know.'

Many echoed the sentiments expressed by the novelist Graham Greene, who describes how he reacted when as a young man he was told he had epilepsy: 'Epilepsy, cancer and leprosy – these are the three medical terms which arouse the greatest fear in the untutored and at twenty-two, one is unprepared for so final a judgement'. He continues, perhaps a trifle melodramatically: 'Was the diagnosis right? With the hindsight of forty years, free from any recurrence, I don't believe it, but I believed it then. I remember the next day standing on an Underground platform and trying to summon the will and the courage to jump' (Greene 1972: 136–37).

People's distress on learning of the diagnosis seemed to be rooted in two related perceptions. First, they had a more or less clearly defined awareness that a doctor's diagnostic utterance, whether delivered in their presence or to a third party (e.g. a parent) some time in the past, had in an important sense *made them into epileptics*. This is realistic enough: a medical – and hence authoritative – diagnosis of epilepsy does indeed confer the social status of 'epileptic'. Second, they saw this new status as a terrible burden. This was because they perceived epilepsy first and foremost as a stigmatizing condition; they felt they had been ascribed a status that would, or could, distance them from or even lead to their rejection by normal people. Sometimes, especially if they were young at the time, they seemed to develop this sense of stigma as a result of what Schneider and Conrad call the 'stigma coaching' of close and influential 'allies' like parents (Schneider and Conrad 1980: 36) and sometimes it seemed to be a residue of the conceptions of epilepsy and epileptics they had once had themselves. Only rarely did their accounts suggest that their perceptions of epilepsy as stigmatizing originated with an actual episode of negative discrimination.

People's perceptions of epilepsy as stigmatizing were clearly anchored in what they understood to be the common perspective on epilepsy within the *lay* community and 84 per cent indicated during the course of the interviews that they regarded laymen as typically ignorant, intolerant, and predisposed to discriminatory practices against epileptics. These internalizations of the lay perspective on epilepsy constituted one of people's two primary 'reference groups' (Shibutani 1962). Their internalizations of the *medical* perspective on epilepsy, of course, constituted the other.

People were often hesitant about accepting that they were 'epileptic' in what they took to be the medical sense of the term, and this despite the fact that, when probed, they generally acknowledged that their doctors possessed an expertise in diagnosis which they manifestly lacked. This seemingly irrational hesitancy was prompted by the realization that one sure consequence of the successful application of the medical label would be that they would have to live thereafter with the burden of being 'epileptic' in what they took to be the lay sense of the term. In short, people saw the *medical* diagnosis as certain to expose them to the harsh and injurious realities of *lay* ignorance, intolerance, and discrimination. It was for this reason that they were prone to resist and even challenge the application of the medical label, overtly or covertly 'negotiating' with their doctors for a less threatening alternative. Very real and obvious medical uncertainties about epileptic phenomena often provided them with an additional incentive: several people, for example, used the fact that no doctor was able to proffer a satisfactory aetiological theory of their seizures – which occurred in no fewer than 73 per cent of cases – to give substance to their denial that they were suffering from epilepsy.

2   *The development of a 'special view of the world'*

Stebbins (1970) has employed a concept of 'subjective career' to refer to an individual's 'recognition of past and future events associated with a particular identity and especially his interpretation of important contingencies as they were or will be encountered. It is his personal view of these happenings as they relate to the important features of his life'. The best way of understanding this, Stebbins continues, is to consider subjective career as a predisposition:

'The usage of the idea of predisposition follows that of Campbell. He limits his statement to acquired states, stressing the importance of the fact that predispositions (or as he calls them, "acquired behavioural dispositions") are enduring and that they remain dormant until activated by situational stimuli. When activated, these products of past experience impinge upon our awareness, equip us with a *special view of the world* and guide behaviour in the immediate present.'

(Stebbins 1970: 35)

Those with epilepsy can be said to have developed a 'special view of the world' in this sense. It will be helpful at this point to distinguish between *enacted* and *felt* stigma. Enacted stigma refers to episodes of discrimination against people with epilepsy on the sole grounds of their social unacceptability or inferiority; this specifically excludes episodes of 'legitimate' discrimination (e.g. banning them from driving trains or from operating heavy industrial machinery). Felt stigma refers, first, to the *shame* associated with being epileptic. People felt ashamed fundamentally because they saw 'being epileptic' as amounting to an infringement against norms relating to 'identity or being' (Goffman 1968: 152). A statement about homosexuality by Warren and Johnson is relevant here: 'Warren's research', they write, 'indicates that among homosexuals, the deviant "sex-act" is not the organizing aspect of their lives: the organizing conception is "being" homosexual, in the full sense of a condition or identity' (Warren and Johnson 1972: 74). This was analogously true of people with epilepsy, in that 'having seizures' was less salient to them than *'being epileptic'*. In line with the earlier discussion, the shame experienced by those with epilepsy may be said, as may felt stigma generally, to be based on a deep sense of ontological inferiority. Second and most important, felt stigma refers to *an oppressive fear of enacted stigma*. The typical epileptic's 'special view of the world' was founded upon these two aspects of felt stigma.

Despite its significance, felt stigma was not omnipresent in people's lives. To make essentially the same point in a slightly different way, the 'special view of the world' characteristic of those with epilepsy only informed and guided their behaviour when 'activated' by 'situational stimuli' or, as they will be referred to below, 'triggers'. When it was activated, however, this 'special view of the world' predisposed them, first, to resist the transition from discreditable to discredited, to try to pass as normal, and second, if they were already discredited, to adopt what Davis has called the stratagem of 'normalization' (Davis 1963: 139) and Goffman 'covering' –

'It is a fact that persons who are ready to admit possession of a stigma (in many cases because it is known about or immediately apparent) may nonetheless make a great effort to keep the stigma from looming large. The individual's object is to reduce tension, that is, to make it easier for himself and the others to withdraw covert attention from the stigma, and to sustain spontaneous involvement in the official content of the interaction.'

(Goffman 1968: 125)

3 *A predisposition to secrecy*

People's primary predisposition was to secrecy and concealment. The evidence for this was considerable and consonant with that of many other studies. When considering the following findings, it must be borne in mind that not all the disclosures were 'voluntary': for example, they were quite often provoked either by 'stigmata' (i.e. clinical manifestations of people's conditions, usually seizures, which led to their exposure as 'epileptics') or by 'stigma cues' (i.e. happenings other than clinical symptoms which similarly led to their exposure as 'epileptics' – slips of the tongue, witnessed drug-taking, absences from work, and so on). The siblings of children with epilepsy were frequently not told of the medical label by parents unless a witnessed seizure made disclosure particularly difficult to avoid. The children of adults with epilepsy were even less likely to be put fully in the picture: 67 per cent of the children living with their families of origin and over the age of sixteen had no knowledge of the diagnosis. Sixty-one per cent of those who had had two or more boy or girl friends after learning of the diagnosis had never disclosed it. Perhaps most remarkably of all, as many as 31 per cent of those who married after onset had made no disclosure of any kind to their future spouses before the wedding day; 36 per cent had made a partial disclosure involving words like 'seizures', 'attacks', 'dizzy spells', and so on; and only 33 per cent had disclosed the diagnosis of epilepsy.

If epilepsy has a perceived focus, it is probably in relation to issues of employability. Past studies have found that most epileptics are reluctant to disclose to employers. For example, Jones (1965) found that only 26 per cent of prospective epileptic employees at a Welsh steel works admitted their condition at a pre-employment 'medical'. Similarly, Aston found that only 7 per cent of the men at a motor works who were suffering from epilepsy prior to employment admitted as much before starting work (see MacIntyre 1976). The present study was unexceptional (Scambler and Hopkins 1981). Fifty-three per cent of those who had had two or more full-time jobs after the onset of their seizures had never disclosed anything at all to an employer. Of those in full-time employment when interviewed, as many as 55 per cent had made no disclosure of any kind to their employer; 17 per cent had mentioned their seizures, often using a more neutral word like 'attacks' or 'turns'; and only 28 per cent had informed their employer that they suffered from epilepsy. Even more significantly, only 17 per cent had disclosed either their seizures or their epilepsy 'voluntarily', and only 5 per cent had done so before starting work. Those who did 'choose' to disclose tended to be having more frequent seizures than those who did not; presumably they reasoned that they would probably have a seizure at work sooner or later and that an anticipatory disclosure was the lesser of two evils (in the event, 57 per cent of those who disclosed 'voluntarily' went on to have seizures at work, compared with only 27 per cent of those who did not). Schneider and Conrad (1980) refer to this as 'anticipatory preventive telling' and write:

> 'To engage in anticipatory preventive telling is to offer a kind of "medical disclaimer" intended to influence others' reactions should a seizure occur. By bringing a blameless, beyond-my-control medical interpretation to such potentially discrediting events, people attempt to reduce the risk that more morally disreputable interpretations might be applied by naive others witnessing one's seizures.'
>
> (Schnieder and Conrad 1980: 41)

4 The relative impacts of felt and enacted stigma

The key argument to emerge from the study was that people's preferred policy of non-disclosure and concealment, which remained feasible for as long as they were in settings where they were discreditable and not discredited, had the function of reducing the opportunities for, and hence rate of, enacted stigma, and that one crucial consequence of this was that felt stigma, and especially the fear of enacted stigma, was typically the source of more personal anguish and unhappiness than was enacted stigma. This argument, of course, is at odds with the orthodox viewpoint cited earlier.

There can be no doubt that the policy of non-disclosure in relation both to seizures and, more importantly, to the diagnosis of epilepsy served to protect people from possible instances of enacted stigma. There can be little doubt also that felt stigma was in its own right a profound and lasting, if intermittent, source of unease, self-doubt and disruption in people's lives. It is instructive to focus on employment again here. A number of married women, sometimes at the urging or insistence of husbands with incomes sufficient for family needs, opted not to seek or pursue their own careers as a result of felt stigma; at the time of interview only 32 per cent of them had full-time jobs, compared with 48 per cent of married women in the British population as a whole. Consider also the implications of the fact that 55 per cent of those of both sexes in full-time work when interviewed had disclosed nothing at all to their employers (and a further 17 per cent had made no mention of the diagnosis). This meant they had acquired at least a temporary, if sometimes quite precarious, immunity from enacted stigma; they had gained a job and a breathing space. However, most of them had paid a psychological price for their silence. Most obviously, they had had to learn to live with the stresses of guarding against the daily risk of exposure through stigmata or stigma cues, which would probably be followed by what Goffman has called a 'showdown': 'He who passes can find himself called to a showdown by persons who have now learned of his secret and are about to confront him with his having been false' (Goffman 1968: 106). Some had also denied themselves opportunities of career advancement because they thought promotion would increase the potential personal cost of exposure and hence the stresses associated with future information management. Felt stigma, in sum, exacted a considerable toll.

Perhaps the most revealing employment statistic of all is that, although only 23 per cent of those who had had at least one full-time job after onset could recount a *single* occasion when they *suspected* they had been victims of enacted stigma at work (even of casual ridicule), and only 14 per cent judged they had actually suffered some kind of career setback as a direct result of enacted stigma, nearly 90 per cent reported experiencing more or less protracted episodes of felt stigma at their various places of work. This is consistent with an observation of Blaxter's in her study of disability. Of the handful of epileptics in her sample she writes:

'Epilepsy came into a special category. In fact, none of the sample's epileptics gave any evidence at all that they had experienced any social stigma, but each one expressed surprise and gratitude at this and all told generalized stories about the problems which epileptics "usually" faced. The condition was "known" to be one against which there was particular prejudice, but in this sample at least, no actual examples of prejudice could be cited by any of the people who spoke in this way.'
(Blaxter 1976: 198–99)

In the absence of any investigations of the prevalence and nature of enacted stigma in relation to epilepsy and employment, the extent to which felt stigma is 'justifiably felt' remains an open question.

5 *Aspects of secondary deviation*

The concept of 'secondary deviation', introduced by Lemert in the 1950s, refers to

'the tendency of the deviator to become "caught up in" a deviant role, to find that it has become highly salient in his overall personal identity (or concept of self), that his behaviour is increasingly organized "around" the role, and that cultural expectations attached to the role have come to have precedence, or increased salience relative to other expectations, in the organization of his activities and general way of life.'
(Schur 1971: 69)

(Interestingly, Schur himself prefers the term 'role-engulfment' to secondary deviation.) The final question in this section is: 'How helpful is this concept of secondary deviation in analysing the experiences of people labelled as "epileptic"?'

It will be helpful to outline and then comment on a recent American typology of modes of adaptation to epilepsy. Schneider and Conrad draw a fundamental distinction between 'adjusted adaptations' and 'unadjusted adaptations'. Of the former they write: 'Adjusted epileptics are in effect persons able to successfully neutralize the actual or perceived negative impact of epilepsy on their lives' (Schneider and Conrad 1981: 214). Three sub-types of adjusted adaptation are described. The first is the *pragmatic* type. The pragmatist 'minimizes' his epilepsy, both to himself and others, but does not invariably try to pass or cover.

'By following what might be called a course of "reason" . . . being open about epilepsy to those who "need to know", e.g., employers, official agencies, close friends and associates, while keeping a knowing eye on the possibility of others' negative judgements were they to know, the pragmatist manages a "normal" existence relatively free of disruption due to epilepsy.'

(Schneider and Conrad 1981: 215)

The second sub-type is the *secret* type. 'Epilepsy is managed here by sometimes elaborate procedures to control and conceal information about what is perceived as a stigmatizing, negative or "bad" quality of self' (Schneider and Conrad 1981: 215). To the extent that these procedures are successful, the individual 'participates, albeit cautiously, in a broad range of social settings, including driving a car (sometimes only at the expense of lying on application and renewal forms), holding a job and having a satisfying informal social life' (Schneider and Conrad 1981: 216). Third, Schneider and Conrad refer to the *quasi-liberated* type.

'This type shares with the pragmatic adaptation a straightforward definition of one's self as "having" epilepsy but goes beyond it in indeed "broadcasting" this fact in an attempt to educate others about epilepsy and "free" one's self of any burdens of secrecy and concealment based on fear of stigma.'

(Schneider and Conrad 1981: 216)

This policy of what is sometimes called 'destigmatization' positively *avows* physical deviance yet challenges the values and norms which attach discreditable meanings and connotations. 'Deviance is shown to be no more than difference and discredit is denied' (Jobling 1977: 83).

With regard to unadjusted adaptations, Schneider and Conrad write:

'While the adapted response to epilepsy is characterized in each case by a sense of agency or control, the unadjusted adaptation is marked by a sense of being "overcome" or "overwhelmed" by epilepsy. People who speak of the condition as having a great negative impact on their lives and who seem to have developed no strategies for managing this impact we call "unadjusted".'

(Schneider and Conrad 1981: 216–17)

They go on to identify one 'extreme' sub-type, which they refer to as the *debilitated* type. This type, they suggest, represents the clearest example of

> 'what Hughes called a "master status" that "floods" one's identity and life with meanings and behaviour that figuratively constipate the self. It is the analogue to Lemert's secondary deviation in that the debilitated response embraces epilepsy as an indelible and irrevocable threat to one's worth; it pursues epilepsy as a deviant, stigmatizing and debilitating blemish or flaw, as a "cross to bear".'
>
> (Schneider and Conrad 1981: 217)

Unfortunately, Schneider and Conrad give no estimates of the proportions in their sample who employed each of the strategies they identify, although they do add the rider that some individuals seemed to have adopted different styles of adaptation at different points in their lives. There are three comments that might be made here in the light of the London study. The first is that the sub-type of adjusted adaptation Schneider and Conrad refer to as the *secret* type seemed in the London study to have been the *first-choice* strategy for most people with epilepsy in respect of most of their various social roles. However, this strategy of secrecy and concealment – regardless of its efficacy – rarely brought them the lasting peace of mind that members of Schneider and Conrad's sample seem to have enjoyed. It seems reasonable to suggest that Schneider and Conrad may be guilty of neglecting, or at least of underestimating, the stresses associated with felt stigma.

To argue that the secret type was the preferred or prime strategy in the London study is not of course to deny that the other sub-types of adjusted adaptation were also represented. Several people had at one time or another and in one role or another employed the *pragmatic* strategy; in other words, they had on occasions selectively and 'voluntarily' disclosed their seizures or epilepsy. Unlike Schneider and Conrad's pragmatists, however, the great majority appeared to have regarded pragmatism as a *second-choice* strategy. They tended to disclose only when their first-choice strategy of secrecy and concealment seemed likely to fail them or to be in some way counter-productive. It has been seen, for example, that only 5 per cent of those engaged in full-time work when interviewed had disclosed 'voluntarily' to their employers before starting work; each of these was suffering *daily* seizures at the time. They had opted for what Schneider and Conrad (1980) have elsewhere called 'preventive telling'. If there were several – intermittent and typically reluctant – pragmatists in the London sample, only 2 per cent seemed ever to have contemplated adopting the *quasi-liberated* strategy. This almost certainly reflects cultural differences in the militancy and organization of pressure and self-help groups for the disabled in the

United States and Britain (for an example of an apparently successful United States self-help group, see Ablon's (1981) account of dwarfism and Little People of America).

The second comment is that in the London study people's epilepsy did not have high salience for them all the time but only periodically. Indeed, most people for most of their waking hours felt and acted 'just like everyone else'. Their epilepsy had high salience for them, in fact, only when untoward circumstances or events, 'triggers', prompted them to engage with or retreat into the 'special view of the world' based on felt stigma. Under the influence of this 'special view of the world' they were likely to adopt the strategy of Schneider and Conrad's secret type. Expressed in the more familiar language of this chapter, people were typically predisposed by their 'special view of the world' to certain stereotyped modes of behaviour – namely, depending on whether they were discreditable or discredited, to attempt to pass or to cover respectively.

There were many species of 'triggers', but not surprisingly the most commonplace and the most potent were those witnessed seizures interpreted as actual or potential stigmata. Seizure frequency was therefore very important. As a buttress to the point that people's epilepsy had high salience for them only periodically, however, it is worth noting that not all seizures were either interpreted as actual or potential stigmata or, indeed, witnessed; and that for many people seizures were fairly infrequent: only 36 per cent had had a seizure in the month prior to interview and 31 per cent had not had a seizure for two years or more.

The third and final comment is that, in the London study, people's epilepsy typically had higher salience for them in some roles – or, following Merton, 'role-sets' – than in others. Merton writes:

'We must note that a particular social status involves, not a single associated role but an array of associated roles . . . This fact of structure can be registered by a distinctive term, role-set, by which I mean that complement of role relationships which persons have by virtue of occupying a particular social status.'

(Merton 1968: 423)

In short, each individual has his 'status-set' and each of these statuses has its distinctive 'role-set'. When people were ascribed the status of 'epileptic' they did indeed discover new and distinctive role relationships (e.g. with general practitioners, neurologists, EEG technicians, and so on). It was typically the case also that their new, 'deviant' status periodically *contaminated* others of their statuses (e.g. wife, mother, friend, employee, and so on) and role-sets. From the accounts rendered it seemed that such contamination was rarely uniformly present across people's status-sets and corresponding role-sets, but rather that, at any given time, it was likely to be more apparent – and people's epilepsy therefore more salient for them – in some than in others. It might be, for example, that an individual had negotiated or otherwise achieved a state of equilibrium within his family but, because the frequency of his seizures had suddenly trebled, was suffering from severe felt stigma in connection with his discreditable position at work. This is not to say, of course, that most people did not from time to time experience black moods of despair and pessimism, when their deviant status of 'epileptic' became a (felt or enacted) master status and they judged themselves truly cursed. At such junctures they became (temporary rather than permanent) candidates for Schneider and Conrad's debilitated sub-type of unadjusted adaptation.

To summarize, when people were diagnosed as epileptic they typically developed a 'special view of the world', underpinned by felt stigma, which predisposed them whenever possible to pass and, failing that, to cover. They generally lived fairly normal lives until prompted by some 'trigger', often a witnessed seizure, to retreat into their characteristic 'special view of the world', which then, to a greater or lesser extent, took over governance of their perceptions and actions. This happened to most people periodically and, when it did happen, their deviant status of 'epileptic' tended to contaminate some, but seldom all, of their other statuses and role-sets. In short, if people were the victims of secondary deviation, they were so periodically rather than continuously and, on most occasions, in respect of some statuses and role-sets rather than across all of them.

Stigma and health policy and practice

There are two broad and related implications of social scientific work on stigma that are worth highlighting here. The first arises from the fact that health policy and practice are deeply embedded in general cultural values. As Scott (1969, 1970) has convincingly shown with reference to blindness, medical theories and models (or 'ideologies') about stigmatizing conditions do not develop in a cultural vacuum but rather reflect – among other things – lay values, beliefs, and attitudes. (Volinn (1983) has made the same point more recently in relation to alcoholism and leprosy.) Scott writes:

'In a sense, this is inevitable. Experts must use their native tongue in order to communicate their constructed meanings to laymen, and the modes of expression that a language affords are grounded in the core values of a culture. Moreover, it is laymen who usually grant legitimacy to expert's claims to special knowledge about stigma; any constructed meanings that are dissonant with lay values, beliefs and attitudes will probably be rejected as nonsensical.'

(Scott 1970: 270)

Doctors and other health workers are of course also likely to be dependent on laymen for resources and for co-operation with treatment and rehabilitation measures.

Scott adds that there is still another, more direct, way in which laymen influence experts' constructions of stigma. Stigma poses problems not only for the person possessing it but also for the community in which that person lives.

> 'Stigma threatens the community and presents it with unpleasant problems it would rather not confront or think about. Old people, poor people, people who are blind or crippled, and those who are crazy make us uneasy; they threaten our sense of mastery of nature, and they are disruptive of routines of daily life. A community's needs relating to stigmata may be to hide them from public view, or at least to dress them up in a way that makes them more palatable to laymen or at least less offensive to them. In writing about mental hospitals, Goffman has stated the point as follows: "Part of the official mandate of the public mental hospital is to protect the community from the dangers and nuisances of certain kinds of misconduct." . . . Such institutions, then, are places to which the unwanted of the community can be sent and where they can be "taken care of".'
>
> (Scott 1970: 273)

Szasz (1966) asks whether the placement of epileptics in 'colonies' was really in their best interests, and adds for good measure 'or their exclusion from jobs, from driving automobiles and from entering the United States as immigrants?' In Britain, as late as 1965, a working party of the BMA recommended that people with epilepsy should not be allowed to immigrate to this country 'for social and economic reasons' (Bagley 1971: 110). Comfort (1967) has made the general, historical case that doctors, deriving spurious authority from a hard-earned technical expertise which sets them apart from laymen, have often made unwarranted moral pronouncements on social or individual problems which have had some apparent connection with physical conditions.

There is an important element of truth in the idea that both the 'treatment' of people with stigmatizing conditions by health workers and discrimination against them by laymen can be seen as responses – the first 'official' and culturally sanctioned and the second 'unofficial' and culturally condemned – to the threat to what was earlier called the social order. Homosexuality provides a particularly good example. Following Plummer, some of the ways in which homosexuality threatens the social order have already been recounted. Indeed, it should not be forgotten that until 1967 in Britain, all male homosexual acts, whether committed publicly or privately, were *illegal*. While it might be justifiably argued that the growing tendency to regard homosexuality as an illness to be 'treated' rather than a crime (or sin) to be 'punished' has been essentially progressive, leading to an increased public tolerance of homosexuals, it remains the case that homosexuality is 'officially' frowned upon. As Freidson puts it: 'Human, and therefore social, evaluation of what is normal, proper, or desirable is as inherent in the notion of illness as it is in notions of morality' (Freidson 1970: 208). In other words, doctors and therapists who make available treatment designed to help homosexuals become non-homosexuals are, wittingly or otherwise, giving medical legitimacy to, and hence reinforcing, negative lay attitudes to homosexuality. Bancroft (1981) has directed attention to the dilemmas over personal and social values that therapists often face in circumstances like these.

If this first implication of work on stigma invites reflection on doctors and other health workers as defenders of the social order, as 'agents of social control', the second has to do with more mundane aspects of the doctor–patient relationship. In the 1950s Parsons (1951) maintained that in modern industrialized societies people are socialized from a very early age into responding 'appropriately' when they feel unwell. They learn, for example, that illness represents a social as well as a personal liability, and that the appropriate – culturally prescribed – response is to seek expert medical help in order to get well and, thenceforth, to defer to 'professional authority'. Haug writes

'Authority in this context is defined as the patient's grant of legitimacy to the professional's exercise of power. The relationship with the physician is asymmetrical; the patient is in a dependent and the physician a super-ordinate status. It is the "competence gap" between doctor and patient which justifies both the professional's authority and the client's trust, confidence and norm of obedience. Although the objective of care is to return the patient to an active, independent status, he is obligated in the model to become temporarily submissive and to accept the doctor's right to tell him what to do.'

(Haug 1976: 23)

Freidson (1961) was perhaps the first to note that Parson's account of the doctor–patient relationship reflects less how doctors and patients *in fact* behave than how *doctors* think they and their patients *ought* to behave. Reacting against this 'bias', he went on to propose that the doctor–patient relationship be analysed within the framework of a 'clash of perspectives'. On the one hand, doctors expect patients to accept and follow professional advice and instruction; and on the other hand, patients seek help on their own terms. In so far as each seeks to gain their own terms, there is likely to be conflict. Freidson stressed that while both doctor and patient are 'theoretically' in accord with the end of their relationship – solving the patient's problem – the means to this end, and even the definition of the problem, are matters of potential difference. In sum, whereas in the Parsonian model of the relationship the accent is on mutuality and reciprocity, Freidson allows for ambivalence and conflicts of interest (see Bloom and Wilson 1972).

Stimson and Webb (1975) have shown that patients routinely develop their own perspectives on illness and that it does not follow from the fact that doctors tend to dominate consultations with their patients at the *interactional* level that the latter are truly acquiescent or 'passive'; behaviour that seems deferential is not necessarily indicative of agreement, satisfaction, or of a readiness to take medical advice (see Chapters 6 and 8). Referring again to the London study of epileptics, the single most important source of the often latent or hidden 'conflict' between the perspectives of doctor and patient was the latter's 'special view of the world', which turned on the perception of epilepsy as stigmatizing. It was this at times overriding perception of epilepsy as an acute social liability, for example, which variously prompted patients to reject the diagnosis of epilepsy, or at least to 'negotiate' for a less virulent alternative; to misinterpret normal EEGs as evidence of premature or mistaken diagnosis; and to defy medical advice about the regular taking of anti-convulsant tablets in order to try to hasten the transition from 'epileptic' to 'normal' status. What is important here is that most people, whether or not it was apparent during doctor–patient consultations, were 'active' in the sense that they both possessed concepts of epilepsy at variance with those utilized by their doctors (i.e. internalized from the lay populace) and assessed and responded to the words and actions of their doctors in the light of these concepts.

Jobling, a social scientist with psoriasis, notes that coming to terms with this skin abnormality 'typically involves both a long career of arduous patienthood ostensibly directed towards symptom control and elimination, and a psychosocial career of personal adjustment and adaptation in an effort, conscious or otherwise, to come to terms with its psychological and social meaning and implications' (Jobling 1977: 73). The same might be said to apply to many other victims of chronic, stigmatizing conditions. It certainly applies to epileptics. Many of those interviewed in the London study, however, took umbrage at what they interpreted as their doctors' preoccupation with the diagnosis and management of disease (itself open to criticism (Hopkins and Scambler 1977)) and manifest lack of interest in issues of 'personal adjustment and adaptation'. This charge that doctors had neither the inclination nor the time to show 'empathy' – and hence offered little or no thoughtful counsel on, for example, strategies for applying for or holding down jobs – was most often directed at 'academic' hospital specialists. West has suggested that such doctors lack a coherent 'stigma ideology' relating to epilepsy: in particular, they have no clear 'set of prescriptions, or 'practice theories', to enable the stigmatized themselves to manage their situation as effectively as possible' (West 1979: 647). One result of this, he contends, is that 'the physician is in danger of legitimating the stigma of epilepsy, not by talking about it, but by *not* talking about it' (West 1979: 652).

An adequate stigma ideology for epilepsy would of necessity be complex. For example, although it was argued earlier that felt stigma can best be defined in terms of a sense of ontological inferiority associated with '*being* epileptic', it must also be acknowledged that occurrences and circumstances like having a seizure, swallowing anti-convulsant tablets two or three times daily, attending a neurological out-patient clinic, declining an alcoholic drink, and being a non-driver, can all be stigmatizing *in their own right*; in other words, they are not only of significance to people as actual or potential stigmata or stigma cues (i.e. as ways in which they might be exposed as 'epileptic'). If '*being* epileptic' was the primary source of people's distress, there were many other secondary sources, some necessarily and some contingently, some ontologically and some morally, related to their conditions; one might credibly refer to a 'family of epilepsy-related stigmas'. Hopper writes in similar vein in her detailed account of the stigmas associated with diabetes in the United States. She concludes that 'as a background, an understanding of the effects of the illness on different groups of people should be part of practitioner education' (Hopper 1981: 16).

Conclusion

The thrust of this chapter has been threefold: to suggest a way of conceptualizing stigma as a threat to the social order; to illustrate some of the ways in which people, whether discredited or discreditable, define and cope with stigmatizing illnesses; and to draw out certain implications of analyses of stigma for health policy and practice. The overall aim has been to encourage or provoke reflection on the part of health workers actively engaged in 'helping' victims of stigmatizing illnesses. It is unlikely, for example, that many have thought of themselves as defenders of the social order, except perhaps in more obvious cases involving the diagnosis and treatment of sexual 'deviance'. Some also might not have noted the paradox that while doctors have it in their power to foist unwanted, stigmatizing identities upon their patients – 'in the case of stigmatizing illnesses, it is the identification and categorization of a person through diagnosis that confers a stigmatizing label' (West 1979: 65) – most, it seems, lack the training, motivation or time to offer sympathetic understanding and support to those they have, in worthy innocence, 'marked'. Issues like these call for a constant monitoring of personal and social values and of their interrelations.

11   Coping with terminal illness

John Hinton

Introduction

Death and dying will affect all of us closely sooner or later, usually through involvement in the last illness of someone close to us, and finally when our own life reaches its end. Some of the readers of this book may also have a professional experience of mortality that overlaps their personal concern. Although dying may be universal and simple in some respects, it is also inseparable from the complexities and desires of living. This review of coping with terminal illness therefore demands both a framework and limits. It will consider in turn *who* is doing the coping, *what* they are coping with and *how* they cope. The *how* will include *how well* people manage, although there can be no indisputable criteria to judge whether it is well or poorly.

Who is coping when a member of a society dies will be given arbitrary limits. The dying person is the key individual, but the family is an integral part of the situation, particularly first-degree relatives. Beyond these central actors are a host of others, many of whom will not be considered to any extent in this chapter. Professional people are bound to be included at some stage; nurses and doctors often influence radically the quality of the terminal illness. Their vocation does not submerge the fact that they are individuals who also have to cope; in fact their personal attitudes to life and death may materially affect their professional behaviour. Nevertheless the reasons and manner of the coping style of medical personnel will not be examined directly here, although the repercussions on patient and family may be noted. Nor will the behaviour of the many others involved in a person's dying. They range from doctor's receptionist to funeral director. Sometimes they have an influence of great individual significance, but, with apologies, there will be no consistent review of the roles of clergy, social worker, neighbour, ambulance man, or ward orderly, nor of the close friend or fellow-patient who may play a major part. The gaps, like so many other omissions in the care of the dying, reflect both immediate convenience and areas where adequate evidence is sadly lacking.

What are the patient and others coping with? First, there are the immediate manifestations of the fatal disease, which are potentially severe when the terminal phase is reached. It should be noted that terminal illness is not synonymous with fatal illness. People may have a fatal disease for months and years without apparent impairment of their living. They may be no more aware of it than anyone with a background recognition of his inherent mortal nature. The question of coping with it does not arise until the condition becomes manifest and its lethal nature subsequently recognized. In the terminal phase, when health is grossly undermined, serious symptoms are to be expected.

As well as the immediate consequences of the disorder that have to be contended with are the secondary effects of being ill. These will include, for example, the resultant need to be confined to bed, perhaps the unwanted effects of treatment or the consequences of leaving home to enter hospital. These changes will make demands on the patient and others. Another type of secondary effect of the illness is the emotional changes which are associated with the primary symptoms, for example the fear of recurring pain. If the emotions become distressful they also need to be coped with.

Third, beyond the enduring of severe illness lies the fact that the individual's life is about to end. The patient may well recognize that he will not live much longer. All the family are facing a final separation and the losses that go with it.

How people cope with terminal illness contains two elements. 'How well' they cope can be considered in terms of the degree of strain they feel or the emotions they display in response to the stress experienced. 'How', implying the strategy or tactics employed, will be viewed in terms of the manoeuvres commonly used to reduce the stress or render the strain tolerable.

What the stresses are

IMMEDIATE EFFECTS OF THE ILLNESS

Information on the effects of a fatal illness in its later stages comes from a number of overlapping sources. The personal observations of those with clinical experience, reinforced by written reports in medical text-books and journals, give foreknowledge of the typical symptoms and signs which accompany particular disorders. A person dying of heart failure or lung cancer may well find it distressingly difficult to breathe; someone with bone cancer is likely to have pain; motor neurone disease will cause increasing physical helplessness. This information on potential suffering is not only very general in nature but progress may well be modified by treatment. A more direct method of evaluating the stresses of the dying is to collect reports derived from consistent observations of patients with terminal disease. Such surveys were sparse until recently and they still tend to focus on certain selected groups. In the last two or three decades the available information has increased. The reports, quite possibly due to an inherent reluctance to intrude into disquieting personal experience, tend to rely on retrospective accounts from those nearby rather than currently gathered observations of dying people. None of the information is scientifically impeccable. However, there is a degree of consistency in the more carefully gathered results to indicate that some period of suffering is a common experience. There is also the implication that except in selected circumstances distress may well occur more often than it should.

An important account of terminal illness is the randomized survey conducted in England and Wales by Cartwright, Hockey and Anderson (1973). The data were based on retrospective accounts, mainly from the nearest surviving relative. They could hardly have been disinterested observers, but their reports largely have the ring of truth. One of the many tables record the symptoms occurring to a 'very distressing degree' during the last year of life in the following percentage of patients: pain 42 per cent, breathing troubles 28 per cent, vomiting 17 per cent, sleeplessness 17 per cent, loss of both bladder and bowel control 12 per cent, loss of appetite 11 per cent, and mental confusion 10 per cent (Cartwright, Hockey and Anderson 1973: 18–24). Other symptoms troubled smaller proportions. Quite a number of people were reported to have been distressed throughout the final year although it is hard to credit that they would have been left at a 'very distressed' level continuously for this time. Ten per cent had no symptoms, and a further 5 per cent had symptoms only in the last month. Whatever the exact truth may be, there is little doubt that the relatives held in their minds a picture of the dying suffering considerably.

These figures are daunting and a potential indictment. They present a worse picture than most of the reports based on current assessments. This may reflect the fact that studies based on patients who are regularly assessed give them the benefits of attention, both the psychological effect of that attention and the reduced chances of neglect. Nevertheless, regular observations of patients' current symptoms have tended to produce a salutary effect on doctors who usually have the impression that they are largely keeping distress at bay in most of their terminally ill patients. For example a conscientious general practitioner reported with some chagrin that 26 per cent of his dying patients had severe or very severe pain at times and the same proportion were equally breathless (Rees 1972). These were peak periods, however, and, judged by the more average level, 8 per cent had severe symptoms. Other prospective investigations have produced results in a similar range; 12 per cent of dying patients in a teaching hospital continued to suffer pain despite treatment (Hinton 1963); so did 14 per cent of an elderly group of people where concurrent disease such as arthritis gave rise to more discomfort than the final illness (Exton-Smith 1961). Cancers tend to receive a disproportionate amount of attention in terminal care studies although they do not necessarily cause most distress. Another investigation in general practice found that 15 per cent of cancer patients dying at home had a significant degree of suffering in their last six weeks of life (Wilkes 1965). Parkes (1980) found that over 20 per cent of people at home with terminal cancer had unsatisfactory relief of pain and a similar proportion were breathless. Although this last thoroughly conducted study indicates that as many as one in five did suffer, the proportion is considerably lower than the very troubling picture painted by the relatives in the first quoted survey.

The problems of assessing subjective feelings are considerable, particularly when they include the distress of dying people. Evaluating physical discomfort with a view to its relief demands a measurement of intensity and this can hardly be exact. It also needs a parallel observation of duration and even for this measure there are problems of defining the duration of terminal illness. Here we are only considering the final phase of the illness, and excluding what may be a lengthy period of life when a patient, although incurable, is not judged to be dying. Moreover, within the terminal illness it is self-evident that isolated peaks of pain are a very different stress from weeks of continued severe pain. The length of the terminal phase has a considerable range. People may die quite suddenly, in moments or days. In Cartwright, Hockey, and Anderson's survey (1973: 16–18) 10 per cent of deaths were unexpected, usually from some circulatory failure and a few through accidents. Data from this and other studies indicate that those who die in hospital mostly do so within a few weeks of admission and usually in less than three months. Those dying outside hospital tend to have a not dissimilar period of about six weeks when the primary effects of the disease cause considerable restrictions and possible distress.

SECONDARY EFFECTS OF THE ILLNESS

The immediate effects of lethal disorders are likely to cause material alterations in the style of living and also affect people's emotional state. The surveys give some indication of gross changes. The 1973 survey in Britain (Cartwright, Hockey, and Anderson 1973: 16–18) showed that about two-thirds of dying people were restricted in their activities for the last three months of their lives. One-fifth of these were confined to bed, while many of the others kept inside the house. It takes little imagination to visualize the stress this may impose on normally active individuals. They may well be incapable of washing, dressing or going to the lavatory independently. Such major difficulties are echoed by a series of lesser frustrations as small actions have to be done by others or with their assistance. Finally, about 60 per cent need to leave home and end their lives in hospital. Most of them are there from one to thirteen weeks.

From this point in the review it becomes increasingly difficult to ascertain the relationship between life changes and feelings. First, it is not always easy to divide emotions from changes in behaviour or events. (In research it may be of cardinal importance to assess them separately.) When they are separable it would be an over-simplification to attribute the psychological changes solely to events in the illness. Emotions are concurrently affected by other factors, including the prospect of life ending, which will be discussed more later. Nevertheless dying people themselves do attribute a great deal of their mental distress to current suffering and privations.

Considerable emotional distress has been recorded. Relatives have reported that about a third of people experience significant depression in their terminal illness, a half of them to a very distressing degree (Cartwright, Hockey, and Anderson 1973: 18–24). Results from a group of hospital patients were similar, over 40 per cent felt depressed and in nearly 20 per cent the lowered mood was obvious to others (Hinton 1963). Suicidal thoughts were by no means rare. Sadness was a commoner emotion than anxiety, but even so about a third of these hospital patients were patently apprehensive.

When an individual is very ill and weak it can be difficult to distinguish exhaustion and physical discomfort from a troubled state of mind. This is not only the problem of cause and effect, but that symptoms such as weakness, loss of weight and appetite, and insomnia are common to bodily and mental changes. In practice enquiry usually allows the physical and mental components to be distinguished so that, for example, two patients with apparently similar fatal physical disease and discomfort can show clearly different levels of morale. Similarly, fatally ill people may be able to explain that their physical state has not altered greatly whereas their disease now worries them or makes them feel low to a different extent. The signs and symptoms of depression and anxiety in terminal illness are essentially those characteristic of these mood states whatever their source but likely to contain the particular fears and sorrows of dying. The sense of apprehension can range from hidden worrying to fears over particular possibilities. It can reach a state of agitation that is only minimally allayed by any reassurance. Depression can range from a little quiet sadness, perhaps tears, to unhappiness and social withdrawal. At its nadir there can be gross misery with suicidal thoughts. It is not uncommon for onlookers to misinterpret the psychological changes. Either the emotions are overlooked because the patient is withdrawn and the severe and fatal physical disease is considered to be the essential focus; or the emotions can be almost dismissed as an inevitable consequence of such a parlous condition. But dying people, given the opportunity, can describe how they feel 'in themselves' as distinct from their physical state and attribute their distress to a source. Some of the sources are aspects of their incurable disease which may be alterable.

Unpleasant physical symptoms are a self-evident basis for psychological distress. Patients can describe for example, how their continued pain has got them down. In parallel, investigations have demonstrated that the longer a painful final illness persists, the greater the prevalence of depression (Hinton 1963). Besides pain, other discomforts such as breathlessness, nausea, and vomiting can cause mental distress. Even when symptoms are eased there can be an anxious awaiting of their return. Suicidal impulses are often linked directly with physical symptoms so that a person feels they would rather die than continue to endure current persistent pain or suffer the return of past agony. Here the pessimistic outlook of depression is not easily distinguished from sombre but justifiable anticipation. Nevertheless, such a situation reinforces the need for competent treatment of physical distress so that any remaining misery can be evaluated.

Disease effects other than physical discomfort are often seen by people as sufficient cause for their mental disquiet. Bodily changes that alter appearance or function may greatly trouble individuals; they may feel that they are no longer the same person or that others could not possibly regard them in the same way. Unless professional familiarity with disease has dulled one's perception it is easy to sympathize with a patient who has, say, become wasted, disfigured by tumours or operations or lost all hair through taking certain drugs. A normally clean and tidy person may be most concerned over a permanent colostomy with the possibility of smelling or over any incontinence of bladder or bowels. General weakness or more defined paralyses may give rise to a wide range of handicaps from difficulty in going far from the house to lying helpless in bed and unable to move, eat, or keep clean without assistance.

Such helplessness has direct and indirect consequences. There are the immediate privations and frustrations of being unable to manage acts previously taken for granted, whether it be cooking a meal for the family or going unobtrusively to the lavatory when one wants to. There is also the further effect on the patient's social position. The mere fact that from earlier in the illness he could be referred to as 'the patient' is a pointer. The status in the family and in society at large is likely to be reduced. A man may lose the importance of his recognized skill or seniority at work and also the sense that he was the earner of money to support his family at home. A woman who ran the household in terms of domestic duties and social matters may now only see herself as a family focus in terms of the sick one to be visited, catered for, and assisted. Such demotion with the prospect of becoming a greater nuisance to others takes much enduring.

Indeed, linked with present symptoms and handicaps are apprehensions over the quality of remaining life. A person who has witnessed the steady or fluctuating downhill progress of his health has cause to be anxious lest his suffering become worse or that he may become more helpless or mentally incompetent. He faces being a liability rather than an asset. He may be only too conscious that the burden is to fall on an equally elderly relative hard put to cope with the strain of nursing an invalid. Hence the anxieties of a dying person lead on from his symptoms and disabilities to an uncertainty about who is going to look after him. The management of future care is very often clear to no one, least of all the patient who may feel lost, sometimes ignored, and threatened with neglect.

So far the stresses that the dying may endure have largely been listed in terms of their own state and prospects. But when interviewing married dying people relieved of any major physical suffering it was notable that the matters that troubled them were about equally divided between concerns for themselves and a matching concern for their spouse and family (Hinton 1979). The experience of terminal illness is a stress shared by relatives and patients. Dying people express concern over the strain on the family and how they will manage; the relatives empathize with the patient. The family's concerns have one important focus, the distress afflicting the patient. Patients are aware that their discomfort troubles the relatives. They may also know that their illness has produced extra work or deprivation for the rest of the family. So all are likely to sympathize and suffer when either experience emotional or physical discomfort. The family's affection also leads them to have equivalent concern that the dying person may become more distressed before he dies. In many respects patient and relatives are the obverse and reverse of the same coin.

Many stresses fall upon the family of a dying person. Relatives are often concerned that the patient's suffering is being underestimated. Sometimes they are right, but their emotional involvement may be misleading. There are complicating factors. Many stoical patients try to minimize their discomfort. Moreover a lay person is often unsure if an unconscious person may not still be in distress. The relatives may also be troubled by their sense of responsibility for the sick patient. Are they doing all they ought, can anything else be done, are they protecting the helpless as much as they should?

Besides this empathic sharing the relatives are being stressed by immediate alterations in their own pattern of life. The surviving spouse may well be elderly because people are more likely to die in old age and so the added tasks for the survivor can prove exhausting. Looking after a dying person at home usually demands, sooner or later, physical efforts, especially when the patient is weak or paralysed. Supporting or lifting a bed-ridden person who needs help with washing or using a bed-pan is no light job. A patient's incontinence may compound the problem. Even if the dying person is not confined to bed, physical assistance and support may well be necessary. If the night's sleep is broken in order to cope with the patient's needs, the family's strength is undermined especially if the sick person is restless and confused. Patients' worries over being a burden on the family are not ill-founded. Material changes within the household of a dying person can be considerable. The family income may have dropped dramatically if the patient was the main wage-earner. If the housewife is ill, others may be clumsy and incompetent substitutes. The initial enthusiasm of helpers over housework is apt to diminish.

When a person is dying at home and needs continuous attention relatives will have their own social life restricted. If there is only one available relative his – or usually her – life may well be confined to coping with the dying individual. There may be no break or rest, day after day. If the patient is in hospital the physical burden may be less but repeated hospital visiting imposes considerable strain, especially if the relative has to rely on public transport. Although the family usually wish to visit the dying, the visits themselves may be stressful. They witness someone they love affected by severe illness and symptoms. The patient may even become quite unlike the individual they knew if mental changes take place. The hospital can be an alien world. And what should be said when facing the end of a life? When visiting time is over it is time to struggle home and try to catch up with neglected housework in a depleted home.

No wonder some people describe the time of looking after a loved and dying person as the most stressful period of their life.

THE FATAL OUTCOME OF THE ILLNESS

Another obvious reason for patients to be troubled during this illness is the fact that it is terminal. If they recognize that their life is about to end they may have intense regret. If they are less well aware of the outlook they may fear that they will not recover. The potential mixture of hope, fear, courage, irritability, and misery is an uneasy state for patients and those who like or love them.

If aware that death is probable, sorrow is a not inappropriate mood. Any significant loss brings unhappiness and depression. Dying people experience a series of losses and foresee yet more. As already noted the dying may be deprived of the ability to enjoy a meal, an activity, or a status. Separation has already begun and some people or places will never be seen again. Those dying in hospital contemplate never returning home or that there will never again be private intimacy between wife and husband. They may have an astringent recognition that the family is already learning how to get along without them. So grief is appropriate in those who recognize that they are dying. Particular aspects of life have now finished forever. The way such endings are regarded depends on the individual and his current perspective. At times their sense of loss can bring deep regret and pain. But a sense of peace or pleasure may attend the recognition that some struggles and unpleasant features of living have now ceased; so balanced against the sense that the remaining sources of enjoyment are reduced and finite may be a relief that, say, a lonely life of continued ill-health need not be endured much longer.

Facing the cessation of living allows final assessments to be made. One individual may consider his life leaves a flavour of pleasure and fulfilment while another may feel the scales tipping towards regret and dissatisfaction. Those who have been dissatisfied with their life were found more likely to be troubled while dying (Hinton 1975). They may feel resentful or guilty over past frustrations or failures in personal relationships. They may have to recognize that hopes which had sustained them during life would now never be fulfilled, perhaps the deprivation of an awaited retirement. But many can look back with pleasure, regarding with equanimity the final weighing in the balance of their own values. They can now leave life with no undue regret.

While the dying individual faces the loss of his existence, the family faces bereavement. In the early part of the fatal illness the disappointments of the patient and the relatives tend to run parallel. The family share many of the curtailments with the patient either in sympathy or in fact. They see what he is missing and some features of their own lives may be similarly reduced. In the terminal illness all share the sense of diminishing time together. But as death approaches patient and family face a different quality of loss and separation. Any future existence for the dying is unknowable except through faith. The future existence for the relatives is partly predictable. They face continued grief and they will mourn. Their immediate future, at least, will be lessened in many social respects, perhaps of status, companionship, income, and even home. The process of bereavement and mourning is a topic in itself. Here it is to be noted that the process of mourning starts before dying becomes death.

How people cope

PRACTICAL PROBLEMS

This chapter so far has considered some of the stresses and the strains of those involved in dying. The ways of coping will now be viewed with regard to, first, the practical measures and, second, the psychological reactions and attitudes. The efficiency of necessary actions during the terminal illness will, of course, radically affect how people feel and respond. In turn, people's emotions and attitudes influence their behaviour, both commissions and omissions. The practical aspects of management include treatment, especially the alleviation of distress. The latter cardinal need will not be reviewed in any detail in this context, but as a principle within the over-all strategy of treatment.

Physical and mental distress can be relieved by an ever-extending range of treatments. For example, pain in a fatal illness can call upon a spectrum of therapies ranging from powerful analgesics (addiction should be no problem here), nerve blocks, radiotherapy, to palliative operations. In theory continued intolerable pain should be rare. In practice, reports have shown it is not (Cartwright, Hockey, and Anderson 1973: 18–24; Parkes 1978). Does this indicate that the available practical methods of coping are not applied effectively or are the claims of therapeutic achievement exaggerated?

The special units, including hospices, expert in pain control nearly always relieve this distress adequately when treatment is closely supervised. This implies that in other circumstances symptomatic treatments may not be applied in the optimal way and, indeed, anecdotal evidence indicates that this can happen. A doctor or nurse may be blamed for not prescribing or administering the best treatment at the right time. The impression is given that some doctors do not devote sufficient time to repeated assessments of a patient's pain or they hesitate unduly to give powerful narcotic drugs in time to prevent pain building up. The demands on the doctor, the nurse, the hospital, or the system may make it difficult to give the ideal treatment promptly. Delay varies from a few minutes before someone carries out a request to many days until a desired report arrives. The distance from the ideal can be forgivably small but greater lapses contribute significantly to the survey reports of continued suffering.

Pain has been used as an example as there is extensive knowledge of its relief. The position is less clear for symptoms such as breathlessness or unpleasant exhaustion where treatments are less effective or may have other drawbacks. Some discomforts and disabilities demand prolonged skilled professional attention to prevent or mitigate symptoms and this degree of care may not be available for the dying. It is clear that distress due to physical symptoms other than pain has often not been wholly relieved. Its incomplete eradication in the dying is not solely due to limitations of professional endeavour or the constraints of available money and labour. Cartwright, Hockey, and Anderson's survey (1973: 87–9) indicated that for a quarter of the symptoms experienced by dying patients no professional help had been sought. In some cases it was because symptoms were brief or minor, but many 'very distressing' symptoms were not reported by the patient or relatives to the doctor or nurse. The families' reticence was influenced by their views on what could or rather could not be done, but this was by no means the total explanation. Some people, for various reasons, choose to cope with troubling symptoms by enduring them.

There is a natural hope that dying need not be attended by any unnecessary physical suffering so anecdotes and reports usually give full attention to the distress which goes unrelieved. Nevertheless in well-provided countries potential physical distress is largely made tolerable. Most studies report that the frequent symptoms of pain, sleeplessness, and constipation are usually alleviated. For those troubled by complaints such as loss of appetite or mental confusion rather less, about half, are improved by treatment. Anxiety can often be relieved when its source is dealt with; alternatively tranquillizing drugs or even the opiates given to relieve pain also specifically reduce the experience of apprehension and agitation. To some extent depression can be helped in a similar fashion although the place of anti-depressant drugs, sometimes of considerable benefit, remains ill-defined in this setting.

The optimal treatment of the above symptoms should not be considered in isolation. For example, physical suffering may well be relieved more efficiently when a person stays in hospital but the patient may strongly prefer that he stays at home despite its drawbacks. This introduces the question of the strategy of terminal care. Ideally various preferred tactics of coping with each of the individual stresses require a balanced synthesis to achieve the best over-all plan. In practice terminal care is often managed by attempting to deal with each particular need as it arises or reaches a crisis level. This *ad hoc* policy has its advantages. It means that no inappropriate rigid programme is adhered to if the illness does not proceed according to a common pattern. It also means that no one need make predictions regarding the course of terminal illness, which postpones the unpleasant necessity to face troubling issues or make difficult decisions. It also has justification when an illness is known to run a fluctuating course or proceed by a series of downward steps which are never quite predictable, as for example, the episodic encroachment of serious vascular disease.

The absence of an over-all policy also has disadvantages. First, if the terminal nature of the illness is not acknowledged, an habitual pattern of treatments or investigations may be conducted with little benefit and some discomfort for the patient. Those responsible for treatment may not give the appropriate priority to the comfort of the dying patient – and the family. Second, even when the illness is recognized as terminal, the *ad hoc* policy may recognize the appropriate solution to each problem as it arises but may not be able to provide it straight away. To do so requires a whole range of immediately available services. That is to say that a proportion of professional staff and various facilities are held in reserve to deal with such requests whenever and whatever their source. In practice, the organization often cannot function on this basis.

Strategically it is advantageous to have an open recognition that some individual, unit or team is responsible for a patient's care which has reached a terminal phase. They should know about what has gone before so that treatments are properly chosen. If the patient's suffering increases rapidly there should be an acknowledged responsibility for arranging more effective or intensive care. Without that there are failures. For example, a particular unit in an acute hospital may have a policy not to re-admit patients whose illness has become terminal and hardship may arise if some palliative treatment is urgently needed. With no recognized alternative arrangement patients may continue in distress while increasingly frantic efforts are made to get help from new sources unable or unwilling to supply it. Pre-arranged provision of assistance and care may spare all concerned much uncertainty and distress, and perhaps justified resentment.

Who should be responsible for terminal care and where should it be given? In Britain the primary source of medical advice is held to be the general practitioner. While the dying patient is in the family doctor's care, he should be advising on immediate treatment, arranging nursing attention and so forth as the situation demands. He should also be able to arrange for the patient's admission to a hospital or some other unit if or when sufficient care cannot be given in the patient's home. Cartwright, Hockey, and Anderson's survey (1973: 82–103) indicated that indeed general practitioners usually did fulfil this role, often very well. These doctors made a series of visits to the patient at home and discussed any difficulties in caring; many relatives were full of praise. For about a third of the patients this continued to be the practitioner's role until the patient died. For the other two-thirds, the family doctor was responsible for the patient until admission to hospital was arranged.

The system has its imperfections. A minority of general practitioners were seen by the family of the patient as not taking enough interest. Some members of the medical profession appeared to underestimate the amount of care that families and friends needed to provide, particularly if they saw little of the patient in his own home. Certain community services were insufficient, particularly night nursing services and some home help facilities. Not infrequently services available were either not sought or even not known about. In turn a proportion of families were seen by the general practitioners as not taking sufficient responsibility for the patient (Cartwright, Hockey, and Anderson 1973: 82–103). Families obviously vary in their ability and willingness to nurse a dying relative. There were indications that a negative evaluation was made more readily by particular doctors, especially if there was a setting of mutual dissatisfaction between family and general practitioner. It also depended on how readily patients could be transferred to hospital. Undoubtedly the family doctor could often meet frustrations in his negotiations with hospitals. Arranging the admission of a dying patient when home conditions were inadequate often proved difficult and sometimes impossible. If the patient was elderly and likely to need a longer period of care the process could be very difficult indeed.

In most areas of western civilization about 60 per cent of people die in hospitals or various institutions. There is considerable debate over whether it is better to die at home or elsewhere and, if a person is to die in some form of institution, what sort it should be. The arguments include points about personal preference, facilities required, attitudes of the caring staff, continuation of care by the same professional team, cost, and so on. The basic requirement is that the available facilities should be able to meet the needs of patient and family. If the family, with support from community services, can look after the patient adequately at home, this is usually preferred. In contrast those living alone have reason usually to spend more of their last days in institutional care. So do women generally, in part because men are thought less able to cope with nursing and additional domestic duties. Moreover the greater longevity of women leads to the added requirement of institutional care of the elderly, solitary, dying woman; the latter words themselves are bleak enough to remind one of the human need. The presence of a daughter or other female relative influences the pattern of care considerably.

About half of the institutional deaths do take place in acute or mixed hospitals. Many approve of this particularly when it provides continuing care following earlier treatment. Some also like to remain in the atmosphere of a hospital geared to curing as it maintains a hope, however forlorn, and is associated with an attitude of being prepared to 'do something'. The doubts arise when the 'doing' is only for its own sake, or when the 'doing' is focused on other patients who may respond while the terminally ill are given too little attention. Certain institutions such as hospices, charitable homes and nursing homes take a special interest in caring for the dying. Some of them, and now some hospitals, work with a home care team who successfully maintain a continuity of care for the dying. The achievements of these specialized units in terms of expert symptom relief and a source of moral support to patient and family have been considerable. There is continuous interplay between the known availability of effective care and the psychological ability to cope with a stressful situation. Uncertain, ineffective treatment and unreliable backing increase the stress. This will engender anxiety and misery which in turn fosters further demands for help. Effective care reduces physical, psychological, and social discomfort. Hence as has been shown, effective home care support enables families to cope longer in looking after the dying at home (Parkes 1980).

PSYCHOLOGICAL AND SOCIAL ASPECTS

Various stresses have been outlined, whether they be the physical symptoms, an unwanted prospect of dying, or an interruption of social links between people. It is normal for experiences and threats of this sort to give rise to a degree of psychological distress. In general a crisis will produce a degree of emotional shock, followed in all tragic situations by various unpleasant feelings or anxiety, resentment, and depression. Ideally, people adapt to radically altered circumstances and eventually achieve a measure of tranquillity. The grief during the last illness is not so different or separate from the grief following bereavement. Kübler-Ross (1970) outlined a series of stages among dying patients; denial and isolation, anger, bargaining, depression, and acceptance. Some individuals do follow a sequence of such reactions when dying, but there is by no means an inevitable smooth passage through a series of predictable stages. Fatal illnesses are often irregular in their progress. Certain emotions or attitudes may be conspicuous in some but absent in others. People can fluctuate to and fro in their reactions, even when their disease or circumstances appear relatively unchanged.

How do normal people cope with emotional pain, which can be intense? As with physical pain some visibly suffer with agitation, tears, misery, and pleas for help. Others do not show any emotion readily because their inclination and fortitude lead them to keep such feelings concealed. This manoeuvre, consciously employed, is not the only way to

encounter severe or intolerable stress without showing mental discomfort. Dying people quite readily reveal in conversation their own ways of
treating the surrounding threats so as to make them more tolerable.
For the sake of convenience these mechanisms will be grouped, first,
according to the way patients negotiate their potential knowledge of
their condition and second, the attitudes they have or adopt to their
degree of awareness.

One crude way of coping with a threat without distress is to ignore it
utterly. This can happen quite unconsciously or there may be degrees of
insight. Such denial is commonplace among people with potentially
lethal disease. The nature of their symptoms, the treatment they have
received, the progressive deterioration, the things they have been told or
not told, the altered attitudes of others, may all clearly indicate they are
likely to die, but their reaction is to ignore it entirely. They appear quite
unaware of their likely fate and may well state their expectations of
improved health. If the conviction although false is entire, there need be
no disturbance of mood, a somewhat unreal calm prevails while there is
no conscious realization of the predicament.

This attitude, of course, is very commonly encouraged or condoned by
relatives, friends, and professionals around them as Glaser and Strauss
recorded (1965: 29–39). The disease may be referred to in euphemistic
terms and the outlook described with unlikely optimism. Any lies are
considered to be nobly white because they protect the patient from any
painful knowledge that he cannot be cured. Clear statements about the
future are avoided apart from misleading comments on treatment or
progress. Such a policy also potentially shields others from facing harsh
reality and embarrassing conversations. The impotence to cure is
decently not mentioned. It is surprising how often this collusion,
conscious or unconscious, is maintained with apparent success and the
primitive coping mechanism of denial avoids much pain.

Often enough, however, the patient's denial is far from absolute.
He may check his own thoughts from pursuing any cue to the outcome of
the illness and he may collude more consciously with others in the
conspiracy of avoidance. Underlying this there may be an evolving
recognition of his truer state, taken at a pace he can manage without
being emotionally overwhelmed. This evolution is not necessarily a
steady progress; it is likely to occur in steps, forward as well as backward.
Commonly there is an ambivalent state, for which the term 'middle
knowledge' has been coined, when a person both recognizes that he is
dying and yet repudiates death (Hackett and Weisman 1962). Again
family and staff may collude in a mutual pretence, now with a more
conscious element. Another less complex attitude is that the illness
could be a fatal one but the patient considers himself among the more
fortunate. Alternatively he may recognize that the disease is to be

considered a fatal one, but death is a long way off and something may turn up.

There are other ways of diluting the impact of defeat and death through an uncontrollable disease in one's own body. A rationalization that makes the illness more comprehensible can help the patient even if others privately regard the explanation as unlikely. A patient's view that his tumour followed a blow may appeal to him more than a medical confession of ignorance or some current respectable but unintelligible theory. A cause that can attribute blame may be seized upon. This can involve various other people – the uncaring attitude of an employer, the neglect or wrong treatment by a doctor, the stresses of an unsatisfactory marital relationship, and so on. Then they can be blamed. The psychological consolation of some rationalizations can shade into less immediately comforting attributions of guilt. It is quite common for people to suspect their illness has arisen through their own past misdemeanours or inadequacy. In so far as it is deserved it is more acceptable, albeit painfully. If disease or death cannot be accepted as inexplicable, then the alternative is to blame oneself or others and react to the justice or injustice involved.

The other extreme of the cognitive aspect of coping is to maximize knowledge rather than reduce it to make it bearable. Some people feel they can manage as long as they are told everything. Many may regard that as a laudable attitude, part of a pathway to full acceptance of dying. Even this rational outlook can, however, be distorted in a less stable adjustment. Some patients need to know all details of every investigation, when the next one is due, why some procedure has been omitted, how some particular organ is faring and what may happen if a particular set of circumstances arise. There is an urge to control the uncontrollable by detailed knowledge. It may accompany a refusal to take certain drugs such as analgesics or sedatives lest they reduce the patient's own alertness and competence.

In terms of awareness, varying degrees of denial are probably the most common defence of psychological equilibrium. As already noted, this is compatible with the commonly held view of those wishing to defend the dying patient from discomfort. The potential collusion is not always an easy one, it may be an imposed view rather than a mutual policy. Commonly at least three-quarters of people in their terminal illness can speak of their awareness that the outcome may be death. Most have largely worked it out themselves. The patient's communication with other people about the outcome depends on both parties. The tendency is for others to be cautious and many, if not most, relatives express the view that patients should not be 'told'. As so many dying patients do come to recognize their fate, it cannot be assumed that the deafening silence about them helps them cope. Some feel lost because they cannot confide, others feel hurt. Paradoxically, a few dying patients can on occasions say they are well aware of the likely fatal outcome and yet not be dissatisfied that others deny the truth because they still gain comfort from the nurses' and doctors' continued avowal that improvement is expected. Other patients keep silent as they do not wish to upset themselves or those who love them by talk of their parting. Nevertheless more dying people criticize the reticence of others rather than commend it.

As many as a third of married patients who know they may be dying have been found to exchange no word to that effect with their spouse (Hinton 1980). Another third had very limited communication about the outcome, perhaps a vague comment or a remark by one that met no truthful acknowledgement from the other. So only a third of married couples where both recognized the likely outcome managed to say much to each other about dying. Those that did, spoke warmly of the benefits of their sharing. Those that did not either indicated that they felt unable to put these thoughts into words or they expressed some regret at this failure to share their feelings. People in the latter predicament often feel it is out of keeping with their previous frank relationship. The prospect of the spouse's death may be seen as a unique justification for silence or they find it too difficult to admit the truth to each other especially if it means confessing to earlier deceit. Reticence over personal death is common enough, however, and even if it does seem an anomaly many people cope well enough in this way. It can mean that other reassurances may appear hollow and future plans, if any, lack reality.

Given that a patient recognizes the serious nature of his illness, his attitude towards the threat affects his feelings. The attitude can range from the adoption of fighting stance to a helpless and excessive surrender. Many are buoyed up by defiance. They intend to survive and wish all those around them to support them in the battle. They wish to submit themselves to any treatment that proffers hope, despite possible discomfort. If orthodox help towards cure is no longer on offer, they may seek the unorthodox which makes claims however unsubstantiated. Unwillingness to give up the struggle for cure is likely to bring its disappointments and may cost much in terms of money, travel, and inconvenience; but for a while it enables the family to cleave to hopes of recovery. This, at times, may be the only acceptable coping strategy.

The individual's sustaining challenge may be modified from the total defeat of death. Not uncommonly the battle may be to live a certain while longer. The goal may be to exceed a supposed prognosis given by a doctor or to an awaited event such as the children leaving school. The target may be to complete something, including the setting of personal affairs in good order. It may be to overcome a disability or fulfil an ambition. It may be a lowly goal but often it is one that helps retain pride, perhaps even just the ability to get to the toilet and manage independently. Anything that reduces a sense of being a burden on others is a desirable aim, and if one object is achieved another may be set. The goals have their intrinsic value, such as the successful enjoyment of a small holiday, and they also keep at bay the anguish of defeat.

Some dying people do surrender their independence relatively early. They are liable to take to their beds in a way that indicates their psychological attitude rather than the weakness of physical disease. Such behaviour can be due to a seriously depressed mood with its associated pessimism and giving up. If this is the case and the depression is relieved, either by pharmacological or psychological means, interest and activity may regenerate. But for some, undue surrender and dependence on others is the attitude they find the least intolerable solution to their predicament; it is a response not easily changed. At least for the patient there is no further need to struggle. Those who try to encourage them to do more may well be resented. The attitude suggests a regression to an excessively child-like dependence, which can drain and irritate others by demands for continuous attention and support.

The majority of dying people do attain a more positive acceptance that their illness is terminal. Some do not. They either use self-protective mechanisms successfully or the remainder of their lives may be permeated by worry and unhappiness. Such people may need help to cope. Apart from the symptomatic treatments of emotional distress noted before, appropriate psychological help may give benefit. Such therapy will not be reviewed in detail here. It can take many forms. A sympathetic sharing of thoughts will tide many over a troubled period; if nothing else it can diminish the social isolation that too frequently affects the dying. It may be appropriate to support the individual in his way of looking at his situation if this is potentially beneficial. There is no universal truth or answer for everyone. Jeremy Taylor's 'Holy Dying' (1651) was long held in esteem with its emphasis on resignation to God, true repentance, and the forgiveness of sins as the way of preparing to die. A rigid application of his guidance would usually be discordant today although for many their faith and the help of the clergy is an essential component of dying.

Professionals may contribute according to their skills and style. Those who view the dying individual as passing through stages may attempt to lead those in discomfort through the remaining stages on to an equable adjustment. In other situations it is pertinent to consider the family rather than the individual alone, so a social worker or psychotherapist may assist them towards mutual adjustment, communication, or the acceptance of separating (Stedeford 1981). The informal support that patients often give each other can be modified to regular group meetings. This has been found to help them cope with their relationships with doctors or family, with their frequent sense of isolation, and even with dying itself (Spiegel, Bloom, and Yalom 1981).

Healthy individuals unfamiliar with serious illness or the declining abilities of age, let alone conceiving their own death, may not comprehend how well many come to face and accept dying. But, during life, people adapt to limitations and reduced achievements as well as gains and advancement. Hence the elderly, the disabled, and the bereaved may still get pleasure from their apparently diminished lives despite any earlier view that such an existence would be intolerable. The same applies to people who have only a very limited life left. If their obvious stresses are relieved, they may still be capable of enjoyment. It helps if there is a sense of fulfilment; that sense depends on the individual's own values. People may derive their greatest satisfaction from their past family life, their career or the children they are leaving behind them or they may place the highest value on their religious faith and view the end of mortal life as entirely fitting. Some have the sense that they need struggle no longer and they can now find peace or believe that their life is now reasonably complete. There may be a conviction that they will rejoin a loved person in immortal existence, or a view that having outlived their strength and their friends, death is due or even overdue. Illness is likely to bring a sense of weakness and change in the body that makes the thought of dying more acceptable than it appears to the fit and lively. Those devoted to the care of the dying, particularly in the hospices, place an emphasis on their patients gaining further fulfilment and pleasure during their remaining life. With good care many people do achieve a positive acceptance of dying and have a peaceful death. In their own fashion families usually reach an acceptance of their separation by death, but they face further grief and mourning.

References

Ablon, J. (1981) Dwarfism and Social Identity: Self-group participation. *Social Science and Medicine* 15(b): 25–30.

Abrams, R. and Finesinger, J. (1953) Guilt Reactions in Patients with Cancer. *Cancer* 6: 474–82.

Acheson, J., Acheson, H., and Tellwright, J. (1968) The Incidence and Pattern of Cerebrovascular Disease in General Practice. *Journal of the Royal College of General Practitioners* 16: 428–36.

Achte, K., Hillbom, E., and Aalberg, V. (1969) Psychoses Following War Brain Injuries. *Acta Scandinavia Psychiatrica* 45: 1–18.

Adelstein, A., Davies, I., and Weatherall, J. (1980) *Perinatal Infant Mortality: Social and Biological Factors 1975–1977*, Studies on Medical and Population Subjects 41. London: HMSO.

Adey, C. (1967) Long Term Prognosis in Closed Head Injury. *Bristol Medicochir. Journal* 82: 58–64.

Adler, M. W., Waller, J. J., Creese, A., and Thorne, S. C. (1978) Randomized Controlled Trial of Early Discharge for Inguinal Hernia and Varicose Veins. *Journal of Epidemiology and Community Health* 32 (2): 136–42.

Ajzen, I. and Fishbein, M. (1980) *Understanding Attitudes and Predicting Social Behaviour*. Englewood Cliffs, NJ: Prentice-Hall.

Albrecht, G. L. (1979) Social Aspects of Medical Care. In G. L. Albrecht and P. C. Higgins (eds) *Health, Illness and Medicine*. Chicago: Rand McNally.

Albrecht, G. L., Walker, V., and Levy, J. (1982) Social Distance from the Stigmatized: A Test of Two Theories. *Social Science and Medicine* 16: 1319–327.

Allport, G. (1958) *The Nature of Prejudice*. New York: Anchor.

Alonzo, A. (1980) Acute Illness Behaviour: A Conceptual Exploration and Specification. *Social Science and Medicine* 14(a): 515–26.

Amara Singham, L. R. (1980) Movement Among Healers in Sri Lanka. *Culture, Medicine and Psychiatry* 4 (1): 71–92.

Anderson, J. L. (1979) Patients' Recall of Information and Its Relation to the Nature of the Consultation. In D. Oborne, M. M. Gruneberg, and J. R. Eiser (eds) *Research in Psychology and Medicine*. London: Academic Press.

Anderson, J. L., Day, J. L., Dowling, M. A. C., and Pettingale, K. W. (1970) The Definition and Evaluation of the Skills Required to Obtain a Patient's History of Illness: The Use of Videotape Recordings. *Postgraduate Medical Journal* 46: 606.

Anderson, J. L., Dodman, S., Kopelman, M., and Fleming, A. (1979) Patient Information Recall in a Rheumatology Clinic. *Rheumatology and Rehabilitation* 18: 18–22.

Anderson, K. O. and Masur, F. T. (1983) Psychological Preparation for Invasive Medical and Dental Procedures. *Journal of Behavioural Medicine* 6 (1): 1–40.

Andrew, J. M. (1970) Recovering from Surgery, with and without Preparatory Instruction, for Three Coping Styles. *Journal of Personality and Social Psychology* 15: 223–26.

Anonymous (1983) *Issues in Race and Education* (editorial). No. 38: Health.

Argyle, M. (1972) *The Psychology of Interpersonal Behaviour*. London: Penguin.

—— (1981) *Social Skills and Health*. London: Methuen.

Argyle, M. and Dean, J. (1965) Eye Contact, Distance and Affiliation. *Sociometry* 28: 289–304.

Ashley, J. (1973) *Journey into Silence*. London: Bodley Head.

Auerbach, S. M. (1973) Trait–State Anxiety and Adjustment to Surgery. *Journal of Consulting and Clinical Psychology* 40: 264–71.

Auerbach, S. M. and Kilman, P. R. (1977) Crisis Intervention with Surgical Patients. *Psychological Bulletin* 84: 1208–217.

Auerbach, S. M., Kendall, P. C., Cuttler, H. F., and Levitt, N. R. (1976) Anxiety, Locus of Control, Type of Preparatory Information and Adjustment to Dental Surgery. *Journal of Consulting and Clinical Psychology* 44: 809–18.

Ausburn, L. (1981) Patient Compliance with Medication Regimens. In J. Sheppard (ed.) *Behavioural Medicine*. Lidcombe, NSW: Cumberland College of Health Sciences.

Baddeley, A. D. (1976) *The Psychology of Memory*. New York: Basic Books.

Bagley, C. (1971) *The Social Psychology of the Child with Epilepsy*. London: Routledge & Kegan Paul.

Bain, D. J. (1976) Doctor–Patient Communication in General Practice Consultations. *British Journal of Medical Education* 10: 125–31.

—— (1977) Patient Knowledge and the Content of the Consultation in General Practice. *British Journal of Medical Education* 11: 347–50.

Balint, M. (1957) *The Doctor, His Patient and the Illness*. London: Tavistock Publications.

Bancroft, J. (1981) Ethical Aspects of Sexuality and Sex Therapy. In S. Bloch and P. Chodoff (eds) *Psychiatric Ethics*. Oxford: Oxford University Press.

Bandura, A. (1977) *Social Learning Theory*. New Jersey: Prentice Hall.

Banton, M. (1977) *The Idea of Race*. London: Tavistock Publications.

—— (1983) *Racial and Ethnic Competition*. Cambridge: Cambridge University Press.

Barofsky, I. (1980) *The Chronic Psychiatric Patient in the Community*. New York: Plenum.

Barrows, H. S., Norman, G. R., Nenfeld, V. R., and Freightner, J. W. (1977) Studies of the Clinical Reasoning Process of Medical Students and Physicians. In *Proceedings of the Sixteenth Annual Conference on Research in Medical Education*. Washington, DC: Association of American Medical Colleges.

Barsky, A. J. (1981) Hidden Reasons Some Patients Visit Doctors. *Annals of Internal Medicine* 94: 492–98.

Barsky, A. J. and Klerman, G. L. (1983) Overview: Hyperchondriasis, Bodily Complaints and Somatic Styles. *American Journal of Psychiatry* 140: 273–83.

Bartley, W. (1977) *Wittgenstein*. London: Quartet Books.

Battistella, R. M. (1971) Factors Associated with Delay in the Initiation of Physicians' Care Among Late Adulthood Persons. *American Journal of Public Health* 61: 1348–361.

Becker, G. (1981) Coping with Stigma: Lifelong Adaptation of Deaf People. *Social Science and Medicine* 15(b): 21–4.

Becker, M. H. (1974) The Health Belief Model and Sick Role Behaviour. *Health Education Monograph* 2: 409–19.

Becker, M. H. and Maiman, L. A. (1975) Sociobehavioural Determinants of Compliance with Health and Medical Care Recommendations. *Medical Care* 13: 10–24.

Becker, M. H., Drachman, R. H., and Kirscht, J. P. (1972) Motivations as Predictors of Health Behaviour. *Health Services Reports* 87: 852–62.

Becker, M. H., Maiman, L. A., Kirscht, J. P., Haefner, D. P., and Drachman, R. (1977) The Health Belief Model and Prediction of Dietary Compliance: A Field Experiment. *Journal of Health and Social Behaviour* 18: 348–66.

Belcher, S. A., Clowers, M. R., Cabanayan, A. C., and Fordyce, W. E. (1982) Activity Patterns of Married and Single Individuals after Stroke. *Archives of Physical Medicine and Rehabilitation* 63: 308–12.

Ben-Sira, Z. (1976) The Function of the Professional's Affective Behaviour in Client Satisfaction: A Revised Approach to Social Interaction Theory. *Journal of Health and Social Behaviour* 17 (1): 3–11.

—— (1980) Affective and Instrumental Components in the Physician–Patient Relationship: An Additional Dimension of Interaction Theory. *Journal of Health and Social Behaviour* 21 (2): 170–80.

Benson, F. (1973) Psychiatric Aspects of Aphasia. *British Journal of Psychiatry* 123: 555–66.

Berger, P. and Luckmann, T. (1966) *The Social Construction of Reality: A Treatise in the Sociology of Knowledge*. New York: Doubleday.

Berkowitz, L. (1980) *A Survey of Social Psychology* (2nd edn). New York: Holt, Rinehart & Winston.

Berrigan, L. P. and Garfield, S. L. (1981) Relationship of Missed Psychotherapy Appointments to Premature Termination and Social Class. *British Journal of Clinical Psychology* 20: 239–42.

Bertakis, K. D. (1977) The Communication of Information from Physician to

Patient: A Method for Increasing Retention and Satisfaction. *Journal of Family Practice* 5: 217–22.

Bhalla, A. and Blakemore, K. (1981) *Elders of the Minority Ethnic Groups*. AFFOR, Nottingham: Russell Press.

Black Health Workers and Patients Group (1983) Psychiatry and the Corporate State. *Race and Class* 25: 49–64.

Blaxter, M. (1976) *The Meaning of Disability: A Sociological Study of Impairment*. London: Heinemann.

—— (1983a) The Causes of Disease: Women Talking. *Social Science and Medicine* 17 (2): 59–69.

—— (1983b) Health Services as a Defence Against the Consequences of Poverty in Industrialised Societies. *Social Science and Medicine* 17: 1139–1148.

Blaxter, M. and Paterson, E. (1982) *Mothers and Daughters*. London: Heinemann Educational.

Bloom, J. R. and Monterossa, S. (1981) Hypertension Labelling and Sense of Well Being. *American Journal of Public Health* 71 (11): 1228–232.

Bloom, S. W. and Wilson, R. N. (1972) Patient–Practitioner Relationships. In M. E. Freeman, S. Levine, and L. G. Reeder (eds) *Handbook of Medical Sociology*. New Jersey: Prentice-Hall.

Bloor, M. (1970) Current Explanatory Models of Pre-Patient Behaviour: A Critique with Some Suggestions on Further Model Development. Unpublished M.Litt thesis University of Aberdeen.

Blumer, D. and Benson, D. F. (1975) Personality Changes with Frontal and Temporal Lobe Lesions. In D. F. Benson and D. Blumer (eds) *Psychiatric Aspects of Neurologic Disease*. New York: Grune & Stratton.

Blumhagen, D. W. (1980) Hypertension: A Folk Illness with a Medical Name. *Culture, Medicine and Psychiatry* 4 (3): 197–227.

Blyth, B. (1981) The Outcome of Severe Head Injuries. *New Zealand Medical Journal* 22 April: 267–69.

Bochner, S. (1983) Doctors, Patients and Their Cultures. In D. Pendleton and J. Hasler (eds) *Doctor–Patient Communication*. London: Academic Press.

Bond, M. R. (1975) Assessment of the Psycho-Social Outcome after Severe Head Injury. In Outcome of Severe Damage to the Central Nervous System. *Ciba Foundation Symposium* 34: 141–53.

Bond, M. R. and Brooks, D. N. (1976) Understanding the Process of Recovery as a Basis for the Investigation of Rehabilitation for the Brain Injured. *Scandinavian Journal of Rehabilitative Medicine* 8: 127–33.

Bonilla, K., Quigly, W., and Bowers, W. (1961) Experiences with Hypnosis on a Surgical Service. *Military Medicine* 126: 364–70.

Boulton, M. G. (1983) *Social Class and the Presentation of Complaints*. Paper presented at joint conference of Royal College of General Practitioners and British Sociological Association at Eynsham Hall, Oxon.

Boulton, M. G. and Williams, A. (1983) Health Education in the General Practice Consultation. *The Health Education Journal* 42 (2): 57–63.

Bradley, N. C. A. (1981) Expectations and Experience of People who Consult in a Training Practice. *Journal of the Royal College of General Practitioners* 31 (28): 420–25.

Bray, G., De Frank, R., and Wolfe, T. (1981) Sexual Functioning in Stroke Survivors. *Archives of Physical Medicine and Rehabilitation* 63: 286–88.

Brennan, M. (1981) Resumption of Work Following Discharge from Hospital. *Irish Medical Journal* 74: 5–7.

Brent Community Health Council (1981) *Black People and the Health Service.*

Breslau, N. and Mortimer, E. A. (1981) Seeing the Same Doctor: Determinants of, Satisfaction with Specialty Care for Disabled Children. *Medical Care* 19 (7): 741–57.

Breslau, N., Jaug, M. R., Burns, A. E., McClelland, C. Q., Reeb, K. G., and Staples, W. I. (1975) Comprehensive Paediatric Care: The Patient Viewpoint. *Medical Care* 13 (7): 562–69.

Brocklehurst, J., Morris, P., Andrews, K., Richards, B., and Laycock, P. (1981) Social Effects of Stroke. *Social Science and Medicine* 15(a): 35–9.

Brody, D. S. (1980) An Analysis of Patient Recall of Their Therapeutic Regimens. *Journal of Chronic Diseases* 33: 57–63.

Brooks, D. N. (1976) Wechsler Memory Scale performance and Its Relationship to Brain Damage after Severe Closed Head Injury. *Journal of Neurology, Neurosurgery and Psychiatry* 39: 593–60.

Brooks, D. N. and McKinlay, W. (1983) Personality and Behavioural Change after Severe Plane Head Injury – a Relative View. *Journal of Neurology, Neurosurgery and Psychiatry* 46: 336–44.

Brotherston, J. (1976) Inequality: Is It Inevitable? In C. Carter and J. Peel (eds) *Equalities and Inequalities in Health.* London: Academic Press.

Bruckner, F. E. and Randle, A. P. M. (1972) Return to Work after Severe Head Injuries. *Rheumatology and Physical Medicine* 11: 344–48.

Buchan, I. C. and Richardson, I. M. (1973) *Time Study of Consultations in General Practice.* Scottish Health Studies No. 27. Scottish Home and Health Department.

Bunker, J. P., Fowles, J., and Schaffarzick, R. (1982) Evaluation of Medical Technology Procedures. *New England Journal of Medicine* 306: 687–92.

Burr, B., Good, J., and Del Vecchio-Good, M. (1978) The Impact of Illness on the Family. In R. B. Taylor (ed.) *Family Medicine: Principles and Practice.* New York: Springer Verlag.

Bury, M. (1982) Chronic Illness as Biographical Disruption. *Sociology of Health and Illness* 4 (2): 167–82.

Byrne, P. S. and Long, B. E. (1976) *Doctors Talking to Patients* London: HMSO.

Calnan, M. (1983) Social Networks and Patterns of Help-seeking Behaviour. *Social Science and Medicine* 17: 25–8.

Caron, H. S. and Roth, H. P. (1968) Patients' Co-operation with a Medical Regimen. *Journal of the American Medical Association* 203: 922–26.

Caron, H. S. and Roth, H. P. (1971) Objective Assessment of Co-operation with an Ulcer Diet: Relation to Antacid Intake and to Assigned Physician. *American Journal of Medical Science* 261: 61–6.

Carpenter, L. and Brockington, I. (1980) A Study of Mental Illness in Asians, West Indians and Africans Living in Manchester. *British Journal of Psychiatry* 137: 201–05.

Carter, A. (1964) *Cerebral Infarction.* New York: Macmillan.

Cartwright, A. (1964) *Human Relations and Hospital Care.* London: Routledge & Kegan Paul.

—— (1967) *Patients and Their Doctors.* London: Routledge & Kegan Paul.

Cartwright, A. and Anderson, R. (1981) *General Practice Revisited: A Second Study of Patients and Their Doctors*. London: Tavistock Publications.

Cartwright, A. and O'Brien, M. (1976) Social Class Variations in Health Care and in the Nature of General Practitioner Consultations. In M. Stacey (ed.) *The Sociology of the NHS*. Sociological Review Monograph 22: University of Keele.

Cartwright, A., Hockey, L., and Anderson, J. L. (1973) *Life before Death*. London: Routledge & Kegan Paul.

Cashmore, E. and Troyna, B. (1983) *Introduction to Race Relations*. London: Routledge & Kegan Paul.

Central Health Services Council (1969) *Advisory Committee on the Health and Welfare of Handicapped Persons: 'People with Epilepsy'*. London: HMSO.

Central Statistical Office (1983) *Social Trends 13*. London: HMSO.

Chapman, C. R. and Cox, G. B. (1976) Anxiety, Pain and Depression Surrounding Elective Surgery: A Multivariate Comparison of Abdominal Surgery Patients with Kidney Donors and Recipients. *Journal of Psychosomatic Research* 21: 7–15.

Chapman, C. R. and Cox, G. B. (1977) Determination of Anxiety in Elective Surgery Patients. In C. G. Spielberger and I. G. Sarason (eds) *Stress and Anxiety*, vol. 4. Washington: Hemisphere.

Chrisman, N. (1977) The Health Seeking Process: An Approach to the Natural History of Illness. *Culture, Medicine and Psychiatry* 1 (4): 351–77.

Clare, A. (1980) Personal communication.

—— (1983) Psychiatric and Social Aspects of Pre-menstrual Complaint. *Psychological Medicine*, Monograph Supplement 4.

Clarke, J. (1983) Sexism, Feminism and Medication: A Decade Review of Literature on Gender and Illness. *Sociology of Health and Illness* 5: 62–82.

Cochrane, A. (1972) *Effectiveness and Efficiency: Random Reflections on the Health Service*. London: Nuffield Provincial Hospitals Trust.

Cochrane, R. (1977) Mental Illness in Immigrants to England and Wales: An Analysis of Mental Hospital Admissions 1971. *Social Psychiatry* 12: 25.

—— (1983) *The Social Creation of Mental Illness*. Harlow: Longman.

Cohen, F. and Lazarus, R. S. (1973) Active Coping Processes, Coping Dispositions and Recovery from Surgery. *Psychosomatic Medicine* 35 (5): 375–87.

Collins, E. and Klein, R. (1980) Equity and the NHS: Self-reported Morbidity, Access and Primary Care. *British Medical Journal* 2: 1111–115.

Comfort, A. (1967) *The Anxiety Makers: Some Curious Pre-occupations of the Medical Profession*. London: Nelson.

Community Relations Commission (1977) *Evidence to the Royal Commission on the National Health Service*.

Consumer's Association (1983) *GPs*. London.

Cook, M. (1970) Experiments on Orientation and Proxemics. *Human Relations* 23: 61–76.

Coughlan, A. and Humphrey, M. (1982) Pre-senile Stroke: Long Term Outcome for Patients and Their Families. *Rheumatology and Rehabilitation* 21: 115–22.

Crandall, L. A. and Duncan, R. P. (1981) Attitudinal and Situational Factors in the Use of Physician Studies by Low-income Persons. *Journal of Health and Social Behaviour* 22: 64–7.

Cromwell, R. I., Butterfield, E. C., Brayfield, F. M., and Curry, J. J. (1977) *Acute Myocardial Infarction: Reaction and Recovery*. St Louis: C. V. Mosby.

Culyer, A. J. (1976) *Need and the National Health Service.* London: Martin Robertson.

Dabbs, J. M. and Leventhal, H. (1966) Effects of Varying the Recommendations in a Fear-arousing Communication. *Journal of Personality and Social Psychology* 4: 5.

Dalrymple, D. G Parbrook, G. D., and Steel, D. F. (1973) Factors Predisposing to Postoperative Pain and Pulmonary Complications. *British Journal of Anaestheology* 45: 21–32, 589–98.

Davis, F. (1963) *Passage Through Crisis.* Indianapolis: Bobbs-Merrill.

—— (1964) Deviance Disavowal: The Management of Strained Interaction by the Visibly Handicapped. In H. Becker (ed.) *The Other Side.* Illinois: Free Press.

Davis, K. (1979) Equal Treatment and Unequal Benefits: The Medicare Program. In G. L. Albrecht and P. C. Higgins (eds) *Health Illness and Medicine.* Chicago: Rand McNally.

Davis, M. S. (1966) Variations in Patients' Compliance with Doctors' Orders: Analysis of Congruence between Survey Responses and Results of Empirical Investigations. *Journal of Medical Education* 41: 1037–048.

Davis, R., Buchanan, B., and Shortliffe, E. (1977) Production Rules as a Representation for Knowledge-based Consultation Program. *Artificial Intelligence* 8: 15–42.

Davis, S. and Aslam, M. (1979) Eastern Treatment for Eastern Health. *Journal of Community Nursing* 2: 16–20.

Dean, G., Walsh, D., Downing, H., and Shelley, E. (1981) First Admissions of Native Born and Immigrants to Psychiatric Hospitals in South-East England 1976. *British Journal of Psychiatry* 139: 512–16.

DeLong, R. D. (1970) *Individual Differences in Patterns of Anxiety, Arousal, Stress – Relevant Information and Recovery from Surgery.* PhD dissertation UCLA.

Department of Health and Social Security (1980) *Inequalities in Health: Report of a Research Working Group.* (The Black Report.) London: HMSO.

De Wolfe, A. S., Barrell, R. P., and Cummings, J. N. (1966) Patient Variables in Emotional Response to Hospitalization for Physical Illness. *Journal Consulting Clinical Psychology* 30: 68–72.

DiMatteo, M. R. and DiNicola, D. D. (1982) *Achieving Patient Compliance.* New York: Pergamon Press.

DiMatteo, M. R., Taranta, A., Friedman, H. S., and Prince, L. M. (1980) Predicting Patient Satisfaction from Physicians' Non-verbal Communication Skills. *Medical Care* 18 (5): 376–87.

Dimond, S. and Beaumont, J. (1974) *Hemisphere Function in the Human Brain.* London: Elek Science.

Dingwall, R. (1976) *Aspects of Illness.* London: Martin Robertson.

Doberneck, R., Griffen, W., Papermaster, A., Bonello, F., and Wangensteen, O. (1959) Hypnosis as an Adjunct to Surgical Therapy. *Surgery* 46: 299–304.

Doll, R. (1973) Monitoring the National Health Service. *Proceedings of the Royal Society of Medicine* 66: 729–40.

—— (1983) Prospects for Prevention. *British Medical Journal* 286 (1): 445–53.

Donaldson, L. and Taylor, J. (1983) Patterns of Asian and Non-Asian Morbidity in Hospitals. *British Medical Journal* 286: 949–51.

Dumas, R. G. and Johnson, B. (1972) Research in Nursing Practice: A Review of Five Clinical Experiments. *Internal Journal of Nursing Studies* 9: 137–49.

Dutton, D. B. (1978) Explaining the Low Use of Health Services by the Poor:

Costs, Attitudes or Delivery Systems? *American Sociological Review* 43: 348–68.

Earthrowl, B. and Stacey, M. (1977) Social Class and Children in Hospital. *Social Science and Medicine* 11: 83–8.

Edgerton, R. (1967) *The Cloak of Competence: Stigma in the Lives of the Mentally Retarded*. Berkeley: University of California Press.

Egbert, L. D., Battit, G. E., Welsh, C. E., and Bartlett, M. K. (1964) Reduction of Post-operative Pain by Encouragement and Instructions of Patients: A Study of Doctor–Patient Rapport. *New England Journal of Medicine* 270: 823–27.

Eisenberg, L. (1977) Disease and Illness: Distinctions between Professional and Popular Ideas of Sickness. *Culture, Medicine and Psychiatry* 1 (1): 9–23.

Eisenbruch, M. (1983) 'Wind Illness' or Somatic Depression? A Case Study in Psychiatric Anthropology. *British Journal of Psychiatry* 143: 323–26.

Elstein, A. S. and Bordage, G. (1979) Psychology of Clinical Reasoning. In G. C. Stone, F. Cohen, N. E. Adler *et al.* (eds) *Health Psychology – A Handbook*. San Francisco: Josey Bass.

Elstein, A. S., Shulman, L. S., and Sprafka, S. A. (1978) *Medical Problem Solving: An Analysis of Clinical Reasoning*. Cambridge: Harvard University Press.

Engel, G. I. (1977) The Need for a New Medical Model: A Challenge for Biomedicine. *Science* 196 (4286): 129–36.

Enterline, P. E., Salter, V., McDonald, A. D., and McDonald, J. C. (1973) The Distribution of Medical Services Before and After 'Free' Medical Care – the Quebec Experience. *New England Journal of Medicine* 289: 1174–178.

Epsom, J. (1969) The Mobile Health Clinic: A Report on the First Year's Work. Mimos. London Borough of Southwark, Health Department.

—— (1978) The Mobile Health Clinic: A Report on the First Year's Work. In D. Tuckett and J. Kaufert (eds) *Basic Readings in Medical Sociology*. London: Tavistock Publications.

Erikson, K. (1964) Notes on the Sociology of Deviance. In H. Becker (ed) *The Other Side*. Illinois: Free Press.

Evans-Pritchard, E. (1937) *Witchcraft, Oracles and Magic Among the Azande*. Oxford: Clarendon Press.

Exton-Smith, A. N. (1961) Terminal Illness in the Aged. *Lancet* 799–801.

Fabrega, H. (1974) *Disease and Social Behaviour*. Cambridge, Massachusetts: MIT Press.

Fahy, T.-J., Irving, M., and Millac, P. (1967) Severe Head Injuries: A Six Year Follow-up. *Lancet:* 475–79.

Feibel, J. H. and Springer, C. J. (1982) Depression and Failure to Resume Social Activities after Stroke. *Archives of Physical Medicine and Rehabilitation* 63: 276–78.

Feinstein, A. R. (1976) 'Compliance Bias' and the Interpretation of Therapeutic Trials. In D. L. Sackett and R. B. Haynes (eds) *Compliance with Therapeutic Regimens*. Baltimore: Johns Hopkins University Press.

Feinstein, A. R., Wood, H. F., Epstein, J. A., Taranta, A., Simpson, R., and Tursky, E. (1959) A Controlled Study of 3 Methods of Prophylaxis against Streptococcal Infection in a Population of Rheumatic Children: II. Results of the First 3 Years of the Study, Including Methods for Evaluating the Maintenance of Oral Prophylaxis. *New England Journal of Medicine* 260: 697–702.

Ferguson, B. F. (1979) Preparing Young Children for Hospitalization: A Comparison of Two Methods. *Pediatrics* 64: 656–64.

Fink, R., Shapiro, S., and Roester, R. (1972) Impact of Efforts to Increase

Participation in Repetitive Screenings for Early Breast Cancer Detection. *American Journal of Public Health* 62: 328–36.

Finlayson, A. and McEwen, J. (1977) *Coronary Heart Disease and Patterns of Living.* London: Croom Helm.

Finnerty, F. A., Mattie, E. C., and Finnerty, F. A. (1973a) Hypertension in the Inner City: I. Analysis of Clinic Drop-outs. *Circulation* 47: 73–5.

Finnerty, F. A., Shaw, L., and Himmelsbach, C. K. (1973b) Hypertension in the Inner City: II. Detection and Follow-up. *Circulation* 47: 76–8.

Fitton, F. and Acheson, H. W. K. (1979) *Doctor–Patient Relationship.* London: HMSO.

Fitzpatrick, R. M. (1983) Cultural Aspects of Psychiatry. In M. Weller (ed) *The Scientific Basis of Psychiatry.* London: Balliere Tindall.

Fitzpatrick, R. M. and Hopkins, A. P. (1981a) Patients' Satisfaction with Communication in Neurological Outpatient Clinics. *Journal of Psychosomatic Research* 25 (5): 329–34.

Fitzpatrick, R. M. and Hopkins, A. P. (1981b) Referrals to Neurologists for Headaches Not Due to Structural Disease. *Journal of Neurology, Neurosurgery and Psychiatry* 44 (12): 1061–067.

Fitzpatrick, R. M. and Hopkins, A. P. (1983) Problems in the Conceptual Framework of Patient Satisfaction Research: An Empirical Exploration. *Sociology of Health and Illness* 5 (3): 297–311.

Fitzpatrick, R. M., Hopkins, A. P., and Harvard-Watts, O. (1983) Social Dimensions of Healing. *Social Science and Medicine* 17 (8): 501–10.

Folstein, M., Maiberger, R., and McHugh, P. (1977) Mood Disorder as a Complication of Stroke. *Journal of Neurology, Neurosurgery and Psychiatry* 40: 1018–020.

Food and Drug Administration (1979) Prescription Drug Products: Patient Labelling Requirements. *Federal Register* 44. 40016–40041.

Fortin, F. and Kirouac, S. (1976) A Randomized Controlled Trial of Pre-operative Patient Education. *International Journal of Nursing Studies* 13: 11–24.

Francis, V., Korsch, B. M. and Morris, M. J. (1969) Gaps in Doctor–Patient Communication. *New England Journal of Medicine* 280: 535–40.

Frankel, G., Ludbrook, J., Dudley, H., Hill, G., and Marshall, V. (1982) *Guide for House Surgeons on a Surgical Unit* (7th edn). London: Heinemann.

Freeman, B., Negrete, V., Davis, M., and Korsch, B. (1971) Gaps in Doctor–Patient Communication: Doctor–Patient Interaction Analysis. *Pediatric Research* 5: 298–311.

Freidson, E. (1961) *Patients' Views of Medical Practice.* New York: Russell Sage Foundation.

—— (1970) *Profession of Medicine: A Study in the Sociology of Applied Knowledge.* New York: Dodd Mead.

—— (1974) Dilemmas in the Doctor–Patient Relationship. In C. Cox and A. Mead (eds) *A Sociology of Medical Practice.* London: Collier Macmillan.

French, K. (1981) Methodological Considerations in Hospital Patient Opinion Surveys. *International Journal of Nursing Studies* 18 (1): 7–32.

Friedlander, M. L., Steinhart, M. J., Daly, S. S., and Snyder, J. (1982) Demographic, Cognitive and Experimental Predictors of Presurgical Anxiety. *Journal of Psychosomatic Research* 26 (6): 623–27.

Fry, A. (1979) *Common Diseases* (2nd edn). London: MTP Press.

Fugl-Meyer, A. and Jaasko, L. (1980) Post-stroke Hemiplegia and Sexual Inter-course. *Scandinavian Journal of Rehabilitative Medicine*, Supplement 7.

Furnham, A. and Pendred, J. (1983) Attitudes towards the Mentally and Physically Disabled. *British Journal of Medical Psychology* 56: 179–87.

Gaines, A. D. (1979) Definitions and Diagnoses: Cultural Implications of Psychiatric Help Seeking and Psychiatrists' Definitions of the Situation in Psychiatric Emergencies. *Culture, Medicine and Psychiatry* 3 (4): 381–418.

Gainotti, G. (1972) Emotional Behaviour and Hemispheric Side of Lesion. *Cortex* 8: 41–55.

Garfinkel, H. (1967) *Studies in Ethnomethodology*. New York: Prentice-Hall.

Gasparrini, W., Satz, P., Heilman, K., and Coolridge, F. (1979) Hemispheric Asymmetries of Affective Processing as Determined by the Minnesota Multiphasic Personality Inventory. Presented at the International Neuro-psychology Society, Sante Fe, New Mexico, 1977. In E. Vallenstein and K. Heilman (eds) *Clinical Neuropsychology*. Oxford: Oxford University Press.

Geltner, L. (1972) Comprehensive Care of Cerebrovascular Accidents. *Clinical Gerontology* 14: 346–53.

Gerstenbrand, F. (1969) Rehabilitation of the Head Injured. In A. Walker, W. Caveness, and M. Critchley *Late Effects of Head Injury*. Springfield: CC Thomas.

Glaser, B. G. and Strauss, A. L. (1965) *Awareness of Dying*. Chicago: Aldine Publishing.

Glasgow, D. (1980) *The Black Underclass*. New York: Jossey Bass.

Goffman, E. (1961) *Encounters*. Indianapolis: Bobbs-Merrill.

—— (1968) *Stigma: Notes on the Management of Spoiled Identity*. Harmondsworth: Penguin.

Goldberg, D. P., Steele, J., Smith, C., and Spivey, L. (1980) Training Family Doctors to Recognize Psychiatric Illness with Increased Efficiency. *Lancet* 2: 521–24.

Good, B. and Good, M. J. (1981) The Meaning of Symptoms: A Cultural Hermeneutic Model for Clinical Practice. In L. Eisenberg and A. Kleinman (eds) *The Relevance of Social Science for Medicine*. Dordrecht, Holland: Reidel.

Good, B. J. (1977) The Heart of What's the Matter. *Culture, Medicine and Psychiatry* 1 (1): 25–58.

Gordis, L. (1979) Conceptual and Methodological Problems in Measuring Patient Compliance. In R. B. Haynes, D. W. Taylor, and D. L. Sackett (eds) *Compliance in Health Care*. Baltimore: Johns Hopkins University Press.

Gordis, L., Desi, L., and Schmerler, H. R. (1976) Treatment of Acute Sore Throats: A Comparison of Pediatricians and General Practitioners. *Pediatrics* 57: 422–24.

Gordis, L., Markowitz, M., and Lilienfield, A. (1969) The Inaccuracy of Using Interviews to Estimate Patient Reliability in Taking Medications at Home. *Medical Care* 7: 49–54.

Gough, H. G. (1977) Doctors' Estimates of the Percentage of Patients Whose Problems Do Not Require Medical Attention. *Medical Education* 11: 380–84.

Granovetter, M. (1973) The Strength of Weak Ties. *American Journal of Sociology* 78: 1360–380.

Gray, L. C. (1980) Consumer Satisfaction with Physician Provided Services: A Panel Study. *Social Science and Medicine* 14a (1): 65–73.

Greenblatt, M., Becerra, R., and Serafetinides, E. (1982) Social Networks and Mental Health: An Overview. *American Journal of Psychiatry* 139: 977–84.

Greene, G. (1972) *A Sort of a Life*. Harmondsworth: Penguin.

Gresham, G., Fitzpatrick, T., Wolf, P., McNamara, P., Kannel, W., and Dawber, T. (1975) Residual Disability in Survivors of Stroke: The Framingham Study. *New England Journal of Medicine* 293: 954–56.

Gresham, G., Phillips, T., Wolf, P., McNamara, P., Kannel, W., and Dawber, T. (1979) Epidemiologic Profile of Long-term Stroke Disability: The Framingham Study. *Archives of Physical Medicine and Rehabilitation* 60: 487–91.

Grosswasser, Z., Mendelson, L., Stern, M., Schechter, I., and Najenson, T. (1977) The Re-evaluation of Prognostic Factors in Rehabilitation after Severe Head Injury. *Scandinavian Journal of Rehabilitative Medicine* 9: 147–49.

Haber, L. and Smith, R. (1971) Disability and Deviance: Normative Adaptations of Role Behaviour. *American Sociological Review* 36: 87.

Hackett, T. P. and Weisman, A. D. (1962) The Treatment of the Dying. In J. H. Masserman (ed.) *Current Psychiatric Therapies: 2*. New York: Grune & Stratton.

Haefner, D. and Kirscht, J. P. (1970) Motivational and Behavioural Effects of Modifying Health Beliefs. *Public Health Reports* 85: 478–84.

Haggerty, R. J. (1968) Community Pediatrics. *New England Journal of Medicine* 278 (1): 15.

Hall, E. T. (1966) *The Hidden Dimension*. New York: Doubleday.

Hammer, M. (1983) 'Core' and 'Extended' Social Networks in Relation to Health and Illness. *Social Science and Medicine* 17: 405–11.

Hamrin, E. (1982) One Year after Stroke: A Follow-up of an Experimental Study. *Scandinavian Journal of Rehabilitative Medicine* 14: 111–16.

Hannay, D. (1980) The 'Iceberg' of Illness and 'Trivial' Consultations. *Journal of the Royal College of General Practitioners* 30: 551–54.

Hartman, P. E. and Becker, M. H. (1978) Non-compliance with Prescribed Regimen among Chronic Hemodialysis Patients: A Method of Prediction and Educational Diagnosis. *Dialysis and Transplantation* 7: 978–89.

Harwood, A. (1971) The Hot–Cold Theory of Disease: Implications for Treatment of Puerto Rican Patients. *Journal of the American Medical Association* 216: 1153–168.

Haug, M. (1976) Issues in General Practitioner Authority in the National Health Service. In M. Stacey (ed.) *The Sociology of the NHS*. Sociological Review Monograph 22.

Hauser, S. T. (1981) Physician–Patient Relationships. In E. Mishler, L. Amara Singham, S. Hauser, R. Liem, S. Osherson, and N. Waxler (eds) *Social Contexts of Health, Illness and Patient Care*. Cambridge: Cambridge University Press.

Haynes, R. B., Sackett, D. L., Taylor, D. W., Gibson, E. S., and Johnson, A. L. (1978) Absenteeism from Work after the Detection and Labelling of Hypertensives. *New England Journal of Medicine* 299: 741–44.

Haynes, R. B., Taylor, D. W., and Sackett, D. L. (1979) *Compliance in Health Care*. Baltimore: Johns Hopkins University Press.

Hayward, J. (1975) *Information: A Prescription against Pain. The Study of Nursing Care Project Reports. Series 2. No. 5*. London: The Royal College of Nursing.

—— (1980) *Management of Acute Head Injuries*. Oxford: Blackwell.

Healey, K. M. (1968) Does Pre-operative Instruction Make a Difference? *American Journal of Nursing* 68: 62–7.

Heiskanen, O. and Sipponen, P. (1970) Prognosis of Severe Brain Injury. *Acta Scandinavia Neurologica* 43: 343–48.

Helfer, R. E. (1970) An Objective Comparison of the Paediatric Interviewing Skills of Freshmen and Senior Medical Students. *Paediatrics* 45: 623–27.

Heller, S., Frank, K., and Kornfield, D. (1974) Psychological Outcome Following Open Heart Surgery. *Archives of Internal Medicine* 135: 908–11.

Helman, C. G. (1978) 'Feed a Cold, Starve a Fever' – Folk Models of Infection in an English Suburban Community. *Culture, Medicine and Psychiatry* 2 (2): 107–37.

—— (1981) 'Tonic', 'Fuel' and 'Food': Social and Symbolic Aspects of the Long-term Use of Psychotropic Drugs. *Social Science and Medicine* 15b (4): 521–34.

Henley, A. (1979) *Asian Patients in Hospital and at Home*. London: King Edward's Hospital Fund for London.

Herbertt, R. M. and Innes, J. M. (1979) Familiarization and Preparatory Information in the Reduction of Anxiety in Child Dental Patients. *Journal of Dentistry in Children* 46: 319–23.

Herzlich, C. (1973) *Health and Illness*. London: Academic Press.

Hibbard, J. and Pope, C. (1983) Gender Roles, Illness Orientation and Use of Medical Services. *Social Science and Medicine* 17: 1107–123.

Higgins, P. (1980) *Outsiders in a Hearing World: A Sociology of Deafness*. Beverly Hills, California: Sage Publications.

Hilbourne, J. (1973) On Disabling the Normal: The Implications of Physical Disability for Other People. *British Journal of Social Work* 3: 497–507.

Hinton, J. M. (1963) The Physical and Mental Distress of the Dying. *Quarterly Journal of Medicine* 32: 1–21.

—— (1975) The Influence of Previous Personality on Reactions to Having Terminal Cancer. *Omega* 6: 95–111.

—— (1979) Comparison of Places and Policies for Terminal Care. *Lancet* 29–32.

—— (1980) Whom Do Dying Patients Tell? *British Medical Journal* 281: 1328–330.

Hitch, P. (1975) *Migration and Mental Illness in a Northern City*. Unpublished PhD thesis, University of Bradford.

Hochstadt, N. J. and Trybula, J. (1980) Reducing Missed Initial Appointments in a Community Health Centre. *Journal of Community Psychology* 8: 261–65.

Hooper, E. M., Comstock, L. M., Goodwin, J. M., and Goodwin, J. S. (1982) Patient Characteristics that Influence Physician Behaviour. *Medical Care* 20: 630–38.

Hopkins, A. and Scambler, G. (1977) How Doctors Deal with Epilepsy. *Lancet* 1: 183–87.

Hopper, S. (1981) Diabetes as a Stigmatized Condition: The Case of Low-income Clinic Patients in the United States. *Social Science and Medicine* 15(b): 11–19.

Horn, E. (1982) A Survey of Referrals from Asian Families to Four Social Services Area Offices. In J. Cheetham (ed.) *Social Work and Ethnicity*. London: Allen & Unwin.

Horwitz, A. (1978) Family, Kin and Friend Networks in Psychiatric Help-seeking. *Social Science and Medicine* 12: 297–304.

Hovland, C. I., Lumsdaine, A. A., and Sheffield, F. D. (1949) The Effects of Presenting 'One Side' Versus 'Both Sides' in Changing Opinions on a Controversial Subject. *Studies in Social Psychology in World War II: vol. III Experiments on Mass Communication*. Princeton, NJ: Princeton University Press.

Hpay, M. (1971) Psychological Effects of Severe Head Injury. *Proceedings of International Symposium on Head Injuries*. Edinburgh: Churchill Livingstone.

Hughes, J. (1982) Emotional Reactions to the Diagnosis and Treatment of Early Breast Cancer. *Journal of Psychosomatic Research* 26: 277–83.

Hulka, B. S., Kupper, L., Cassel, J., Efird, R., and Brudette, J. (1975a) Medication Use and Misuse: Physician–Patient Discrepancies. *Journal of Chronic Diseases* 28: 7–21.

Hulka, B. S., Kupper, L., Cassel, J. C., and Mayo, F. (1975b) Doctor–Patient Communication and Outcomes among Diabetic Patients. *Journal of Community Health* 1: 15–27.

Hulka, B. S., Kupper, L. L., Daly, M. B., Cassel, J. C., and Schoen, F. (1975c) Correlates of Satisfaction and Dissatisfaction with Medical Care. *Medical Care* 13 (7): 648–58.

Hull, D. (1979) Migration, Adaptation and Illness: A Review. *Social Science and Medicine* 13(a): 25–36.

Humphrey, M. and Oddy, M. (1978) Social Costs of Head Injuries. *New Society*, 31 August.

Hunt, E. B. and MacLeod, C. M. (1979) Cognition and Information Processing in Patient and Physician. In G. C. Stone, F. Cohen, N. E. Adler *et al.* (eds) *Health Psychology – A Handbook*. San Francisco: Josey Bass.

Hunt, P. (ed.) (1966) *Stigma: The Experience of Disability*. London: Chapman.

Hutchinson, E. and Acheson, E. (1975) *Strokes: Natural History, Pathology and Surgical Treatment*. London: Saunders.

Ignu, U. (1979) Stages in Health Seeking: A Descriptive Model. *Social Science and Medicine* 13(a): 445–56.

Illsley, R. (1980) *Profession or Public Health?* London: Nuffield Provincial Hospitals Trust.

Ingham, J. and Miller, P. (1979) Symptom Prevalence and Severity in a General Practice. *Journal of Epidemiology and Community Health* 33: 191–98.

Inui, T., Yourtee, E. L., and Williamson, J. W. (1976) Improved Outcomes in Hypertension after Physician Tutorials. *Annals of Internal Medicine* 84: 646–51.

James, W. H., Woodruff, A. B., and Werner, W. (1965) Effect of Internal and External Control upon Changes in Smoking Behaviour. *Journal of Consulting Psychology* 29: 184–86.

Jamieson, K. and Kelly, D. (1973) Crash Helmets Reduce Head Injuries. *Medical Journal of Australia* 2: 806.

Janis, I. L. (1958) *Psychological Stress – Psychoanalytic and Behavioural Studies of Surgical Patients*. New York: J. Wiley.

—— (1969) *Stress and Frustration*. New York: Harcourt, Brace & Jovanovich.

Janzen, J. M. and Prins, G. (eds) (1981) *Causality and Classification in African Medicine and Health. Special Issue: Social Science and Medicine* 158 (3).

Jefferys, M. (1977) What Are Health Services for: Whom Do They Serve? *New Universities Quarterly* 30 (2): 181–92.

Jobling, R. (1977) Learning to Live with It: An Account of a Career of Chronic Dermatological Illness and Patienthood. In A. Davis and G. Horobin (eds) *Medical Encounters: The Experience of Illness and Treatment*. London: Croom Helm.

Johnson, D. T. and Spielberger, C. D. (1968) The Effects of Relaxation Training and the Passage of Time on Measures of State and Trait Anxiety. *Journal of Clinical Psychology* 24: 20–3.

Johnson, J. E. (1966) The Influence of Purposeful Nurse–Patient Interaction on the Patient's Post-operative Course. In ANA *Exploring Progress in Medical and Surgical Nursing Practice*. New York: American Nurses' Association.

—— (1975) Stress Reduction through Sensation Information. In I. G. Sarason and C. D. Spielberger (eds) *Stress and Anxiety*, vol. 2. Washington: Hemisphere.

Johnson, J. E., Dabbs, J. M., and Leventhal, H. (1970) Psychosocial Factors in the Welfare of Surgical Patients. *Nursing Research* 19: 18–29.

Johnson, J. E., Leventhal, H., and Dabbs, J. M. (1971) Contribution of Emotional and Instrumental Response Processes in Adaption to Surgery. *Journal of Personality and Social Psychology* 20: 55–64.

Johnson, J. E., Morrisey, J. E., and Leventhal, H. (1973) Psychological Preparation for an Endoscopic Examination. *Gastrointestinal Endoscopy* 19: 180–82.

Johnston, M. (1976) Communication of Patient's Feelings in Hospital. In A. E. Bennet (ed.) *Communication between Doctors and Patients*. Oxford: Oxford University Press.

—— (1980) Anxiety in Surgical Patients. *Psychological Medicine* 10: 145–52.

—— (1982) Recognition of Patients' Worries by Nurses and by Other Patients. *British Journal of Clinical Psychology* 21 (4): 255–61.

—— (1984a) Pre-operative Emotional States and Post-operative Recovery. In F. G. Guggenheim (ed.) *Psychological Aspects of Surgery*, vol. 12 of Advances in Psychosomatic Medicine. Basel: Karges (in press).

—— (1984b) Dimensions of Recovery from Surgery. *Journal of Applied Psychology*. In press.

Johnston, M. and Carpenter, L. (1980) Relationship between Pre-operative Anxiety and Post-operative State. *Psychological Medicine* 10: 361–67.

Jones, J. (1965) Employment of Epileptics. *Lancet* 2: 486–89.

Jourard, S. M. (1966) An Exploratory Study of Body Accessibility. *British Journal of Social and Clinical Psychology* 5: 221–31.

Joyce, C. R. B., Caple, G., Mason, M., Reynolds, E., and Mathews, J. A. (1969) Quantitative Study of Doctor–Patient Communication. *Quarterly Journal of Medicine* 38: 183–94.

Kahn, R. L. and Cannell, C. F. (1957) *The Dynamics of Interviewing: Theory, Technique and Cases*. New York: John Wiley.

Kaplan, R. M., Atkins, C. J., and Lenhard, L. (1982) Coping with Stressful Sigmoidoscopy: Evaluation of Cognitive and Relaxation Preparations. *Journal of Behavioural Medicine* 5 (1): 67–82.

Kasl, S. and Cobb, S. (1966) Health Behaviour, Illness Behaviour and Sick Role Behaviour. *Archives of Environmental Health* 12: 246–66.

Katon, W. and Kleinman, A. (1981) Doctor–Patient Negotiation and Other Social Science Strategies in Patient Care. In L. Eisenberg and A. Kleinman (eds) *The Relevance of Social Science for Medicine*. Dordrecht, Holland: Reidel.

Katon, W., Kleinman, A. M., and Rosen, G. (1982) Depression and Somatization: A Review. *American Journal of Medicine* 72: 127–35.

Kegeles, S. S. (1969) A Field Experiment Attempt to Change Beliefs and Behaviour of Women in an Urban Ghetto. *Journal of Health and Social Behaviour* 10: 115–24.

Kelley, H. H. (1950) The Warm–Cold Variable in First Impressions of Persons. *Journal of Personality* 18: 431–39.

260 *The Experience of Illness*

Kendon, A. (1967) Some Functions of Gaze Direction in Social Interaction. *Acta Psychologia* 26: 22–63.

Kessel, N. (1979) Reassurance. *Lancet* 2: 1128–133.

Kessel, N. and Coppen, A. (1963) The Prevalence of Common Menstrual Symptoms. *Lancet* 3: 61–4.

Kincey, J., Bradshaw, P., and Ley, P. (1975) Patients' Satisfaction and Reported Acceptance of Advice in General Practice. *Journal of the Royal College of General Practitioners* 25 (157): 558–66.

Kinney, M. R. (1977) Effects of Pre-operative Teaching upon Patients with Differing Modes of Response to Threatening Stimuli. *International Journal of Nursing Studies* 14: 49–59.

Kinsella, G. and Duffy, F. (1979) Psychological Readjustment in the Spouses of Aphasic Patients. *Scandinavian Journal of Rehabilitative Medicine* 11: 129–32.

Kirscht, J. P., Becker, M. H., Haefner, D. P., and Maiman, L. A. (1978) Effects of Threatening Communications and Mothers' Health Beliefs on Weight Change in Obese Children. *Journal of Behavioural Medicine* 1: 147–57.

Kirscht, J. P. and Rosenstock, I. M. (1977) Patient Adherence to Antihypertensive Medical Regimens. *Journal of Community Health* 3: 115–24.

Kleinman, A. M. (1980) *Patients and Healers in the Context of Culture.* Berkeley: University of California Press.

Kleinman, M., Eisenberg, L., and Good, B. J. (1978) Culture, Illness and Care. *Annals of Internal Medicine* 88: 251–58.

Knudson-Cooper, M. (1981) Adjustment to Visible Stigma: The Case of the Severely Burned. *Social Science and Medicine* 15(b): 31–44.

Korsch, B. M., Gozzi, E. K., and Francis, V. (1968) Gaps in Doctor–Patient Communications: 1. Doctor–Patient Interaction and Patient Satisfaction. *Paediatrics* 42: 855–71.

Krausz, E. (1972) *Ethnic Minorities in Britain.* London: Paladin.

Kronenfeld, J. J. and Wasner, C. (1982) The Use of Unorthodox Therapies and Marginal Practitioners. *Social Science and Medicine* 16 (11): 1119–126.

Kübler-Ross, E. (1970) *On Death and Dying.* London: Tavistock Publications.

Kurtze, J. (1969) *Epidemiology of Cerebrovascular Disease.* Berlin: Springer Verlag.

Labi, M. (1980) Psycho-social Disability in Physically Restored Long-term Stroke Survivors. *Archives of Physical Medicine and Rehabilitation* 61 (12): 561–65.

LaCrosse, M. B. (1975) Nonverbal Behaviour and Perceived Counsellor Attractiveness and Persuasiveness. *Journal of Counselling Psychology* 22: 563–66.

Langer, E. J., Janis, I. L., and Wolfer, J. A. S. (1975) Reduction of Psychological Stress in Surgical Patients. *Journal of Experimental Social Psychology* 11: 155–65.

Larsen, D. E. and Rootman, I. (1976) Physician Role Performance and Patient Satisfaction. *Social Science and Medicine* 10 (1): 29–32.

Larsen, K. M. and Smith, C. K. (1981) Assessment of Nonverbal Communication in the Patient–Physician Interview. *Journal of Family Practice* 12 (3): 481–88.

Last, J. (1963) The Iceberg: Completing the Clinical Picture in General Practice. *Lancet* 2: 28–31.

Lawrence, C. (1979) The Nervous System and Society in the Scottish Enlightenment. In B. Barnes and S. Shapin (eds) *Natural Order.* London: Sage.

Lawrence, L. and Christie, D. (1979) Quality of Life after Stroke – A Three Year Follow-up. *Age and Ageing* 8 (3): 167–72.

Lazare, A., Eisenthal, S., Frank, A., and Stoeckle, J. (1978) Studies on the Negotiated Approach to Patienthood. In E. B. Gallagher (ed.) *The Doctor–Patient Relationship In the Changing Health Scene*. Washington, DC: DHEW Publishers No. (NIH) 78–183, pp. 119–39.

Le Grand, J. (1982) *The Strategy of Equality*. London: Allen & Unwin.

—— (1978) The Distribution of Public Expenditure: The Case of Health Care. *Economica* 45: 125–42.

Leventhal, H., Hochbaum, G., and Rosenstock, I. (1960) Epidemic Impact on the General Population in Two Cities: The Impact of Asian Influenza on Community Life: A Study in Five Cities. *Public Health Service Publication 766*. Washington, DC: Government Printing Office.

Levesque, L. and Charlebois, M. (1977) Anxiety, Locus of Control and the Effect of Pre-operative Teaching on Patients' Physical and Emotional State. *Nursing Papers* 8: 11–26.

Levin, H. S., Grossman, R., and Kelly, P. (1976) Aphasic Disorder in Patients with Closed Head Injury. *Journal of Neurology, Neurosurgery and Psychiatry* 39: 1062–070.

Lewin, W. (1968) Rehabilitation after Head Injury. *British Medical Journal* 1: 465–70.

Ley, P. (1973) The Measurement of Comprehensibility. *Journal of the Institute of Health Education* 11: 17–20.

—— (1976) Towards Better Doctor–Patient Communication: Contributions from Social and Experimental Psychology. In A. E. Bennett (ed.) *Communications between Doctors and Patients*. London: Nuffield Provincial Hospitals Trust.

—— (1977) Psychological Studies of Doctor–Patient Communication. In S. Rachman (ed.) *Contributions to Medical Psychology*, vol. 1. Oxford: Pergamon Press.

—— (1978) Psychological and Behavioural Factors in Weight Loss. In G. A. Bray (ed.) *Recent Advances in Obesity Research*, vol. 2. London: Newman Publishing.

—— (1979a) Improving Communications: Effects of Altering Doctor Behaviour. In D. J. Oborne, M. M. Gruneberg, and J. R. Eiser (eds) *Research in Psychology and Medicine*. London: Academic Press.

—— (1979b) The Psychology of Compliance. In D. J. Oborne, M. M. Gruneberg, and J. R. Eiser (eds) *Research in Psychology and Medicine*, vol. 2. London: Academic Press.

—— (1979c) Memory for Medical Information. *British Journal of Social and Clinical Psychology* 18: 245–56.

—— (1980) Practical Methods for Improving Communication. In L. Morris, M. Mazis, and L. Barofsky (eds) *Product Labelling and Health Risks*, Cold Spring Harbour, NY: Banbury Reports.

—— (1981) Professional Non-compliance: A Neglected Problem. *British Journal of Clinical Psychology* 20: 151–54.

—— (1982) Satisfaction, Compliance and Communication. *British Journal of Clinical Psychology* 21: 241–54.

Ley, P. and Spelman, M. S. (1965) Communications in an Out-patient Setting. *British Journal of Social and Clinical Psychology* 4: 114–16.

Ley, P. and Spelman, M. S. (1967) *Communicating with the Patient*. London: Staples Press.

Ley, P., Whitworth, M. A., Skilbeck, C. E., Woodward, R., Pinset, R. J. F. H., Pike, L. A., Clarkson, M. E., and Clark, P. B. (1976) Improving Doctor–Patient Communication in General Practice. *Journal of the Royal College of General Practitioners* 26: 720–24.

Lezak, M. (1978) Living with Characterologically Altered Brain-Injured Patients. *Journal of Clinical Psychiatry* 39: 592–98.

Lezak, M. (1982) Coping with Head Injury in the Family. In G. Broe and R. Tate (eds) *Brain Impairment. Proceedings of the Fifth Annual Brain Impairment Conference.* Sydney: Postgraduate Committee in Medicine of the University of Sydney.

Lezak, M. (1983) *Neuropsychological Assessment.* New York: Oxford University Press.

Lezak, M., Cosgrove, J., O'Brien, K., and Wooster, N. (1980) *Relationships between Personality Disorder, Social Disturbances and Physical Disability Following Traumatic Brain Injury.* Presented at 8th International Neuropsychology Society meeting, San Francisco.

Lindeman, C. A. and Aernam, R. V. (1971) Nursing Intervention with the Presurgical Patient: The Effects of Structure and Unstructured Pre-operative Teaching. *Nursing Research* 20: 319–32.

Lindeman, C. A. and Stetzer, S. L. (1973) Effect of Pre-operative Visits by Operating Room Nurses. *Nursing Research* 22: 4–16.

Linder-Pelz, S. (1982) Toward a Theory of Patient Satisfaction. *Social Science and Medicine* 16 (5): 577–82.

Linn, M. W., Linn, B. S., and Stein, S. R. (1982) Beliefs about Causes of Cancer in Cancer Patients. *Social Science and Medicine* 16 (7): 835–40.

Lipton, H. L. and Svarstad, B. L. (1974) Parental Expectations of a Multidisciplinary Clinic for Children with Developmental Disabilities. *Journal of Health and Social Behaviour* 15 (2): 157–66.

Lishman, W. A. (1968) Brain Damage in Relation to Psychiatric Disability after Head Injury. *British Journal of Psychiatry* 114: 375–410.

—— (1978) *Organic Psychiatry. The Psychological Consequences of Cerebral Disorder.* Oxford: Blackwell.

Littlewood, R. and Lipsedge, M. (1982) *Aliens and Alienists: Ethnic Minorities and Psychiatry.* Harmondsworth: Penguin.

Liu, W. and Duff, R. (1972) The Strength of Weak Ties. *Public Opinion Quarterly* 36: 361–66.

Lloyd, M. (1974) Medical Authoritarianism and Its Effect on Health Care. *Medical Journal of Australia* 2 (11): 413–16.

Lock, M. (1982) Models and Practice in Medicine: Menopause as Syndrome or Life Transition. *Culture, Medicine and Psychiatry* 6 (3): 261–80.

Locker, D. and Dunt, D. (1978) Theoretical and Methodological Issues in Sociological Studies of Consumer Satisfaction with Medical Care. *Social Science and Medicine* 12 (4): 283–92.

London, P. S. (1967) Some Observations on the Course of Events after Severe Injury of the Head. *Annals of the Royal College of Surgeons of England* 41: 460–69.

Lonsdale, S. (1981) Job Protection for the Disabled. *Low Pay Report* 6.

—— (1984) *Work and Inequality.* London: Longman.

Lonsdale, S. and Walker, A. (1983) *Labour Market Policies towards People with Disabilities in the UK.* Paper presented to International Institute of Management, Berlin.

Lucente, F. E. and Fleck, S. (1972) A Study of Hospitalization Anxiety in 408 Medical and Surgical Patients. *Psychosomatic Medicine* 34: 304–12.

Lundholm, J., Jepsen, B., and Thornval, G. (1975) The Late Neurological, Psychological and Social Aspects of Severe Traumatic Coma. *Scandinavian Journal of Rehabilitative Medicine* 7: 97–100.

Lundy, J. R. (1972) Some Personality Correlates of Contraceptive Use among Unmarried Female College Students. *Journal of Personality* 80: 9–14.

MacCormack, C. (1980) Health Care Problems of Ethnic Minority Groups. *Mimms Magazine* 15 July: 53–60.

MacIntyre, I. (1976) Epilepsy and Employment. *Community Health* 7: 195–204.

McKinlay, J. (1972) Some Approaches and Problems in the Study of the Use of Services: An Overview. *Journal of Health and Social Behaviour* 13: 115–52.

—— (1973) Social Networks, Lay Consultation and Help-seeking Behaviour. *Social Forces* 53: 275–92.

—— (1975) Who Is Really Ignorant – Physician or Patient? *Journal of Health and Social Behaviour* 16 (1): 3–11.

—— (1981) Social Network Influences on Morbid Episodes and the Career of Help Seeking. In L. Eisenberg and A. Kleinman (eds) *The Relevance of Social Science for Medicine.* Dordrecht, Holland: D. Reidel Publishing.

McKinlay, W., Brooks, D., Bond, M., Martinage, D., and Marshall, M. (1981) The Short Term Outcome of Severe Blunt Head Injury as Reported by Relatives of the Injured Person. *Journal of Neurology, Neurosurgery and Psychiatry* 44: 527–33.

Maguire, G. P., Julier, D. L., Hawton, K. E., and Bancroft, J. H. (1974) Psychiatric Morbidity and Referral on Two General Medical Wards. *British Medical Journal* 1: 268–70.

Maguire, P. and Rutter, D. R. (1976) Teaching Medical Students to Communicate. In A. E. Bennett (ed.) *Communication between Doctors and Patients.* London: Oxford University Press for the Nuffield Provincial Hospitals Trust.

Maher, E. (1982) Anomic Aspects of Recovery from Cancer. *Social Science and Medicine* 16: 907–12.

Manchester Law Centre (1982) *From Ill Treatment to No Treatment: The New Health Regulations: Black People and Internal Controls.* Manchester: Manchester Free Press.

Mankoff, M. (1971) Societal Reaction and Career Deviance: A Critical Analysis. *Sociological Quarterly* 12: 214–18.

Mann, L. and Janis, I. L. (1968) A Follow-up Study on the Long-term Effects of Emotional Role Playing. *Journal of Personality and Social Psychology* 8: 339–42.

Manno, B. and Marston, A. R. (1972) Weight Reduction as a Function of Negative Covert Reinforcement (Sensitisation) Versus Positive Covert Reinforcement. *Behaviour Research and Therapy* 10: 201–07.

Marks, I. (1981) Cure and Care of Neuroses. *Theory and Practice of Behavioural Psychotherapy.* Chichester: John Wiley.

Marks, J. N., Goldberg, D. P., and Hillier, V. F. (1979) Determinants of the Ability of General Practitioners to Detect Psychiatric Illness. *Psychological Medicine* 9: 337–45.

Markson, E. W. (1971) Patient Semiology of a Chronic Disease. *Social Science and Medicine* 5 (4): 159–67.

Marquis, K. H. (1970) Effects of Social Reinforcement on Health Reporting in the Household Interview. *Sociometry* 33: 203–15.

Marsh, G. M. (1977) 'Curing' Minor Illness in General Practice. *British Medical Journal* 2: 1267–269.

Marshall, J. (1976) *The Management of Cerebrovascular Disease*. Oxford: Blackwell.

Martinez-Urrutia, A. (1975) Pain and Anxiety in Surgical Patients. *Journal of Consulting and Clinical Psychology* 43 (4): 437–42.

Mathews, A. and Ridgeway, V. (1981) Personality and Surgical Recovery: A Review. *British Journal of Clinical Psychology* 20: 243–60.

Mathews, A. and Ridgeway, V. (1984) Psychological Preparation for Surgery. In A. Steptoe and A. Mathews (eds) *Health Care and Human Behaviour*. London: Academic Press.

Mayou, R. (1976) The Nature of Bodily Symptoms. *British Journal of Psychiatry* 129 (1): 55–6.

Mazzuca, S. (1982) Does Patient Education in Chronic Disease Have Therapeutic Value? *Journal of Chronic Diseases* 35 (7): 521–29.

Mechanic, D. (1969) Illness and Cure. In J. Kosa, A. Antonowsky, and I. Zola (eds) *Poverty and Health*. Cambridge, Massachusetts: Harvard University Press.

—— (1978) *Medical Sociology*. London: Collier Macmillan.

Mechanic, D. and Volkart, E. (1961) Stress, Illness Behaviour and the Sick Role. *American Sociological Review* 20: 51–8.

Melamed, B. and Siegel, L. (1975) Reduction in Anxiety in Children Facing Hospitalization and Surgery by Use of Filmed Modelling. *Journal of Consulting and Clinical Psychology* 43: 511–21.

Melamed, B., Hawes, R., Heiby, E., and Guck, J. (1975a) Use of Filmed Modelling to Reduce Unco-operative Behaviour of Children during Dental Treatment. *Journal of Dental Research* 54: 801–979.

Melamed, B., Weinstein, D., Hawes, R., and Katin-Borland, M. (1975b) Reduction of Fear-Related Dental Management: Problems with Use of Filmed Modelling. *Journal of the American Dental Association* 90: 822–26.

Melamed, B., Yurcheson, R., Fleece, L., Hutcherson, S., and Hawes, R. (1978) Effects of Filmed Modelling on the Reduction of Anxiety Related Behaviours in Individuals Varying in Level of Previous Experience in the Stress Situation. *Journal of Consulting and Clinical Psychology* 46: 1357–467.

Merton, R. (1968) *Social Theory and Social Structure*. New York: Free Press.

Miller, H. and Stern, G. (1965) The Long Term Prognosis of Severe Head Injury. *Lancet* 1: 225–29.

Miller, R. L., Brickman, P., and Bolen, D. (1975) Attribution Versus Persuasion as a Means for Modifying Behaviour. *Journal of Personality and Social Psychology* 31: 3.

Miller, W. B. (1978) Psychiatry and Physical Illness: The Psychosomatic Interface. In C. Rosenbaum and J. Beebe (eds) *Psychiatric Treatment: Crisis/Clinic/Consultation*. New York: McGraw Hill.

Moos, R. (1977) *Menstrual Distress Questionnaire Manual*. California: Stanford University Press.

Morisky, D. E., Lavine, D. M., Green, L. W., Shapiro, S., Russell, R. P., and Smith, C. R. (1983) Five Year Blood Pressure Control and Mortality Following Health Education for Hypertensive Patients. *American Journal of Public Health* 73 (2): 153–63.

Morrell, D. and Wale, C. (1976) Symptoms Perceived and Recorded by Patients. *Journal of the Royal College of General Practitioners* 31: 746–50.

Morris, L. A. and Halperin, J. (1979) Effects of Written Drug Information on Patient Knowledge and Compliance: A Literature Review. *American Journal of Public Health* 69: 47–52.

Mumford, E., Schlesinger, H. J. and Glass, G. V. (1982) The Effects of Psychological Intervention on Recovery from Surgery and Heart Attacks: An Analysis of the Literature. *American Journal of Public Health* 72 (2): 141–51.

Najenson, J., Mendelson, L., Schechter, I., David, C., Mintz, N., and Grosswasser, Z. (1974) Rehabilitation after Severe Head Injury. *Scandinavian Journal of Rehabilitative Medicine* 6: 5–14.

Najman, J. M. and Levine, S. (1981) Evaluating the Impact of Medical Care and Technologies on the Quality of Life: A Review and Critique. *Social Science and Medicine* 15 (2): 102–16.

Nathanson, C. (1977) Sex, Illness and Medical Care: A Review of Data, Theory and Method. *Social Science and Medicine* 11: 13–25.

Newman, S. P. (1981) *Family Effects of Cerebrovascular Disease.* Talk to Irish College of Speech Therapists, Dublin.

—— (1984) Individual and Family Responses to Stroke and Head Injury. *Journal of Applied Psychology.* In press.

Oddy, M. and Humphrey, M. (1980) Social Recovery during the Year Following Severe Head Injury. *Journal of Neurology, Neurosurgery and Psychiatry* 43: 798–802.

Oddy, M., Humphrey, M., and Uttley, D. (1978a) Stresses upon the Relatives of Head-injured Patients. *British Journal of Psychiatry* 133: 507–13.

Oddy, M., Humphrey, M., and Uttley, D. (1978b) Subjective Impairment and Social Recovery after Closed Head Injury. *Journal of Neurology, Neurosurgery and Psychiatry* 41: 611–16.

Office of Population Censuses and Surveys (1978a) *Occupational Mortality.* Decennial Supplement, 1970–1972, England and Wales. London: HMSO.

—— (1978b) *Royal Commission on the National Health Service: Patients' Attitudes to the Hospital Service.* London: HMSO.

Ogionwo, W. (1973) Socio-psychological Factors in Health Behaviour: An Experiment Study on Methods and Attitude Change. *International Journal of Health Education* 16: 1–16.

Oliver, M. (1983) Disability, Adjustment and Family Life – Some Theoretical Considerations. In A. Brechin, P. Liddiard, and J. Swain (eds) *Handicap in a Social World.* Sevenoaks: Hodder & Stoughton.

Panting, A. and Merry, P. H. (1972) Long Term Rehabilitation of Severe Head Injuries and Social and Medical Support for the Patient's Family. *Injury* 2: 33.

Parbrook, G. C., Steel, D. F., and Dalrymple, D. G. (1973) Factors Predisposing to Post-operative Pain and Pulmonary Complications. *British Journal Anaestheology* 45: 21–32, 589–98.

Park, L. D. and Lipman, R. S. (1964) A Comparison of Patient Dosage Deviation Reports with Pill Counts. *Psychopharmacologia* 6: 299–302.

Parkes, C. M. (1972) *Bereavement: Studies of Grief in Adult Life*. London: Tavistock Publications.

—— (1978) Home or Hospital? Terminal Care as Seen by Surviving Spouses. *Journal of the Royal College of General Practitioners* 28: 19–30.

—— (1980) Terminal Care: Evaluation of an Advisory Domiciliary Service at St. Christopher's Hospice. *Postgraduate Medical Journal* 56: 685–89.

Parkin, F. (1979) *Marxism and Class Theory: A Bourgeois Critique*. London: Tavistock Publications.

Parsons, T. (1951) *The Social System*. London: Routledge & Kegan Paul.

Pendleton, D. A. and Bochner, S. (1980) The Communication of Medical Information in General Practice Consultations as a Function of Patients' Social Class. *Social Science and Medicine* 14(a): 669–73.

Peterson, L. and Shigetomi, C. (1981) The Use of Coping Techniques to Minimize Anxiety in Hospitalized Children. *Behaviour Therapy* 12: 1–14.

Phares, E. J. (1976) *Locus of Control in Personality*. Morristown, NJ: General Learning Press.

Pickett, C. and Clum, G. (1982) Comparative Treatment Strategies and Their Interaction with Locus of Control in the Reduction of Post-surgical Pain and Anxiety. *Journal of Consulting and Clinical Psychology* 50 (3): 439–41.

Pill, R. and Stott, N. C. H. (1982) Concepts of Illness Causation and Responsibility: Some Preliminary Data from a Sample of Working Class Mothers. *Social Science and Medicine* 16 (1): 43–52.

Pillsbury, B. (1978) 'Doing the Month': Confinement and Convalescence of Chinese Women after Childbirth. *Social Science and Medicine* 12: 11–22.

Plaja, A. O., Cohen, L. M., and Samora, J. (1968) Communication between Physicians and Patients in Outpatient Clinics. *Milbank Memorial Fund Quarterly* 46 (2): 161–213.

Plummer, K. (1975) *Sexual Stigma: An Interactionist Account*. London: Routledge & Kegan Paul.

Pope, C. R. (1978) Consumer Satisfaction in a Health Maintenance Organization. *Journal of Health and Social Behaviour* 19 (3): 291–303.

Pritchard, P. (1983) Patient Participation. In D. Pendleton and J. Hasler (eds) *Doctor–Patient Communication*. London: Academic Press.

Pyrczak, D. and Roth, D. M. (1976) The Readability of Directions on Non-prescription Drugs. *Journal of the American Pharmaceutical Association* 16: 242–43, 267.

Rack, P. (1982) *Race, Culture and Mental Disorder*. London: Tavistock Publications.

Radius, S. M., Becker, M. H., Rosenstock, I. M., Drachman, R. H., Schuberth, K., and Teets, K. (1978) *The Journal of Asthma Research* 15 (3): 133–49.

Rains, A. J. H. and Ritchie, H. D. (1981) *Bailey and Love's Short Practice of Surgery* (18th edn). London: H. K. Lewis.

Ramsay, M. A. E. (1972) A Survey of Pre-operative Fear. *Anaesthesia* 27 (4): 396–401.

Raphael, W. (1969) *Patients and Their Hospitals: A Survey of Patients' View of Life in General Hospitals*. London: King Edward's Hospital Fund.

Rapoport, J. (1979) Patients' Expectations and Intention to Self-medicate. *Journal of the Royal College of General Practitioners* 29 (205): 468–72.

Raw, M. (1981) Giving Up Smoking. In R. M. Greenhalgh (ed.) *Smoking and Arterial Disease.* London: Pitman Medical.

Raw, M., Jarvis, M. J., Feyerabend, C., and Russell, M. A. H. (1980) Comparison of Nicotine Chewing-gum and Psychological Treatments for Dependent Smokers. *British Medical Journal* 1: 481–82.

Reeder, S., Marcus, A., and Seeman, T. (1978) The Influence of Social Networks on the Use of Health Services. Unpublished paper, UCLA.

Rees, W. D. (1972) The Distress of the Dying. *British Medical Journal* 2: 105–07.

Reid, I. (1981) *Social Class Differences in Britain.* London: Grant McIntyre.

Reif, L. (1973) Ulcerative Colitis: Strategies for Managing Life. *American Journal of Nursing* 73: 261–64.

Reynolds, M. (1978) No News Is Bad News: Patients' Views about Communication in Hospital. *British Medical Journal* 1: 1673–676.

Rex, J. and Tomlinson, S. (1979) *Colonial Immigrants in a British City: A Class Analysis.* London: Routledge & Kegan Paul.

Richardson, J. (1971) The Late Management of Industrial Head Injuries. In *Proceedings of an International Symposium on Head Injuries.* Edinburgh: Churchill Livingstone.

Rickels, K. and Briscoe, E. (1970) Assessment of Dosage Deviation in Outpatient Drug Research. *Journal of Clinical Pharmacology* 10: 153–60.

Ridgeway, V. and Mathews, A. (1982) Psychological Preparation for Surgery: A Comparison of Methods. *British Journal of Clinical Psychology* 21: 271–80.

Roberts, A. (1979) *Severe Accidental Head Injury. An Assessment of Long Term Prognosis.* London: Macmillan.

Robinson, R. and Benson, D. R. (1981) Depression in Aphasic Patients: Frequency. Severity and Clinical-pathological Correlations. *Brain and Language* 14: 282–91.

Robinson, R. and Price, T. (1982) Post-stroke Depressive Disorders: A Follow up Study of 103 Patients. *Stroke* 13 (5): 635–41.

Robinson, R. and Szetela, B. (1981) Mood Change Following Left Hemispheric Brain Injury. *Annals of Neurology* 9: 447–53.

Rodda, B., Miller, M., and Bruten, J. (1971) Prediction of Anxiety and Depression Patterns among Coronary Patients Using a Markov Process Analysis. *Behavioural Science* 16: 482–89.

Rogers, D. E., Blendon, R. J., and Moloney, T. W. (1982) Who Needs Medicaid? *New England Journal of Medicine* 307: 13–18.

Romm, F. J., Hulka, B. S., and Mayo, F. (1976) Correlates of Outcomes in Patients with Congestive Heart Failure. *Medical Care* 14 (9): 765–66.

Rosenbaum, M. and Najenson, J. (1976) Changes in Life Patterns and Symptoms of Low Mood as Reported by Wives of Severely Brain-injured Soldiers. *Journal of Consulting and Clinical Psychology* 44: 881–88.

Rosenstock, I. (1966) Why People Use Health Services. *Milbank Memorial Fund Quarterly* 44: 94–127.

—— (1975) Prevention of Illness and Maintenance of Health. In J. Kosa and I. K. Zola (eds) *Poverty and Health.* Cambridge, Massachusetts: Harvard University Press.

Rosenstock, I. and Kirscht, J. (1979) Why People Seek Health Care. In G. Stone, F. Cohen, and N. Adler (eds) *Health Psychology – A Handbook: Theories,*

Applications and Challenges of a Psychological Approach to the Health Care System. San Francisco: Jossey-Bass.

Ross, C. E., Wheaton, B., and Duff, R. S. (1981) Client Satisfaction and the Organization of Medical Practice: Why Time Counts. *Journal of Health and Social Behaviour* 22 (3): 243–55.

Roter, D. (1979) Altering Patient Behaviour in Interaction with Providers. In D. J. Oborne, M. M. Gruneberg, and J. R. Eiser (eds) *Research in Psychology and Medicine*, vol. 2. London: Academic Press.

Rotter, J. B. (1954) *Social Learning and Clinical Psychology.* Englewood Cliffs, NJ: Prentice Hall.

—— (1966) Generalized Expectancies for Internal Versus External Control of Reinforcement. *Psychology Monographs* 80: 1.

Rowbotham, G., McIver, I., and Dickson, J. (1954) Analysis of 1400 Cases of Acute Injury to the Head. *British Medical Journal* 1: 726.

Royal College of General Practitioners (1981) *Health and Prevention in Primary Care.* London: Royal College of General Practitioners.

Royal Commission on the National Health Service (1979) London: HMSO.

Rundall, T. G. and Wheeler, J. R. (1979) The Effect of Income on Use of Preventive Care: An Evaluation of Alternative Explanations. *Journal of Health and Social Behaviour* 20: 397–406.

Runnymede Trust and Radical Statistics Group (1980) *Britain's Black Population.* London: Heinemann.

Russell, M. A., Wilson, C., Taylor, C., and Baker, C. D. (1979) Effect of General Practitioners' Advice against Smoking. *British Medical Journal* 281 (1): 231–35.

Rutter, D. R. and Maguire, G. (1976) History Taking for Medical Students: II. Evaluation of a Training Programme. *Lancet* 1: 558–60.

Sacco, R., Wolf, P., Kannel, W., and McNamara, P. (1982) Survival and Recurrence Following Stroke: The Framingham Study. *Stroke* 13 (3): 290–95.

Sackett, D. L. (1976) The Magnitude of Compliance and Non-compliance. In D. L. Sackett and R. B. Haynes (eds) *Compliance with Therapeutic Regimes.* Baltimore: John Hopkins University Press.

Sackett, D. L. and Snow, J. C. (1979) The Magnitude and Measurement of Compliance. In R. B. Haynes, D. W. Taylor, and D. L. Sackett (eds) *Compliance in Health Care.* Baltimore: John Hopkins University Press.

Safilios-Rothschild, C. (1970) *The Sociology and Social Psychology of Disability and Rehabilitation.* New York: Random House.

Sainsbury, S. (1970) *Registered as Disabled.* Occasional Papers on Social Administration No. 35. London: Bell.

Salloway, J. and Dillon, P. (1973) A Comparison of Family Networks and Friend Networks in Health Care Utilization. *Journal of Comparative Family Studies* 4: 131–42.

Saltzer, E. B. (1978) Cognitive Moderators of the Relationship between Behavioural Intentions and Behaviour. *Journal of Personality and Social Psychology* 41 (2): 260–71.

Samora, J., Saunders, L., and Larson, M. (1961) Medical Vocabulary Knowledge among Hospital Patients. *Journal of Health and Human Behaviour* 2: 83–9.

Sapira, J. D. (1972) Reassurance Therapy. *Annals of Internal Medicine* 77: 603–04.

Scambler, A. and Scambler, G. (1984) Menstrual Symptoms, Attitudes and Consulting Behaviour. Unpublished manuscript.

Scambler, A., Scambler, G., and Craig, D. (1981) Kinship and Friendship Networks and Women's Demand for Primary Care. *Journal of the Royal College of General Practitioners* 26: 746–50.

Scambler, G. (1983) *'Being Epileptic': Sociology of a Stigmatizing Condition.* Unpublished PhD thesis, University of London.

Scambler, G. and Hopkins, A. (1977) How Doctors Deal with Epilepsy. *Lancet* 1: 183–86.

Scambler, G. and Hopkins, A. (1981) Social Class, Epileptic Activity and Disadvantage at Work. *Journal of Epidemiology and Community Health* 34: 129–33.

Schacter, S. (1975) Cognition and Peripheralist–Centralist Controversies in Motivation and Emotion. In M. S. Gazzaniga and C. Blakemore (eds) *Handbook of Psychobiology.* London: Academic Press.

Schmitt, F. and Wooldrige, P. (1973) Psychological Preparation of Adult Surgical Patients. *Nursing Research* 22 (2): 108–16.

Schneider, J. and Conrad, P. (1980) In the Closet with Illness: Epilepsy, Stigma Potential and Information Control. *Social Problems* 28: 32–44.

Schneider, J. and Conrad, P. (1981) Medical and Sociological Typologies: The Case of Epilepsy. *Social Science and Medicine* 15(a): 211–19.

Schur, E. (1971) *Labelling Deviant Behaviour: Its Sociological Implications.* New York: Harper & Row.

Scott, R. (1969) *The Making of Blind Men.* New York: Russell Sage Foundation.

—— (1970) The Construction of Conceptions of Stigma by Professional Experts. In J. Douglas (ed.) *Deviance and Respectability: The Social Construction of Moral Meanings.* New York: Basic Books.

—— (1972) A Proposed Framework for Analyzing Deviance as a Property of Social Order. In R. Scott and J. Douglas (eds) *Theoretical Perspectives on Deviance.* New York: Basic Books.

Scott-Palmer, J. and Skevington, S. M. (1981) Pain during Childbirth and Menstruation: A Study of Locus of Control. *Journal of Psychosomatic Research* 25 (3): 151–55.

Seeman, M. and Evans, J. (1962) Alienation and Learning in a Hospital Setting. *American Sociological Review* 27: 772–83.

Segall, A. and Roberts, L. W. (1980) A Comparative Analysis of Physician Estimates and Levels of Medical Knowledge among Patients. *Sociology of Health and Illness* 2 (3): 317–34.

Shaines, N. (1961) A Re-evaluation of Some Aspects of Femininity through a Study of Menstruation. *Comparative Psychiatry* 2: 20–26.

Shibutani, T. (1962) Reference Groups and Social Control. In A. Rose (ed.) *Human Behaviour and Social Processes: An Interactionist Approach.* London: Routledge & Kegan Paul.

Shipley, R. H., Butt, J. H., Horwitz, B., and Farbry, I. (1978) Preparation for a Stressful Medical Procedure: Effect of Amount of Stimulus Pre-exposure and Coping Style. *Journal of Consulting and Clinical Psychology* 46: 499–507.

Shipley, R. H., Butt, J. H., and Horwitz, E. (1979) Preparation to Re-experience a Stressful Medical Examination: Effect of Repetitious Videotape Exposure and Coping Style. *Journal of Consulting and Clinical Psychology* 47: 485–92.

Siegel, L. and Peterson, L. (1980) Stress Reduction in Young Dental Patients through Coping Skills and Sensory Information. *Journal of Consulting and Clinical Psychology* 48: 785–87.

Sime, M. (1976) Relationship of Pre-operative Fear, Type of Coping and Information Received about Surgery to Recovery from Surgery. *Journal of Personality and Social Psychology* 34: 716–24.

Skuse, D. H. (1975) Attitudes of the Psychiatric Outpatient Clinic. *British Medical Journal* 2: 469–71.

Smith, D. (1977) *Racial Disadvantage in Britain*. Harmondsworth: Penguin.

—— (1980) *Overseas Doctors in the National Health Service*. London: Heinemann.

Snow, L. F. (1974) Folk Medical Beliefs and Their Implications for Care of Patients. *Annals of Internal Medicine* 81: 82–96.

Snow, L. F. and Johnson, S. (1977) Modern Day Menstrual Folklore: Some Clinical Implications. *Journal of the American Medical Association* 237: 2736–739.

Spiegel, D., Bloom, J. R., and Yalom, I. (1981) Group Support for Patients with Metastatic Cancer. *Archives of General Psychiatry* 38: 527–33.

Spielberger, C. D., Auerbach, S. M., Wadsworth, A. P., Dunn, T., and Taulbee, E. S. (1973) Emotional Reactions to Surgery. *Journal of Consulting and Clinical Psychology* 40 (1): 33–8.

Spielberger, C. D., Gorsuch, R. L., and Lushene, R. E. (1970) *Manual for the State-Trait Anxiety Inventory*. Palo Alto: Consulting Psychologists Press.

Stacey, M. (1976) The Health Service Consumer: A Sociological Misconception. In M. Stacey (ed.) *The Sociology of the NHS, Sociological Review Monograph No. 22*. Keele: University of Keele.

Stallones, R. (1975) Epidemiology of Cerebrovascular Disease. *Journal of Chronic Diseases* 18: 859–72.

Stanton, F. and Baker, K. H. (1942) Interviewer Bias and the Recall of Incompletely Learned Materials. *Sociometry* 5: 123–34.

Steadman, J. and Graham, J. (1970) Head Injuries: An Analysis and Follow up Study. *Proceedings of the Royal Society of Medicine* 63: 23–8.

Stebbins, R. (1970) Career: The Subjective Approach. *Sociological Quarterly* 11: 32–49.

Stedeford, A. (1981) Couples Facing Death. *British Medical Journal* 283: 1033–036, 1098–101.

Steffenson, M. and Colker, L. (1982) Intercultural Misunderstandings about Health Care: Recall of Descriptions of Illness and Treatment. *Social Science and Medicine* 16: 1949–954.

Steffy, R. A., Meichenbaum, D., and Best, J. A. (1970) Aversive and Cognitive Factors in the Modification of Smoking Behaviour. *Behaviour Research and Therapy* 8: 115–25.

Stevenson, I. N. (1980) Editorial comment. *Social Science and Medicine* 14B (1): 1.

Stewart, D. C. and Sullivan, T. J. (1983) Illness Behaviour and the Sick Role in Chronic Disease. The Case of Multiple Sclerosis. *Social Science and Medicine* 16 (15): 1397–404.

Stiles, W. B., Putnam, S. M., Wolf, M. H., and James, S. A. (1979) Interaction Exchange Structure and Patient Satisfaction with Medical Interviews. *Medical Care* 17 (6): 667–79.

Stimson, G. V. (1974) Obeying Doctor's Orders: A View from the Other Side. *Social Science and Medicine* 8 (2): 97–104.

Stimson, G. V. and Webb, B. (1975) *Going to See the Doctor: The Consultation Process in General Practice*. London: Routledge & Kegan Paul.

Stoeckle, J. D. and Barsky, A. J. (1981) Attributions: Uses of Social Science Knowledge in the 'Doctoring' of Primary Care. In L. Eisenberg and A. M. Kleinman (eds) *The Relevance of Social Science for Medicine*. Dordrecht, Holland: Reidel.

Stone, G. (1979a) Psychology and the Health System. In G. Stone, F. Cohen, and N. Adler (eds) *Health Psychology – A Handbook: Theories, Applications and Challenges of a Psychological Approach to the Health Care System*. San Francisco: Jossey-Bass.

—— (1979b) Patient Compliance and the Role of the Expert. *Journal of Social Issues* 35 (1): 34–59.

Straits, B. and Sechrest, L. (1963) Further Support of Some Findings about the Characteristics of Smokers and Non-smokers. *Journal of Consulting Psychology* 27: 282.

Straus, R. (1957) The Nature and Status of Medical Sociology. *American Sociological Review* 22: 200–04.

Strauss, A. and Glaser, B. (1975) *Chronic Illness and the Quality of Life*. St. Louis, Missouri: Mosby.

Suchman, E. A. (1964) Sociomedical Variations among Ethnic Groups. *American Journal of Sociology* 70: 319–31.

—— (1967) Health Attitudes and Behaviour. A Model for Research on Community Health Campaigns. *Journal of Health and Social Behaviour* 8: 197–209.

Svarstad, B. (1976) Physician–Patient Communication and Patient Conformity with Medical Advice. In D. Mechanic (ed.) *The Growth of Bureaucratic Medicine*. New York: Wiley.

Szasz, T. (1966) Whither Psychiatry? *Social Research* 33: 439–62.

Tapia, F. (1972) Teaching Medical Interviewing: A Practical Technique. *British Journal of Medical Education* 6: 133–6.

Tash, R. H., O'Shea, R. M., and Cohen, L. K. (1969) Testing a Preventive Symptomatic Theory of Dental Health Behaviour. *American Journal of Public Health* 59: 514–21.

Taylor, J. (1847) *The Rule and Exercises of Holy Dying (1651)*. London: Pickering.

Tessler, R. and Mechanic, D. (1975) Consumer Satisfaction with Prepaid Group Practice. *Journal of Health and Social Behaviour* 16 (1): 95–113.

Thomas, K. B. (1978) The Consultation and the Therapeutic Illusion. *British Medical Journal* 1: 1327–328.

Thompson, J. A. and Anderson, J. L. (1982) Patient Preferences and the Bedside Manner. *Medical Education* 16: 17–21.

Thomsen, I. V. (1974) The Patient with Severe Head Injury and His Family. *Scandinavian Journal of Rehabilitative Medicine* 6: 180–83.

Tobis, J. S., Puri, K. B., and Sheridan, J. (1982) Rehabilitation of the Severely Brain-injured Patient. *Scandinavian Journal of Rehabilitative Medicine* 14: 83–8.

Townsend, P. (1979) *Poverty in the United Kingdom*. Harmondsworth: Penguin.

Townsend, P. and Davidson, N. (1982) *Inequalities in Health*. Harmondsworth: Penguin.

Trimble, M. (1981) *Neuropsychiatry*. Chichester: John Wiley.

Tuckett, D. (ed.) (1976) *An Introduction to Medical Sociology*. London: Tavistock Publications.

Tudor Hart, J. (1981) A New Kind of Doctor. *Journal of the Royal Society of Medicine* 74: 871–83.

Unterhalter, B. (1979) Compliance with Western Medical Treatment in a Group of Black Ambulatory Hospital Patients. *Social Science and Medicine* 13(a): 621–30.

Vallenstein, E. and Heilman, K. (1979) Emotional Disorders Resulting from Illness in the Central Nervous System. In E. Vallenstein and K. Heilman (eds) *Clinical Neuropsychology*. Oxford: Oxford University Press.

Varlaam, A., Dragoumis, M., and Jefferys, M. (1972) Patients' Opinions of Their Doctors – A Comparative Study of Patients in a Central London Borough Registered with Single-handed and Partnership Practices in 1969. *Journal of the Royal College of General Practitioners* 22 (125): 811–16.

Vaughn, C. E. and Leff, J. P. (1976) The Influence of Family and Social Factors in the Course of Psychiatric Illness. *British Journal of Psychiatry* 129: 125–37.

Verby, J. E., Holden, P., and Davis, R. H. (1979) Peer Review of Consultations in Primary Care: The Use of Audiovisual Recordings. *British Medical Journal* i: 1686–688.

Vernon, D. T. W. and Bigelow, D. W. (1974) Effects of Information about a Potentially Stressful Situation on Responses to Stress Impact. *Journal of Personality and Social Psychology* 29: 50–9.

Visintainer, M. A. and Wolfer, J. A. (1975) Psychological Preparation for Surgical Pediatric Patients: The Effect on Children's and Parents' Stress Responses and Adjustment. *Pediatrics* 56: 187–202.

Volicer, B. J. and Bohannon, M. W. (1975) A Hospital Stress Rating Scale. *Nursing Research* 24: 352–59.

Volinn, I. (1983) Health Professionals as Stigmatizers and Destigmatizers of Diseases: Alcoholism and Leprosy and Examples. *Social Science and Medicine* 17: 385–93.

Wakeman, R. and Kaplan, J. (1978) An Experimental Study of Hypnosis in Painful Burns. *American Journal Clinical Hypnosis* 21: 3–12.

Waldron, I. (1983) Sex Differences in Illness Incidence, Prognosis and Mortality: Issues and Evidence. *Social Science and Medicine* 17: 1107–123.

Wallis, S. (1981) Bengali Families in Camden. In J. Cheetham, W. James, M. Loney, B. Mayor, and W. Prescott (eds) *Social and Community Work in a Multiracial Society*. London: Harper & Row.

Wallsten, T. S. (1978) *Three Biases in the Cognitive Processing of Diagnostic Information*. Unpublished paper, Psychometric Laboratory, University of North Carolina, Chapel Hill.

Wallston, K. A., Wallston, B. S., and DeVellis, R. (1978) Development of the Multi-dimensional Health Locus of Control (MHLC) Scales. *Health Education Monographs* 6 (2): 160–70.

Ware, J. E. and Snyder, M. K. (1975) Dimensions of Patient Attitudes Regarding Doctors and Medical Care Services. *Medical Care* 13 (8): 669–79.

Warren, C. and Johnson, J. (1972) A Critique of Labelling Theory from Its Phenomenological Perspective. In R. Scott and J. Douglas (eds) *Theoretical Perspectives on Deviance*. New York: Basic Books.

Wason, P. C. and Johnson-Laird, P. N. (1972) *Thinking and Reasoning*. Harmondsworth: Penguin.

Watson, J. (1977) The Chinese: Hong Kong Villagers in the British Catering

Trade. In J. Watson (ed.) *Between Two Cultures: Migrants and Minorities in Britain.* Oxford: Basil Blackwell.

Weddell, R., Oddy, M., and Jenkins, P. (1980) Social Adjustment after Rehabilitation: A Two Year Follow-up of Patients with Severe Head Injury. *Psychological Medicine* 10: 257–63.

Weidman, H. (1979) The Transcultural View: Prerequisite to Interethnic (Intercultural) Communication in Medicine. *Social Science and Medicine* 13(b): 85–7.

Weighill, V. E., Hodge, J., and Peck, D. F. (1983) Keeping Appointments with Clinical Psychologists. *British Journal of Clinical Psychology* 22: 143–44.

Weiner, C. (1975) The Burden of Rheumatoid Arthritis: Tolerating the Uncertainty. *Social Science and Medicine* 9: 97–104.

Weiss, O. F., Sriwatanakul, K., Weintraub, M., and Lasagna, L. (1983) Reduction of Anxiety and Post-operation Analgesic Requirements by Audiovisual Instruction. *Lancet* 1 (8): 43–4.

West, P. (1979) *An Investigation into the Social Construction and Consequences of the Label 'Epilepsy'.* Unpublished PhD thesis, University of Bristol.

Westbrook, M. and Viney, L. (1983) Psychological Reactions to the Onset of Chronic Illness. *Social Science and Medicine* 16: 899–905.

Whisnant, L. and Zegans, L. (1965) A Study of Attitudes towards Menarche in White Middle-class American Girls. *American Journal of Psychiatry* 132: 809–14.

White, G. M. (1982) The Role of Cultural Explanations in 'Somatization' and 'Psychologization'. *Social Science and Medicine* 16 (16): 1519–530.

White, R. (1979) What's in a Name? Problems in Official and Legal Uses of 'Race'. *New Community* 7: 333–49.

Wilkes, E. (1965) Terminal Cancer at Home. *Lancet* 1: 799–801.

Wilkinson, L. (1979) *Classical Attitudes to Modern Issues.* London: William Kimber.

Williams, A. F. (1972) Factors Associated with Seat Belt Use in Families. *Journal of Safety Research* 4 (3): 133–38.

Williams, R. G. (1983) Concepts of Health: An Analysis of Lay Logic. *Sociology* 17: 185–205.

Wilson, J. F. (1981) Behavioural Preparation for Surgery: Benefit or Harm? *Journal Behavioural Medicine* 4 (1): 79–102.

Wilson-Barnett, J. (1976) Patients' Emotional Reactions to Hospitalization: An Explanatory Study. *Journal of Advanced Nursing* 1: 351–58.

—— (1984) Interventions to Alleviate Patients' Stress – A Review. *Journal of Applied Psychology.* In press.

Wilson-Barnett, J. and Carrigy, A. (1978) Factors Influencing Patients' Emotional Reactions to Hospitalization. *Journal of Advanced Nursing* 3: 221–29.

Winefield, H. R. (1982) Reliability and Validity of the Health Locus of Control Scale. *Journal of Personality Assessment* 46 (6): 614–19.

Wolfer, J. and Davis, C. (1970) Assessment of Surgical Patients: Pre-operative Emotional Condition and Post-operative Welfare. *Nursing Research* 19: 402–14.

Woods, N., Dery, G., and Most, A. (1982) Recollections of Menarche, Current Menstrual Attitudes and Perimenstrual Symptoms. *Psychosomatic Medicine* 44: 285–93.

Young, A. (1981) When Rational Men Fall Sick: An Inquiry into Some Assumptions Made by Medical Anthropologists. *Culture, Medicine and Psychiatry* 5 (4): 317–35.

Zola, I. K. (1973) Pathways to the Doctor: From Person to Patient. *Social Science and Medicine* 7 (9): 677–89.

—— (1981) Structural Constraints in the Doctor–Patient Relationship: The Case of Non Compliance. In L. Eisenberg and A. Kleinman (eds) *The Relevance of Social Science for Medicine*. London: Reidel.

Name index

Subject index